AF567082

Technological Advances in the Treatment of Type 1 Diabetes

Frontiers in Diabetes

Vol. 24

Series Editors

M. Porta Turin

F.M. Matschinsky Philadelphia, Pa.

Technological Advances in the Treatment of Type 1 Diabetes

Volume Editors

Daniela Bruttomesso Padua

Giorgio Grassi Turin

43 figures, 30 in color, and 27 tables, 2015

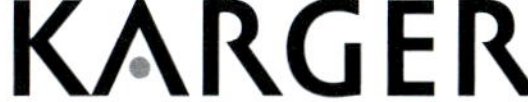

Basel · Freiburg · Paris · London · New York · Chennai · New Delhi · Bangkok · Beijing · Shanghai · Tokyo · Kuala Lumpur · Singapore · Sydney

Frontiers in Diabetes
Founded 1981 by F. Belfiore, Catania

Daniela Bruttomesso, PhD
Department of Clinical and Experimental Medicine, Diabetology and Metabolism
University of Padua
Via Giustiniani 2
IT-35128 Padua (Italy)

Giorgio Grassi, MD
Endocrinology, Diabetology and Metabolism
A.O. Città della Salute e della Scienza
Corso Bramante 88
IT-10126 Turin (Italy)

Library of Congress Cataloging-in-Publication Data

Technological advances in the treatment of type 1 diabetes / volume editors, Daniela Bruttomesso, Giorgio Grassi.
p. ; cm. -- (Frontiers in diabetes ; vol. 24)
Includes bibliographical references and index.
ISBN 978-3-318-02336-7 (hard cover : alk. paper) -- ISBN 978-3-318-02337-4 (electronic version)
I. Bruttomesso, Daniela, editor. II. Grassi, Giorgio (Physician), editor. III. Series: Frontiers in diabetes ; v. 24. 0251-5342
[DNLM: 1. Diabetes Mellitus, Type 1--therapy. 2. Blood Glucose Self-Monitoring. 3. Hypoglycemia--prevention & control. 4. Insulin--therapeutic use. 5. Insulin Infusion Systems. W1 FR945X v.24 2014/ WK 810]
RC661.I6
616.4'622--dc23
2014030005

Bibliographic Indices. This publication is listed in bibliographic services.

Disclaimer. The statements, opinions and data contained in this publication are solely those of the individual authors and contributors and not of the publisher and the editor(s). The appearance of advertisements in the book is not a warranty, endorsement, or approval of the products or services advertised or of their effectiveness, quality or safety. The publisher and the editor(s) disclaim responsibility for any injury to persons or property resulting from any ideas, methods, instructions or products referred to in the content or advertisements.

Drug Dosage. The authors and the publisher have exerted every effort to ensure that drug selection and dosage set forth in this text are in accord with current recommendations and practice at the time of publication. However, in view of ongoing research, changes in government regulations, and the constant flow of information relating to drug therapy and drug reactions, the reader is urged to check the package insert for each drug for any change in indications and dosage and for added warnings and precautions. This is particularly important when the recommended agent is a new and/or infrequently employed drug.

www.karger.com
Printed in Germany on acid-free and non-aging paper (ISO9706) by Kraft Druck, Ettlingen
ISSN 0251–5342
e-ISSN 1662–2995
ISBN 978–3–318–02336–7
e-ISBN 978–3–318–02337–4

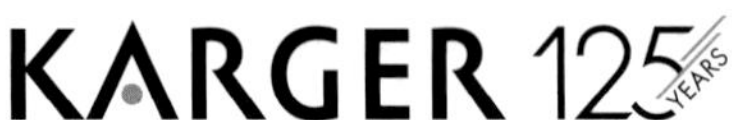

Contents

Preface

All technologies, including the most innovative, are always built on other existing technologies and adapted to new targets. The progress is relentless and unstoppable, like the evolution of living species. As in other fields, medical technology is presently experiencing a momentous time.

This review aims to provide an update of developments that promise to revolutionize the treatment of diabetes. It concerns hospital and outpatient care, intensive insulin therapy, blood glucose monitoring, and innovative steps towards the construction of a real artificial pancreas. 'Better care of diabetes through technology' could be the motto of this review.

We thank all of our colleagues who contributed to the book, but our thoughts are for the patients who, we hope, will benefit from the developments reported here.

Giorgio Grassi, MD, Turin

Preface

Bruttomesso D, Grassi G (eds): Technological Advances in the Treatment of Type 1 Diabetes.
Front Diabetes. Basel, Karger, 2015, vol 24, pp 1–10 (DOI: 10.1159/000363460)

Glucose Control in Diabetes: Targets and Therapy

Geremia B. Bolli · Francesca Porcellati · Paola Lucidi · Carmine G. Fanelli

Department of Medicine, University of Perugia Medical School, Perugia, Italy

Abstract

In 1993, the Diabetes Control Complications Trial (DCCT) study established that chronic hyperglycemia initiates and progresses to microvascular complications such as retinopathy in type 1 diabetes mellitus (T1DM). The milestone message from DCCT has been that early near-normalization of blood glucose in recent-onset T1DM with glycated hemoglobin (HbA_{1C}) <7.0% prevents the appearance and delays progression of microvascular complications. To achieve this, the physiological model of insulin substitution is needed with basal insulin for the fasting state and prandial insulin at each carbohydrate meal. This can be achieved with continuous subcutaneous insulin infusion (CSII), the gold-standard approach to substituting basal insulin, or multiple daily insulin injections (MDI) using long-acting insulin analogues as basal insulin (glargine or degludec once a day, detemir twice a day) with very similar results. Neutral protamine Hagedorn should be totally dismissed in the treatment of T1DM. It does not really matter whether CSII or MDI is used, as long as HbA_{1C} is maintained <7.0% in each treatment. Unfortunately, only a minority of T1DM patients reach this target. To increase the success of intensive treatment, education of diabetologists, the diabetes team, and the diabetic subjects on how to use insulin, diet, and physical exercise are strongly needed.

The Question of Origin of Microangiopathy in Diabetes Mellitus

History

In 1993, the Diabetes Control Complications Trial (DCCT) [1] provided us with the ideal targets of intensive treatment of type 1 diabetes mellitus (T1DM). The DCCT was a milestone study which answered in a clear and definitive manner the long-asked question of whether the microvascular complications of diabetes are due to chronic hyperglycemia or rather to a genetic predisposition. The debate among opinion leaders had been going on for decades since the late vascular complications of diabetes were discovered in the early 1940s and 1950s in subjects with T1DM treated with insulin for 10–15 years. From its introduction in the clinics in 1922, it was clear that insulin saves lives, but, as life was prolonged, the surprise was the appearance of complications. The reason diabetic retinopathy was only first recognized in the 1940s was the simple fact that diabetic subjects did not live long enough to develop this complication before the discovery of insulin.

Today's young doctors and specialists have been living the 'post-DCCT era' and use the targets of DCCT to best prevent complications by aiming at near-normoglycemia. However, they may not necessarily be familiar with the recent hot discussion concerning the origin of chronic vascular complications of diabetes. As early as in 1968, Siperstein et al. [2] introduced the hypothesis that microangiopathy in patients with diabetes was inherited and not acquired after many years of uncontrolled hyperglycemia. On the other hand, large epidemiological observations [3] and experimental evidence in animals [4] have suggested that chronic hyperglycemia is behind the development of microangiopathy, especially retinopathy. In 1983, there was a debate in the *New England Journal of Medicine* between those in favor of the genetic versus the metabolic (hyperglycemia) hypothesis to explain microangiopathy in diabetes [5]. Clearly, only a randomized, controlled, intervention trial comparing the effect of near-normal versus elevated blood glucose on appearance and progression of microangiopathy in subjects with T1DM could ultimately answer this key question and end the decades-long controversy. This trial was the DCCT [1]. The DCCT was designed to ultimately guide diabetologists and subjects with T1DM alike on how to control hyperglycemia and at which level to keep it long term in order to prevent later complications and/or progression of complications. A few years later in 1998, the results of another trial on blood glucose control and complications, this time in subjects with T2DM, were reported in the UK Prospective Diabetes Study (UKPDS) [6].

The Trials of Glucose Control on Microangiopathy: The Common Messages from the DCCT and UKPDS

The core messages from the DCCT and UKPDS should be emphasized because they are, and will always be, relevant for everyday practice in the diabetic clinic. Whenever we sit in front of our patients with T1DM or T2DM and have to establish a treatment strategy of blood glucose management, we base our decisions on the messages from the DCCT and UKPDS.

First, the chronic elevation of blood glucose, not genetics, is responsible for microangiopathy (and macroangiopathy). Figures 1 and 2 present results on risk for developing retinopathy, and similar results have also been obtained for neuropathy and nephropathy. Genetics may explain the variance of effects of chronic hyperglycemia in different individuals who develop different degrees (severity) of micro/macroangiopathy. Microangiopathy, however, does not develop when blood glucose is normal, it

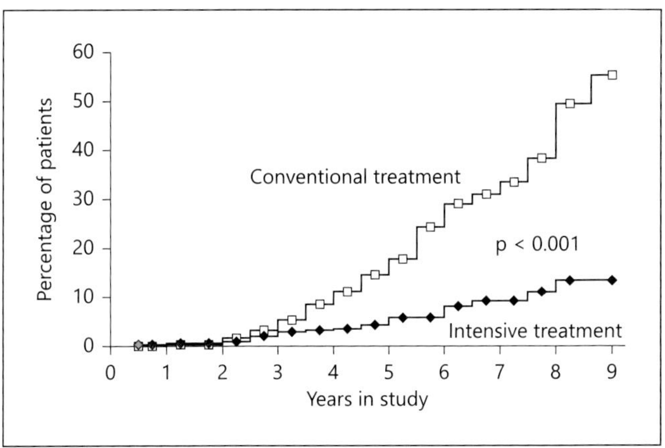

Fig. 1. Cumulative incidence of retinopathy (3-step progression) in the DCCT study, primary prevention cohort [1]. When near-normoglycemia is established and early clinical onset of T1DM and HbA_{1C} is at or below 7.0%, corresponding to a mean blood glucose of 140 mg/dl (intensive treatment), retinopathy appears at the end of 9 years only in a small percentage of subjects. In contrast, in subjects in whom blood glucose is maintained elevated (220 mg/dl, HbA_{1C} about 9.0%), retinopathy appears already after 3 years and nearly all subjects are affected after a few years. Reproduced with permission from the *New England Journal of Medicine*.

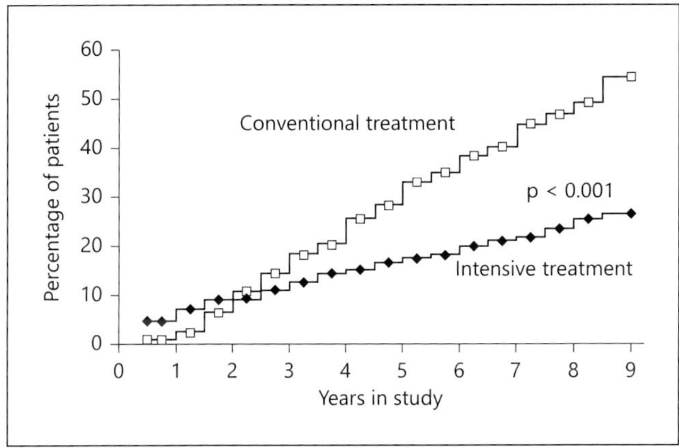

Fig. 2. Cumulative incidence of retinopathy (3-step progression) in the DCCT study, secondary intervention cohort [1]. These are subjects with retinopathy at baseline already after a few years of T1DM. When near-normoglycemia is established and HbA_{1C} is at or below 7.0%, corresponding to mean blood glucose of 140 mg/dl (intensive treatment), retinopathy progresses less as compared to the standard group in which blood glucose is maintained elevated (220 mg/dl, HbA_{1C} about 9.0%). Reproduced with permission from *New England Journal of Medicine*.

develops only after years of hyperglycemia. Thus, chronic hyperglycemia is the necessary and nearly always sufficient condition for the development of microangiopathy (although there is a restricted minority of individuals genetically protected by hyperglycemia who do not develop complications). As mentioned earlier, genetics by itself cannot result in microangiopathy as long as blood glucose is normal – genetics can only modulate the negative effects of chronic hyperglycemia. Second, the prospective benefit of lowering mean blood glucose over time is relevant to subjects with new diabetes onset (and thus no complications at baseline), as well as to those presenting with initial complications due to several years of diabetes. Third, lowering blood glucose, this time in T2DM as shown by the UKPDS [6], is as beneficial as it is in T1DM on appearance and progression of microangiopathy. Fourth, in the extension of the DCCT (EDIC), subjects have been monitored for nearly 20 years with no additional intervention [7]. Interestingly, in the intensive group, glycated hemoglobin (HbA_{1C}) increased from 7.0 to 8.0%, whereas in the control group it decreased from 9.0 to 8.0%. So, in the EDIC follow-up of DCCT, HbA_{1C} is quite similar between the two groups of the DCCT study. The surprising observation has been that the originally intensive group continues to benefit from the antecedent good glycemic control of the DCCT with less microangiopathy despite deterioration of blood glucose. In contrast, the original control group continues to develop more microangiopathy despite improved glycemic control. Fifth, the EDIC study has also examined cardiovascular events (macroangiopathy) in addition to microangiopathy. After 15 years of follow-up, the original intensive group presented lower numbers of cardiovascular events and greater survival.

Taken together, the above findings are the basis of our current understanding on how to treat diabetic subjects with T1DM to prevent microangiopathy. In subjects with new-onset T1DM, the goal is achieving (quickly) and maintaining near-normoglycemia (for decades) to prevent microangiopathy which otherwise appears after a few years, and to prevent macroangiopathy 10–20 years later. In subjects with several years of T1DM and already established complications, it is still important to lower hyperglycemia and maintain HbA_{1c} at about 7.0% to prevent the progression of microangiopathy. The same applies to T2DM and suggests that hyperglycemia is a common vascular poison to microvessels regardless of the origin of hyperglycemia (T1DM, T2DM, or secondary diabetes; fig. 3). The benefits of lowering blood glucose extend after 10–15 years to macroangiopathy as well, which, again, is true for both T1DM [7] and T2DM [8].

Blood Glucose Targets

The current blood glucose targets that we have adopted for the treatment of diabetes mellitus are derived from evidence of protection against onset or progression of microangiopathic complications in the DCCT (for T1DM) [1] and UKPDS (for T2DM) [6]. As previously stated, the relationship between long-term elevation of blood glucose and risk for developing microvascular complications is remarkably similar in the

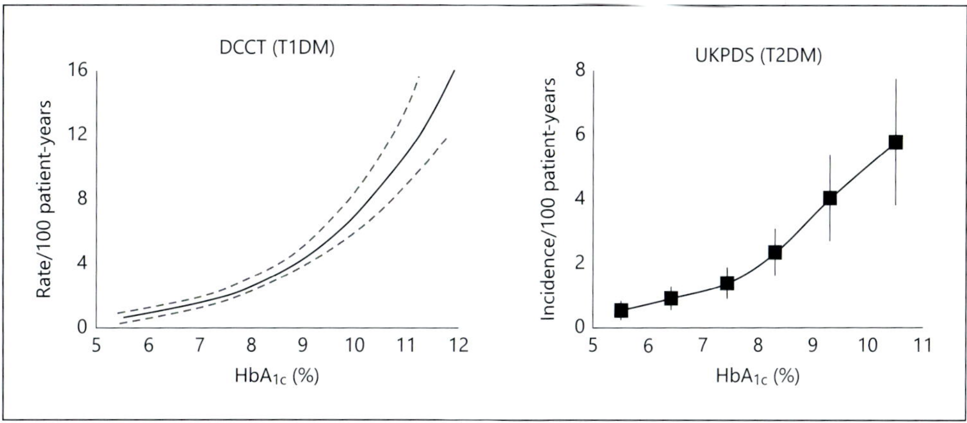

Fig. 3. Similarly beneficial effects of long-term control of blood glucose on microangiopathy in the DCCT study (T1DM) and UKPDS study (T2DM) [1, 6]. Reproduced with permission from the *New England Journal of Medicine* and *The Lancet*.

Table 1. Recommended glycemic targets based on the DCCT and UKPDS trials on intensive treatment to prevent primarily long-term micro- and macroangiopathic complications and limit hypoglycemia in T1DM and T2DM

	Blood glucose, mg/dl; HbA_{1c}, %		A1C (%)
	fasting	2-hour postprandial	
Intensive treatment[1]	>80; <110	>100; <160	>6.5; <7.0
Nonintensive treatment[2]	>120; <150	>150; <200	>7.0; <8.0

[1] New-onset diabetes, age <75 years, no comorbidities.
[2] Long-term diabetes (>30 years), age >75 years, and/or comorbidities.

two types of diabetes. As shown in figure 3, there is no threshold effect of hyperglycemia on complications, i.e. the lower the mean blood glucose attained over time, the better (lower risk of developing retinopathy and microangiopathy). The glycemic thresholds are presented in table 1.

Intensive and Nonintensive Treatment

Glycemic targets should be differentiated between intensive and nonintensive treatment (table 1). Intensive treatment is indicated in new-onset diabetes, especially in young subjects. Additionally, if life expectancy is estimated to be long, even in subjects who have late-onset diabetes (i.e. at 50–60 and even 70 years of age), intensive treatment should

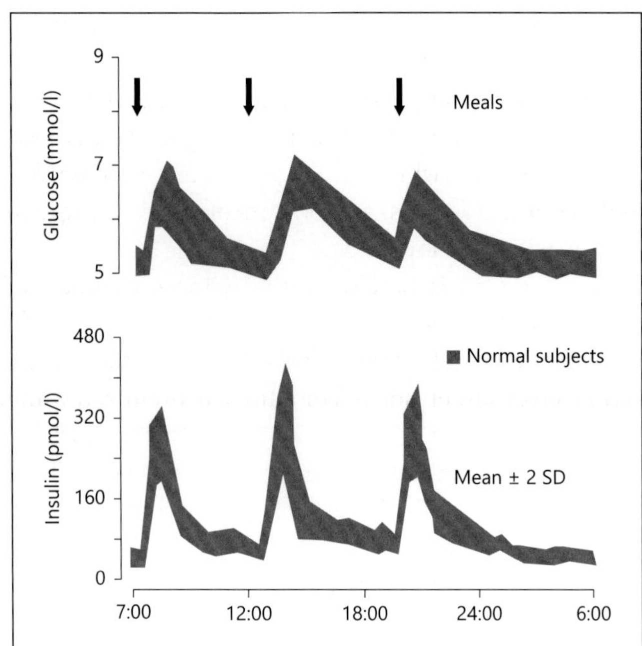

Fig. 4. Physiology of glucose homeostasis in normal nondiabetic subjects [9]. Reproduced with permission from *Diabetes Care.*

also be considered. Nonintensive treatment on the other hand is indicated in elderly subjects (>75 years), and in general whenever life duration is expected to be only a few years.

Comorbidities play a role in the decision whether to aim for intensive or nonintensive treatment. In the presence of established microangiopathic complications (e.g. proliferative retinopathy or end-stage renal disease), it is perhaps not useful to aim for intensive treatment given the nonreversibility of these complications. However, the decision whether to aim for intensive or nonintensive treatment should be made on a case-by-case basis. For example, there might cases with severe complications in the kidney, but not so in the eye. In this case, intensive treatment would be indicated to prevent retinopathy even in the presence of advanced nephropathy.

How to Treat People with Type 1 Diabetes: Intensively or Nonintensively

The Common Basis of Intensive and Nonintensive Treatment

Several studies have established the physiology of glucose homeostasis in normal nondiabetic subjects (fig. 4) [9]. In normal nondiabetic subjects, plasma glucose is always maintained in a narrow range. Despite nocturnal fasting or ingestion of large carbohydrate meals, plasma glucose never decreases below 70 mg/dl or increases above 125–130 mg/dl. This fine equilibrium where both hypoglycemia and hyperglycemia are avoided is made possible by the fine physiology of the pancreatic β-cells which secrete insulin in a dynamic mode, with a progressive decrease between meals and nocturnal fasting, as well as rapid increases to elevated peaks immediately after a carbohydrate meal (fig. 4).

To be as close as possible to glucose homeostasis, we need to mimic the fine insulin dynamics of the physiological model (fig. 4). This is best made today with replacement of 'basal' insulin (which ideally should maintain normoglycemia in the interprandial and nocturnal periods) and boluses of rapid-acting insulin any time there is meal ingestion with carbohydrates.

Basal insulin is best delivered with continuous subcutaneous insulin infusion (CSII), an approach invented in 1976 by Pickup et al. [10] to overcome the poor performance of basal insulin available at that time, i.e. neutral protamine Hagedorn (NPH; given either isolated or admixed-premixed with rapid-acting insulin). The superiority of CSII in the NPH era was indisputable with lower mean blood glucose and less hypoglycemia as shown by several trials [11]. The 'egg of Columbus' of CSII was simply not to use NPH, but to rely on microboluses of rapid-acting insulin as basal insulin. These are given every few minutes resulting into a continuous infusion calculated in units/hour which could be varied depending on the subject need. The unique advantage of CSII is that the basal insulin need is met by replacement with rapid-acting insulin which has a pharmacokinetic and pharmacodynamic variability much lower as compared to NPH, as shown by Binder et al. [12] in 1984.

However, after 2000, long-acting insulin analogues (glargine, detemir, and recently degludec) have progressively replaced NPH. These analogues differ considerably among themselves in terms of insulin molecule modifications, mode of action, pharmacokinetics, and pharmacodynamics, but have a common aspect superior to NPH (fig. 5) [13]. Notably, since insulin glargine and detemir do not have the action peak commonly observed 4–6 h after the injection of NPH [13], they can both protect from nocturnal hypoglycemia. In addition, glargine and detemir (soluble insulins) are both less variable than the insoluble NPH [14]. Insulin degludec is nearly peakless as insulin detemir, but has a longer duration of action [15]. Today, the long-acting insulin analogue glargine is widely used in T1DM and the results indicate that it is very competitive with respect to CSII [16, 17].

Prandial insulin is given as a bolus of a rapid-acting analogue (lispro, aspart, glulisine) a few minutes before a carbohydrate meal in amounts related to the carbohydrate content of the meal. However, the time interval between injection and meal ingestion should be flexible depending on the preprandial blood glucose concentration. Large fatty meals (e.g. pizza) or long meals (wedding, parties, etc.) require a second or third bolus administration 2–4 h after the start of the meal.

Figure 6 summarizes the CSII and multiple daily insulin injection (MDI) options for insulin replacement in T1DM. There is no superiority of one approach over the other – they only must be used according to the appropriate principles. In individual subjects, it may be more convenient to use CSII instead of injecting insulin 6 or 7 times/day. Other subjects, however, may find CSII an inconvenient external, mechanical appendix to their body and refuse the idea. Other subjects may appreciate the high flexibility of CSII which best meets the insulin physiological needs, whereas other subjects

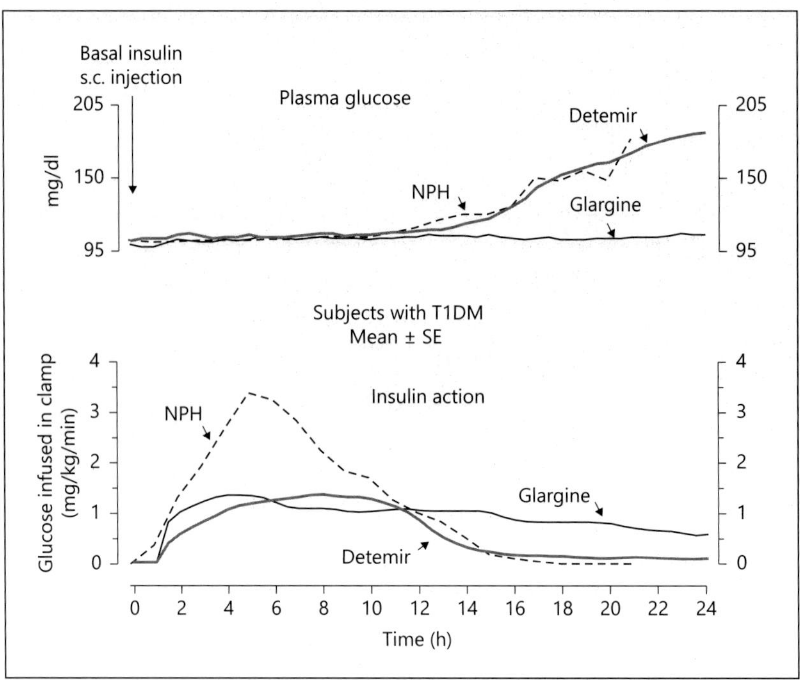

Fig. 5. Pharmacodynamics of basal insulins NPH, glargine, and detemir [13]. With NPH, there is an early peak of action 4–6 h after subcutaneous injection and loss of activity after 12–14 h with an increase in plasma glucose. With glargine and detemir, there is no postinjection peak, with a rather flat action profile which decreases the risk of nocturnal hypoglycemia as compared to NPH. The duration of action of glargine is longer than that of detemir. Degludec (not shown) has a pharmacodynamics action profile similar to glargine and a duration of action that is likely longer. Reproduced with permission from *Archives of Physiology and Biochemistry.*

may find it easier to increase the number of daily subcutaneous injections to mimic CSII exactly. Finally, CSII is nearly 4 times more expensive than MDI [17]. Thus, use of CSII should be proposed to all subjects who for different reasons cannot achieve near-normoglycemia or suffer from disabling hypoglycemia; however, after a short-term trial it should be continued long term only in those subjects in whom HbA_{1C} decreases and hypoglycemia were prevented.

How to Manage Multiple Daily Insulin Injections and Continuous Subcutaneous Insulin Infusion in Intensive and Nonintensive Treatment

The question here is how to reach the targets of table 1 in intensive or nonintensive treatment. The model of insulin replacement should be identical (basal bolus) in intensive and nonintensive treatment, i.e. the same MDI or CSII should be used by young subjects who need to prevent long-term complications and by elderly subjects in whom the primary goal is prevention of hypoglycemia by maintaining higher mean blood glucose values (table 1). The only difference between intensive and noninten-

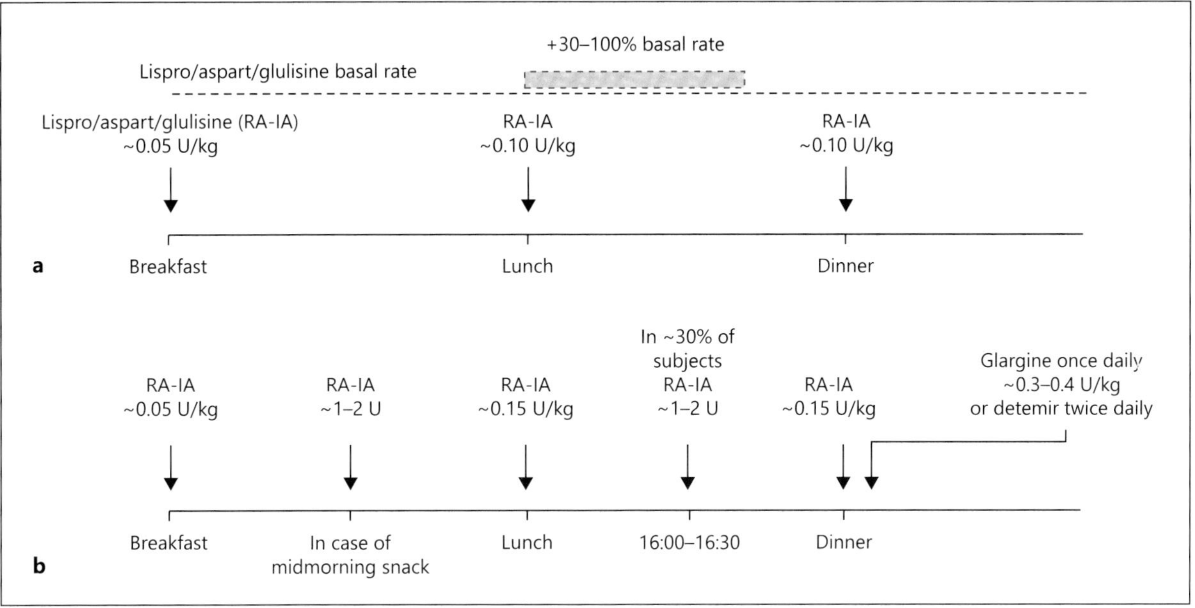

Fig. 6. The regimens of physiological insulin delivery as either CSII (**a**, the 'gold standard' of basal insulin) or MDI (**b**). RA-IA = Rapid acting insulin analogue.

sive treatment is titration to different blood glucose targets before and after meals, not different strategies of insulin replacement (table 1).

Conclusions

After more than 90 years of use of insulin in diabetes, we have only recently learned how to prevent long-term vascular complications, both micro- and macrovascular. This has become possible because we now understand the physiology of glucose homeostasis, which is the model to be mimicked in insulin replacement. Also, we have evidence of the beneficial effects of long-term near-normalization of blood glucose from large long-term trials [1, 6].

However, today only a minority of subjects with T1DM or T2DM are at desirable blood glucose targets. Therefore, the question we have to answer today is not 'if', 'when', or 'which' patient we should treat at the targets indicated in table 1, but rather 'what' we need to do to be more successful with our patients in reaching these targets.

Education of diabetologists and members of the diabetes team (nurses, educators, and dieticians), education of patients to blood glucose monitoring, physiological insulin replacement with either MDI or CSII and continuing close interaction between patient and the diabetes team, are among the key needs which are required to maintain the targets long term and thus prevent late vascular complications of diabetes.

References

1 The Diabetes Control and Complication Trial Research Group: The effect of intensive treatment of diabetes on the development and progression of long-term complications in insulin-dependent diabetes mellitus. N Engl J Med 1993;329:977–986.

2 Siperstein MD, Unger RH, Madison LL: Studies of muscle capillary basement membranes in normal subjects, diabetic, and prediabetic patients. J Clin Invest 1968;47:1973–1999.

3 Pirart J: Diabetes mellitus and its degenerative complications: a prospective study of 4400 patients observed between 1947 and 1973. Diabetes Care 1978; 1:168–188, 252–263.

4 Engerman R, Bloodworth J Jr, Nelson S: Relationship of microvascular disease in diabetes to metabolic control. Diabetes 1977;26:760–769.

5 Siperstein MD: Diabetic microangiopathy and the control of blood glucose. N Engl J Med 1983;309: 1577–1579.

6 UK Prospective Diabetes Study (UKPDS) Group: Intensive blood-glucose control with sulphonylureas or insulin compared with conventional treatment and risk of complications in patients with type 2 diabetes (UKPDS 33). Lancet 1998;352:837–853.

7 The Diabetes Control and Complications Trial/Epidemiology of Diabetes Interventions and Complications (DCCT/EDIC) Study Research Group: Intensive diabetes treatment and cardiovascular disease in patients with type 1 diabetes. N Engl J Med 2005;353: 2643–2653.

8 Holman RR, Paul SK, Bethel MA, Matthews DR, Neil HA: 10-year follow-up of intensive glucose control in type 2 diabetes. N Engl J Med 2008;359:1577–1589.

9 Ciofetta M, Lalli C, Del Sindaco P, Torlone E, Pampanelli S, Lepore M, Di Loreto C, Brunetti B, Bolli GB: Contribution of postprandial versus interprandial blood glucose to HbA_{1c} in type 1 diabetes on physiologic intensive therapy with lispro insulin at mealtime. Diabetes Care 1999;22:795–800.

10 Pickup JC, Keen H, Stevenson RW, Parsons JA, Alberti KG, White M, Kohner EM: Insulin via continuous subcutaneous infusion. Lancet 1978;2:988–989.

11 Pickup JC, Sutton AJ: Severe hypoglycaemia and glycaemic control in type 1 diabetes: meta-analysis of multiple daily insulin injections compared with continuous subcutaneous insulin infusion. Diabet Med 2008;25:765–774.

12 Binder C, Lauritzen T, Faber O, Pramming S: Insulin pharmacokinetics. Diabetes Care 1984;7:188–199.

13 Rossetti P, Porcellati F, Fanelli CG, Perriello G, Torlone E, Bolli GB: Superiority of insulin analogues versus human insulin in the treatment of diabetes mellitus. Arch Physiol Biochem 2008;114:3–10.

14 Heise T, Nosek L, Rønn BB, Endahl L, Heinemann L, Kapitza C, Draeger E: Lower within-subject variability of insulin detemir in comparison to NPH insulin and insulin glargine in people with type 1 diabetes. Diabetes 2004;53:1614–1620.

15 Jonassen I, Havelund S, Hoeg-Jensen T, Steensgaard DB, Wahlund PO, Ribel U: Design of the novel protraction mechanism of insulin degludec, an ultra-long-acting basal insulin. Pharm Res 2012;29:2104–2114.

16 Bruttomesso D, Crazzolara D, Maran A, Costa S, Dal Pos M, Girelli A, Lepore G, Aragona M, Iori E, Valentini U, del Prato S, Tiengo A, Buhr A, Trevisan R, Baritussio A: In type 1 diabetic patients with good glycaemic control, blood glucose variability is lower during continuous subcutaneous insulin infusion than during multiple daily injections with insulin glargine. Diabet Med 2008;25:326–332.

17 Bolli GB, Kerr D, Reena T, Torlone E, Gazagnes S, Vitacolonna E, Selam JL, Home PD: Comparison of a multiple daily insulin injection regime (basal once-daily glargine plus mealtime lispro) and CSII (lispro) in type 1 diabetes: a randomized open parallel multicenter study. Diabetes Care 2009;32:1170–1176.

Geremia B. Bolli, MD
Department of Medicine, Hospital Santa Maria Della Misericordia
Ellisse Building, Floor +1, Room No. 17
IT–06156 Perugia (Italy)
E-Mail geremia.bolli@unipg.it

Bruttomesso D, Grassi G (eds): Technological Advances in the Treatment of Type 1 Diabetes.
Front Diabetes. Basel, Karger, 2015, vol 24, pp 11–22 (DOI: 10.1159/000363461)

Pregnancy and Diabetes

Annunziata Lapolla · Maria Grazia Dalfrà
Department of Medicine, University of Padua, Padua, Italy

Abstract
Achieving good metabolic control during the period prior to conception is the key to reducing congenital malformations that can occur in pregnancies complicated by diabetes. Various different glycated hemoglobin (HbA_{1c}) levels (the gold standard for ascertaining metabolic control in diabetes) and glucose levels have been recommended. The current guidelines and latest studies on the best levels to obtain in diabetic women before and during pregnancy are reported here and discussed. Finally, the optimal therapeutic approach and the possible benefits and risks related to the use of the new insulin analogues in pregnancy will be analyzed.

Even today, pregnancy in diabetic women is a high-risk condition for both the mother and fetus [1]. The prevalence of type 2 diabetes is continuously rising worldwide and more women of reproductive age have diabetes. This means there are more pregnancies complicated by type 2 diabetes, a condition that shares the same risks for mother and fetus as type 1 diabetes [2].

There is plenty of evidence that neonatal conditions in pregnancy complicated by diabetes, such as congenital malformations, hypoglycemia, hypocalcemia, hyperbilirubinemia, macrosomia, intrauterine growth retardation, respiratory distress syndrome, polycythemia, and hypertrophic myocardiopathy are caused by hyperglycemia [3]. According to the Pedersen hypothesis, maternal hyperglycemia leads to fetal hyperglycemia, which causes fetal hyperinsulinemia, fetal overgrowth, and macrosomia [4]. Fetal hyperinsulinemia also induces increased metabolism and tissue hypoxia, which are responsible for other neonatal complications. These risks can be reduced by optimal glycemic control both prior to conception and during pregnancy. This can be achieved by means of comprehensive preconception care and strict follow-up dur-

Table 1. Prepregnancy counseling in women with preexisting diabetes

	ADA 2008	NICE 2008
Multidisciplinary team need	yes	–
Empowerment of the women in the management of diabetes before and during pregnancy	yes	yes
Evaluation and treatment of retinopathy	yes	yes
Evaluation and treatment of nephropathy	yes	yes
Evaluation and treatment of neuropathy	yes	–
Evaluation and treatment of CVD	yes	–
Evaluation and treatment of hypertension	–	–
Evaluation and modification of all medications	yes	–
Stop ACE	yes	yes
Stop ARBs	yes	yes
Stop diuretics	yes	
Stop β-blockers		yes
Stop statins	yes	yes
Metabolic control evaluation		
HbA_{1c} preconception target, %	<7.0	<6.1
Self-monitoring of blood glucose	7–8 times/day	7–8 times/day
Insulin	yes	yes
Folic acid supplementation	600 μg/day	5 mg/day (from preconception –12 g.w.)
Advise of congenital malformation risk if metabolic control is poor or pregnancy is not planned	yes	yes
Advise of need of a effective contraception during planning period	yes	yes
Dietary advice	yes	yes

CVD = Cardiovascular disease; ACE = angiotensin-converting enzyme; ARBs = angiotensin-II receptor blockers; g.w. = gestational week.

ing pregnancy. A recent systematic review and meta-analysis on the effectiveness and safety of prepregnancy care in reducing the rate of congenital malformations and perinatal mortality among women with pregestational diabetes showed that preconception care reduced the rate of congenital malformations from 7.4 to 1.9%, making it similar to the figures reported for the background population. The review underscored the importance of integrating preconception care in the routine management of diabetic women of reproductive age [5]. Nonetheless, unplanned pregnancies still occur in about 2 in 3 women with diabetes, which explains the high rate of malformations among their babies [2, 6]. It is imperative to provide diabetes care and education in women of childbearing age before conception. This needs to be done by multidisciplinary teams including diabetologists, gynecologists, family physicians, nurses skilled in diabetes, dieticians, and other specialists where necessary. The diabetic women must also become active members of this team in order to achieve the goal of a healthy pregnancy and newborn (table 1).

Maternal Metabolism during Pregnancy

A number of changes in metabolism occur during pregnancy to provide fuel for the growing fetoplacental unit [7, 8]. Glucose reaches the fetus by means of a facilitated diffusion, amino acids are actively transported to the fetus against a concentration gradient, glycerol and ketones are delivered to the fetus proportionally with maternal levels, and free fatty acids are provided by the placenta.

Insulin sensitivity does not change during the first trimester, while it decreases as the pregnancy progresses, falling by about 50% in late pregnancy [8]. These changes are triggered by a gradual increase in the hormones of the fetoplacental unit (hormone placental lactogen, estrogens, progesterone, human chorionic somatropin) and they are essential to normal fetal growth. Postprandial hyperglycemia enhances glucose transfer to the fetus. Because insulin resistance is more evident in skeletal muscle than in adipose tissue, nutrients are preferentially diverted to maternal fat synthesis so that a condition of 'facilitated anabolism' occurs during meals. In late pregnancy, in a fasting state (when glucose and insulin levels are low), maternal lipolysis is enhanced because the insulin is unable to suppress lipolysis in adipose tissue. This leads to an increase in free fatty acids, used as an alternative fuel for the mother, while carbohydrate oxidation is reduced, thus sparing glucose for the fetus. This enhanced lipolysis is due to placental hormones: in the second half of pregnancy, hormone placental lactogen reduces insulin sensitivity and glucose tolerance, and enhances lipolysis and proteolysis. The passage through the placenta of glucose, thanks to a facilitated diffusion, and of actively transported amino acids gives rise to maternal hypoglycemia, hypoalaninemia, and hyperketonemia (due to the enhanced lipolysis). These changes under fasting conditions have been termed 'accelerated starvation' [7–9]. Normal pregnancy is therefore characterized by low fasting plasma glucose levels, and by larger and longer-lasting glucose excursions after meals.

In normal pregnant women, both first- and second-phase insulin responses increase to compensate for this reduction, and this is associated with β-cell hypertrophy and hyperplasia. In pregnant women with type 1 diabetes, the complete absence of exogenous insulin interferes with the proper balance of accelerated starvation and facilitated anabolism, which explains the marked daily excursions in blood sugar levels.

Glucose turnover was recently assessed by stage of gestation (early vs. late) with a view to clarifying the mechanism behind postprandial hyperglycemia in pregnant women with type 1 diabetes. The rate of systemic glucose appearance and glucose disposal was measured in 10 type 1 pregnant women having standardized meals. There were no changes in fasting glucose appearance and disposal in early gestation, whereas there was a higher hepatic insulin resistance and a lower insulin sensitivity in late gestation. Interestingly, there was delayed glucose disposal in late gestation. So, postprandial glucose control is impaired by a significantly slower glucose disposal in late pregnancy. Early prandial insulin dosing may help to accelerate glucose disposal and have the potential to ameliorate postprandial hyperglycemia in late pregnancy [10].

Pregnancy-induced lipolysis also exposes pregnant type 1 diabetic women to the risk of developing ketoacidosis if insulin is not administered correctly.

Target of Metabolic Control

All the clinical practice guidelines agree that diabetic women who want to become pregnant should be assessed by a multidisciplinary team that undertakes a complete preconception analysis of medical and obstetric history, assesses and treats their diabetic complications, reviews their ongoing medication, and monitors their metabolic control and blood glucose management [11–13].

Although glucose levels play a pivotal part in maternal and fetal outcomes of pregnancy complicated by diabetes, the current clinical recommendations for target levels to reach during pregnancy vary greatly. They are based on results obtained in small samples of normal pregnant women and they have never been tested prospectively and compared. This explains why fetal complications (e.g. macrosomia) may still develop, even if these glucose targets are reached during a diabetic pregnancy. A recent review of data collected from 12 studies on normal, nonobese, pregnant women (taking into account the methods used and the strengths and weaknesses of the studies) has clearly shown that glucose concentrations during normal pregnancy are lower than the currently recommended therapeutic targets for diabetic pregnancies [14]. The authors suggested values of 71 ± 8 mg/dl (1 SD) for fasting, 109 ± 13 mg/dl for 1 h after meals, 99 ± 10 mg/dl for 2 h after meals, and 88 ± 10 mg/dl for the mean glucose concentration as a pattern of normal glycemia in nonobese, nondiabetic pregnant women (fig. 1). Prospective studies evaluating lower therapeutic targets for fasting and postprandial glycemia are consequently urgently needed to test any positive impact they might have in reducing maternal and fetal complications in diabetic pregnancy.

As for glycemic control, all the guidelines recommend a target glycated hemoglobin (HbA_{1c}) as close to normal as possible before pregnancy, with no significant hypoglycemia. Although HbA_{1c} levels are normally lower in pregnancy [15] (fig. 2), most laboratories do not report pregnancy-specific reference ranges. The guidelines generally suggest a lower HbA_{1c} target (<6.0%) during pregnancy because the outcome is better if the HbA_{1c} levels remain within the normal range in early pregnancy [16]. HbA_{1c} should be tested, using the International Federation of Clinical Chemistry (IFCC) standardized methods, at the first visit during pregnancy, then monthly until target levels are reached, and then every 2–3 months thereafter [11].

As for the prepregnancy glycemic target, the American Diabetes Association (ADA) suggests a blood glucose level between 4.4 and 6.1 mmol/l before meals, and below 8.6 mmol/l 2 h after meals. All the guidelines indicate that blood glucose levels should be kept as normal as possible, avoiding hypoglycemic episodes. To achieve this

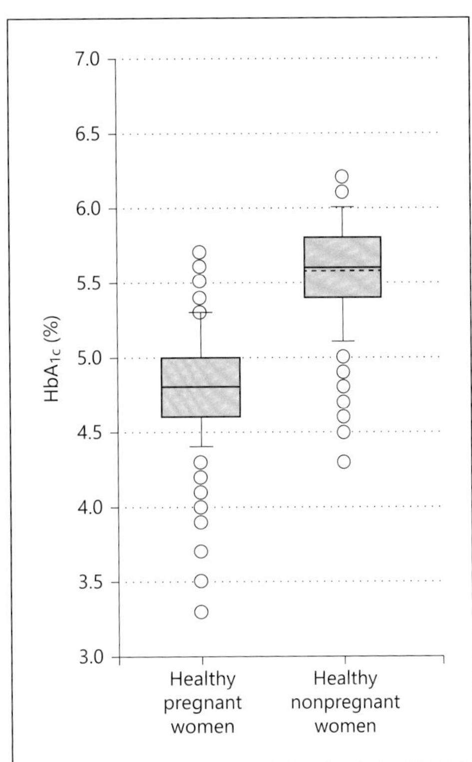

Fig. 1. Reference range of HbA_{1c} in pregnant and nonpregnant women (median value 4.8 and 5.6%, respectively) [15].

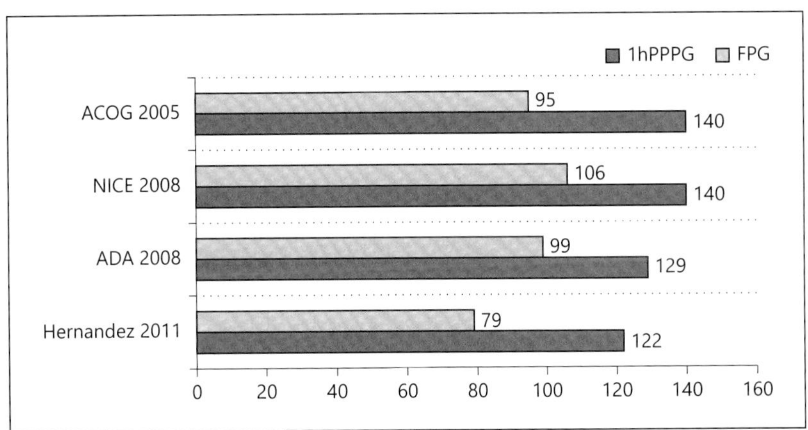

Fig. 2. Glycemic targets recommended by the International Scientific Societies and new targets suggested and derived from the mean pattern of glycemia across 12 studies (weighted mean values +1 SD) [14].

Table 2. Glycemic targets recommended during pregnancy in women with preexisting diabetes

	ADA 2008	AGOC 2005	NICE 2008
FPG			
mg/dl	60–99	<95	63–106
mmol/l	3.3–5.5	<5.3	3.5–5.9
1hPPPG			
mg/dl	100–129	<130–140	<140
mmol/l	5.5–7.2	<7.2–7.8	<7.8
2hPPPG			
mg/dl		<120	
mmol/l		<6.7	
HbA_{1c}, %	<6.0	<6.0	<6.0

FPG = Fasting plasma glucose; 1hPPPG = 1-hour postprandial plasma glucose; 2hPPPG = 2-hour postprandial plasma glucose.

result, it is important to improve the patient's awareness about hypoglycemia and its treatment.

For women who already have type 1 or type 2 diabetes when they become pregnant, the ADA consensus statement [17] recommends preprandial, bedtime, and overnight glucose levels between 60 and 99 mg/dl (3.3–5.4 mmol/l), postprandial levels of 100–129 mg/dl (5.4–7.1 mmol/l), and mean daily glucose levels <110 mg/dl, if they can be achieved without any hypoglycemic episodes. The American College of Obstetricians and Gynaecologists (AGOG) suggests fasting glucose levels <95 mg/dl (<5.3 mmol/l), and 1- and 2-hour postprandial levels <130–140 mg/dl (<7.2–7.8 mmol/l) and <120 mg/dl (6.7 mmol/l), respectively. The National Institute for Health and Clinical Excellence (NICE) recommends fasting glucose levels between 63 and 106 mg/dl (3.5–5.9 mmol/l) and 1-hour postprandial glucose levels <140 mg/dl (<7.8 mmol/l) (table 2). A recent Cochrane review assessed the effects of different intensities of glycemic control in diabetic pregnant women, based on 3 trials (totaling 223 pregnant type 1 diabetic women). Two of them compared very strict fasting glucose limits (3.33–5.0 mmol/l) with less strict glycemic targets (4.45–6.38 mmol/l), and showed very few differences between the two groups, although there were more hypoglycemic episodes in women under the stricter regime. One trial (involving 60 women) compared strict (≤5.6 mmol/l fasting glucose), moderate (5.6–6.7 mmol/l fasting glucose), and permissive glycemic control (6.7–8.9 mmol/l fasting glucose), and found significantly higher rates of preeclampsia, cesarean section, and large babies in the least strictly controlled group [18].

It thus seems that strict glycemic control alone is unable to optimally reduce the fetal and maternal complications related to diabetic pregnancies; however, the Cochrane review had some limitations: only 3 small trials were judged suitable for inclusion in the analysis, no trials were available on type 2 pregnant women, only glucose measurements were considered, and there were no details on patients' compliance and formal education or their understanding of how to monitor their own blood glucose levels appropriately. We consequently agree with the authors' conclusions, that 'Future trials comparing interventions, rather than control targets, may be more feasible particularly for pregnant women with type 2 diabetes' [18].

But how should metabolic control be measured in these women? The ADA recommendations clearly state that self-monitoring of blood glucose is a key aspect of diabetes management before and during pregnancy, and that it has to be done daily before and after meals, at bedtime and occasionally from 2:00 to 4:00 a.m. Compared to postprandial blood glucose measurement 2 h after meals, blood glucose measurement 1 h after meals is more useful since it may capture glucose peaks even though, given the individual differences, it would be useful for each patient to identify the time of their own postprandial peak.

The accuracy of self-monitoring of blood glucose depends on the method used and the user's ability, so it is very important for healthcare providers to carefully assess a woman's capacity to use the instrument correctly, both at the initial visit and at regular intervals thereafter. It is also essential for women to be able to interpret the results correctly and adjust their food intake, insulin therapy, and exercise to reach the therapeutic goals agreed with the healthcare providers. Patients should use meters calibrated to measure plasma glucose with a memory capacity and, last but not least, be able to contact the healthcare providers quickly to discuss any problem concerning the management of their diabetes.

Continuous glucose monitoring systems include a device that measures glucose levels in subcutaneous interstitial tissue fluids continuously throughout the day. They provide useful information on the magnitude and duration of any glucose peak, which could be useful in the management of diabetic pregnancies. Despite some promising results obtained with this method [19], it is a relatively inconvenient and expensive tool, so NICE has called for randomized controlled trials assessing its efficacy before it can be recommended for use in the routine management of pregnancies complicated by diabetes. On the other hand, the ADA recommends its use as a supplemental tool in selected patients with type 1 diabetes (e.g. in women with little hypoglycemia awareness).

The role of glycemic variability in terms of its detrimental impact on chronic diabetic complications has recently been emphasized. There are contrasting reports concerning the perfect timing to intensify glycemic control: some studies found glycemia at conception and during the first trimester to be particularly important; others focus on the importance of glucose levels in the second and third trimesters. Considering fetal growth for example, fasting glucose levels have been shown to explain only 12%

of the variation in birth weight, while postprandial plasma glucose about 40%. It would therefore seem that the parameters currently used to monitor metabolic control in diabetes are unable to predict fetal growth, probably because they are incapable of assessing a patient's glucose levels on a continuous basis. In a recent paper analyzing glycemic variability, we measured mean amplitude of glycemic excursion, mean glycemia, continuous overlapping net glycemic action, standard deviation, high blood glucose index, low blood glucose index, and interquartile range in type 1 women affected by gestational diabetes mellitus (GDM) and normal pregnant women, and compared fetal growth. We found higher mean birth weights and ponderal index, though not significant, in diabetic women than in pregnant controls. In type 1 patients, the ponderal index related to high blood glucose index in the first trimester, continuous overlapping net glycemic action 1 and interquartile range in the second, and to mean glycemia and standard deviation in the third. In GDM patients, the ponderal index related to mean glycemia and high blood glucose index in the second trimester. Exposure to glycemic variability and hyperglycemia thus seems to be important in determining fetal overgrowth in diabetic pregnant women [20]. Moreover, although HbA_{1c} remains one of the key markers to monitor metabolic control (especially if a standardized procedure is adopted), it cannot reflect the marked glucose variability that often occurs in diabetic pregnancies [21].

Pregnant diabetic women also need to be taught to measure their ketonuria when they are ill and/or when their blood glucose levels exceed 200 mg/dl, given the high fetal mortality rate associated with maternal ketoacidosis [17].

Insulin Therapy during Pregnancy

There are typical changes in insulin requirements during pregnancy [8, 9]. During the first trimester, the placental passage of glucose and gluconeogenic substrates causes maternal hypoglycemia, so a reduction of about 10% in the dosage required before conception is common. Blood glucose control during this period is also less stable, with a tendency for low fasting plasma glucose, high postprandial excursions, and nocturnal hypoglycemia. Pregnancy-induced nausea and vomiting can also predispose women to hypoglycemia. During the second and third trimesters, the gradually increasing production of placental anti-insulin hormones causes a progressive increase in insulin requirements. From the 24th gestational week onwards, glucose excursions tend to decrease. In the last month of pregnancy, there may be a decline in insulin requirements, particularly during the night, because maternal glucose and amino acid transfer to the fetus through the placenta continues at an ever-increasing rate as the fetus grows – especially at night when the fetus is feeding. Some patients experience a 20–30% reduction in their insulin requirements. All these changes lead both to a greater demand for short-acting insulin to cover meals, and to the need to optimize doses of intermediate-acting insulin to guarantee a constant basal rate [22].

In this scenario, the particular characteristics of the new insulins currently on the market can be of great help in attaining desirable metabolic control in pregnancy.

Three different rapid-acting insulin analogues are now available (lispro, aspart, and glulisine), all of which have been obtained using the recombinant DNA technique and substituting or deleting one or more amino acids in regions that do not affect binding to the insulin receptor. Their particular characteristics make these analogues more able to mimic postprandial physiological insulin secretion and their earlier waning reduces the risk of postprandial hypoglycemia. Given these features, rapid-acting insulin analogues could become the front-line treatment in diabetic pregnancy, provided they prove to be safe (in terms of their teratogenicity, embryo toxicity, immunogenicity, transplacental passage, and mitogenicity) as well as effective.

Studies on animals have shown no teratogenic effects on the fetus after insulin lispro injection at a dosage 4 times the average dose of human insulin. This analogue, however, shows a greater homology with insulin growth factor 1 (IGF-1) than with human insulin, and studies on placental transfer were unable to detect insulin lispro in the umbilical cord of infants after its intravenous administration in mothers during labor. Clinical studies on type 1 diabetes and GDM found no differences in the frequency of preterm delivery, preeclampsia, or other neonatal morbidities between pregnancies treated with lispro versus regular human insulin. In GDM patients, insulin lispro was able to normalize 1-hour postprandial glucose levels better than regular human insulin, and this was associated with normal anthropometric characteristics in the newborn [22, 23].

Insulin aspart shows a receptor affinity comparable with that of insulin lispro, whereas its affinity with the IGF-1 receptor is the same as that of human insulin. In GDM patients, aspart was more effective than human insulin in reducing postprandial glucose concentrations. A randomized multicenter clinical trial designed to assess the safety and efficacy of insulin aspart for type 1 diabetic patients in pregnancy reported a comparable fetal outcome and a trend towards fewer fetal losses and preterm deliveries than in women treated with human insulin [22, 23]. No data on the safety and efficacy of insulin glulisine in pregnancies complicated by diabetes are available yet [23].

Two long-acting insulin analogues are available, but have different structures. Glargine is obtained by adding two molecules of arginine to the C-terminal of the B chain in the human insulin molecule and replacing aspartic acid with glycine in position A21. These structural changes result in a shift in the isoelectric point from pH 5.4 to 6.7, a lower insulin solubility when injected subcutaneously, and a capacity for dimerization, which give rise to a longer-lasting action, a more limited glucose variability, and a lower risk of nocturnal hypoglycemia by comparison with neutral protamine Hagedorn (NPH) insulin.

The safety of glargine in pregnancy has not been fully demonstrated, and contrasting data on the binding of this insulin to the IGF-1 and the consequent mitogenic stimulation have raised concerns [21, 22]. A recent meta-analysis examining papers

Table 3. Insulin analogues and pregnancy: FDA categories

Insulin	Categories
Aspart	B
Lispro/lispro N-protamine	B
Glulisine	C
Detemir	B
Glargine	C

published on the topic found no significant differences in the efficacy and safety-related outcome between glargine and NPH insulin during pregnancy [24].

Insulin detemir is a long-acting insulin analogue, an acylated derivative of human insulin [LysB29(*N*-tetradecanoyl)des(B30) human insulin], in which a combination of increased self-association and albumin binding contributes to a protracted action, providing a more reproducible absorption and a prolonged action profile, and a lower risk of nocturnal hypoglycemia in comparison to NPH insulin.

These long-acting insulin analogues could be useful for managing pregnancy complicated by pregestational diabetes, mainly to contain the nocturnal hypoglycemia that can occur in such cases due to the need to obtain and maintain a strict glycemic target.

Animal reproduction studies in rabbits and rats have revealed no differences between insulin detemir and human insulin in regard to embryo toxicity and teratogenicity. A low affinity of insulin detemir for the IGF-1 receptor has also been demonstrated. A first report on the use of insulin detemir in human pregnancy in a small cohort of women found that it seems to help improve glycemic control and does not appear to have any adverse effects on maternal or fetal outcome in type 1 diabetic women [25]. A randomized controlled noninferiority trial comparing the efficacy and safety of insulin detemir versus NPH insulin in pregnant women with type 1 diabetes has since been published [26]. The results indicate that insulin detemir induces lower fasting plasma glucose levels, but not lower HbA_{1c} levels, in late pregnancy by comparison with NPH insulin, while the hypoglycemia rates were similar.

The intermediate-acting insulin analogue LysPro N-protamine has recently become available. The pharmacokinetic characteristics of this insulin are very similar to those of NPH insulin over a period of approximately 15 h, achieving a maximum insulin concentration approximately 6 h after injection. There are no clinical data on its use in pregnancy, but in general we can assume that the same concerns apply as for insulin lispro [23]. Indications for the use of these insulins are given in table 3.

In women with diabetes already before pregnancy, insulin therapy needs to be provided with intensified regimens, using multiple doses of subcutaneous long- and short-acting insulin. Algorithms should be used to adjust premeal insulin doses in these patients in order to correct glucose values outside the target range. The prandial insulin doses need to be matched not only with the premeal glucose values, but also with carbohydrate intake and physical activity. The insulin should be injected in the abdomen and/or hips to obtain the best absorption rate. In women with type 2 diabetes, the initial daily insulin doses should be calculated from 0.7 to 1.0 units/kg of actual body weight, then the dose needs to be adjusted on the basis of glucose levels. It is important to remember that obese pregnant women may require higher insulin doses and that insulin requirements may double or triple during pregnancy.

As for the use of insulin pumps (continuous subcutaneous insulin infusion) in pregnancy, despite recent innovations, continuous subcutaneous insulin infusion has not been proven superior to multiple daily insulin injection, but it can be useful in pregnant women suffering from hypoglycemia (especially at night and/or in cases of the dawn phenomenon). However, considering the potential risk of marked hyperglycemia and ketoacidosis in the event of insulin delivery failure due to kinking of the catheter, women need to be trained to use this device correctly [17].

References

1 Platt MJ, Stanisstreet M, Casson IF, Howard CV, Walkinshaw S, Pennycook S, McKendrick O: St Vincent's Declaration 10 years on: outcomes of diabetic pregnancies. Diabet Med 2002;19:216–220.

2 Lapolla A, Dalfrà MG, Fedele D: Pregnancy complicated by type 2 diabetes: an emerging problem. Diabetes Res Clin Pract 2008;80:2–7.

3 Reece EA, Homko C: Why do diabetic women deliver malformed infants? Clin Obstet Gynecol 2000; 43:32–45.

4 Pedersen J: Weight and length at birth of infants of diabetic mothers. Acta Endocrinol 1954;16:330–342.

5 Wahabi HA, Alzeidan RA, Esmaeil SA: Prepregnancy care for women with pre-gestational diabetes mellitus: a systematic review and meta-analysis. BMC Public Health 2012;12:792–804.

6 Lapolla A, Dalfrà MG, DiCianni G, Bonomo M, Parretti E, Mello G; Scientific Committee of the GISOGD Group: A multicenter Italian study on pregnancy outcome in women with diabetes. Nutr Metab Cardiovasc Dis 2008;18:291–297.

7 Freinkel N, Phelps R, Metzger BE: The mother in pregnancies complicated by diabetes; in Rifkin H, Porte D Jr (eds): Diabetes Mellitus. Theory and Practice, ed 4. New York, Elsevier, 1990, pp 634–650.

8 Di Cianni G, Miccoli R, Volpe L, Lencioni C, Del Prato S: Intermediate metabolism in normal pregnancy and in gestational diabetes. Diabetes Metab Res Rev 2003;19:259–270.

9 Buchanan TA: Metabolic changes during normal and diabetic pregnancy; in Reece EA, Coustan DR (eds): Diabetes Mellitus in Pregnancy. New York, Churchill Livingstone, 1995, pp 59–77.

10 Murphy HR, Elleri D, Allen JM, Harris J, Simmons D, Rayman G, Temple RC, Umpleby AM, Dunger DB, Haidar A, Nodale M, Wilinska ME, Hovorka R: Pathophisiology of postprandial hyperglycemia in women with type 1 diabetes during pregnancy. Diabetologia 2012;55:282–293.

11 American Diabetes Association: Standards of medical care in diabetes – 2013. Diabetes Care 2013; 36(Suppl 1):S11–S65.

12 NICE Guideline Development Group: Management of diabetes from preconception to the postnatal period: summary of NICE guidance. BMJ 2008;336: 714–717.

13 ACOG Practice Bulletin: Clinical management guidelines for obstetrician-gynecologists: pregestational diabetes mellitus. Obstet Gynecol 2005;105: 675–685.

14 Hernandez TL, Friedman JE, Van Pelt RE, Barbour LA: Patterns of glycemia in normal pregnancy: should the current therapeutic targets be challenged? Diabetes Care 2011;34:1660–1668.

15 Mosca A, Paleari R, Dalfrà MG, DiCianni G, Cuccuru I, Pellegrini G, Malloggi L, Bonomo M, Granata S, Ceriotti F, Castiglioni MT, Songini M, Tocco G, Masin M, Plebani M, Lapolla A: Reference intervals for haemoglobin A_{1c} in pregnant women: data from an Italian multicentric study. Clin Chem 2006;52:1138–1143.

16 Suhonen L, Hiilesmaa V, Teramo K: Glycaemic control during early pregnancy and fetal malformations in women with type 1 diabetes mellitus. Diabetologia 2000;43:79–82.

17 Kitzmiller JL, Block JM, Brown FM, Catalano PM, Conway DL, Coustan DR, Gunderson EP, Herman WH, Hoffman LD, Inturrisi M, Jovanovic LB, Kjos SI, Knopp RH, Montoro MN, Ogata ES, Paramsothy P, Reader DM, Rosenn BM, Thomas AM, Kirkman MS: Managing preexisting diabetes for pregnancy: summary of evidence and consensus recommendations for care. Diabetes Care 2008;31:1060–1079.

18 Middleton P, Crowther CA, Simmonds L, Muller P: Different intensities of glycaemic control for pregnant women with pre-existing diabetes. Cochrane Database Syst Rev 2010;9:CD008540.

19 Murphy HR, Rayman G, Lewis K, Kelly S, Johal B, Duffield K, Fowler D, Campbell PJ, Temple RC: Effectiveness of continuous glucose monitoring in pregnant women with diabetes: randomised clinical trial. BMJ 2008;25:337–344.

20 Dalfrà MG, Sartore G, DiCianni G, Mello G, Lencioni C, Ottanelli S, Sposato J, Valgimigli F, Scuffi C, Scalese M, Lapolla A: Glucose variability in diabetic pregnancy. Diabetes Technol Ther 2011;13:853–859.

21 Lapolla A, Dalfrà MG, Fedele D: Pregnancy complicated by diabetes: what is the best level of HbA_{1c} for conception? Acta Diabetol 2010;47:187–192.

22 Lapolla A, Dalfrà MG, Fedele D: Insulin therapy in pregnancy complicated by diabetes: are insulin analogs a new tool? Diabetes Metab Res Rev 2005;21: 241–252.

23 Torlone E, Di Cianni G, Mannino D, Lapolla A: Insulin analogs and pregnancy: an update. Acta Diabetol 2009;46:163–172.

24 Lepercq J, Lin J, Hall GC, Wang E, Dain MP, Riddle MC, Home PD: Meta-analysis of maternal and neonatal outcomes associated with the use of insulin glargine versus NPH insulin during pregnancy. Obstet Gynecol Int 2012;2012:649070.

25 Lapolla A, DiCianni G, Bruttomesso D, Dalfrà MG, Fresa R, Mello G, Napoli A, Romanelli T, Sciacca L, Stefanelli G, Torlone E, Mannino D: Use of insulin detemir in pregnancy: a report on 10 type 1 diabetic women. Diabet Med 2009;26:1179–1183.

26 Mathiesen ER, Hod M, Ivanisevic M, Duran Garcia S, Brøndsted L, Jovanovic Damm P, McCance DR; Detemir in Pregnancy Study Group: Maternal efficacy and safety outcomes in a randomized, controlled trial comparing insulin detemir with NPH insulin in 310 pregnant women with type 1 diabetes. Diabetes Care 2012;35:2012–2017.

Prof. Annunziata Lapolla
Department of Medicine
Via Giustiniani 2
IT–35100 Padova (Italy)
E-Mail annunziata.lapolla@unipd.it

Bruttomesso D, Grassi G (eds): Technological Advances in the Treatment of Type 1 Diabetes.
Front Diabetes. Basel, Karger, 2015, vol 24, pp 23–30 (DOI: 10.1159/000363462)

Management of Hyperglycemia in Hospitalized Patients: Critical Care Setting

Giorgio Grassi[a] · Matteo Bonomo[b]

[a]Department of Internal Medicine, Division of Endocrinology, Diabetes and Metabolism, Città della Salute e della Scienza, Torino, and [b]Diabetes Unit, Niguarda Ca Granda Hospital, Milano, Italy

Abstract

Increased blood glucose (BG) levels is common in critically ill patients both with and without a previous history of diabetes. Morbidity and mortality related to hyperglycemia is an important issue when managing BG in critically ill patients. Thus far, however, the characteristics of patients who may benefit from intensive insulin therapy remain to be clearly defined, as does the effect of different BG algorithms, the method of measuring BG, and the influence of different nutritional strategies. Intensive care units (ICUs) around the world have adopted insulin infusion protocols to achieve stringent BG targets in critically ill patients. Different insulin algorithms have been developed with variable effectiveness. Most of those algorithms require considerable training and experience. Computer decision support systems might improve the outcomes of patients in the ICU. Intensive insulin infusion managed using software-guided programs achieves tighter glycemic control and equal or fewer hypoglycemic episodes than paper protocols. The measurement of BG concentrations in the ICU is performed intermittently in the majority of ICUs, using either arterial blood gas analyzers, glucose meters, or central laboratory. Blood gas analyzers are considered the best compromise between accuracy and practicality. Real-time continuous glucose monitoring (RTCGM) offers interesting possibilities: automatic measurement of large numbers of BG values and alarms that warn whenever 'outlier' values are reached. Data published to date from some randomized studies in ICUs have indicated a lower incidence of hypoglycemia when RTCGM is used in adults under mechanical ventilation and after cardiac surgery; however, until further studies provide sufficient evidence for its accuracy and safety, the use of RTCGM alone in not recommended.

The 2001 study by Van den Berghe et al. [1] concerning the target of blood glucose (BG) in the surgical intensive care unit (ICU; 80–110 mg/dl) related to morbidity and mortality had a deep impact on the management of BG in critically ill patients.

Increased BG levels are common in critically ill patients both with and without a previous history of diabetes [2]. BG levels above 80 mg/dl are positively associated with increasing mortality among critically ill patients without diabetes [3]. The relation between increasing mean BG levels above 80 mg/dl and mortality among diabetic patients is less clear [4].

In critically ill patients, an association exists between even mild or moderate hypoglycemia and mortality [5]. Furthermore, glucose variability is greater in patients with hypoglycemia [6].

Since all three domains of glycemic control (hyperglycemia, hypoglycemia, and glucose variability) are related to mortality and morbidity in critically ill patients [7], insulin treatment should minimize glucose excursions.

It is appropriate that the timing of glycemic control and insulin therapy are under the control of a protocol to increase safety. ICUs around the world have adopted insulin infusion protocols to achieve stringent BG targets in critically ill patients (89–110 mg/dl). Several subsequent studies [8, 9], however, have questioned the efficacy and safety of targeting strict euglycemia and raised the concern of high rates of hypoglycemia produced by these stringent limits. The results of an updated meta-analysis do not support widespread adoption of intensive insulin therapy in critically ill patients. The characteristics of patients who may benefit from intensive insulin therapy, different BG control algorithms and glucose targets, method of measuring BG, and nutritional strategies remain to be clearly defined [10].

The most important aspects related to the control of hyperglycemia in the critical care setting are insulin algorithms and protocols to control high BG, the technology for glucose measurement, the mode of glucose monitoring (intermittent vs. continuous), and timing and reporting of glucose control.

Treatment of Hyperglycemia

Guidelines for hospital management of hyperglycemia have recommended insulin as the preferred treatment modality for a variety of reasons [11, 12]. It is highly effective, easy to titrate, and has very few contraindications. There is a rationale for treatment with metformin, in consideration of insulin resistance due to stress, but little supporting evidence [13]. Preadmission metformin therapy is associated with reduced mortality in critically ill patients with type 2 diabetes and the mortality benefit persists after controlling for other variables since the use of a statin is also associated with reduced risk of death [14]. A favorable effect when metformin was continued during admission was also detected in postcardiac surgery patients [15]. It is not possible to draw conclusions from these observations, but they raise a possible role for metformin during intensive care in patients with diabetes.

Different insulin algorithms have been developed with variable effectiveness [16–18]; most of those algorithms require considerable ICU team training and experience. The time commitment for the management of frequent BG testing and insulin infusion protocol for the team is high. The autonomy of choice given to the operator may vary from algorithms that leave more space to the human factor and protocols that completely replace human feedback. Protocols differ in the degree of dynamism, the attention given to the change in BG levels between the two determinations, the use of boluses, the input of variables such as the type of nutrition, and the possible intake of food by mouth.

In recent years, several algorithms have been proposed that can be managed directly by the nursing staff and require the adjustment of insulin dosing on the basis of BG values measured every 1–2 h. Studies comparing the different algorithms are lacking and so it is not possible to recommend a specific protocol. However, the most recent dynamic algorithms which base insulin dosing on absolute BG values and on glycemic trend look promising.

Computer-Based Protocols

Computer decision support systems might improve the outcomes of patients in ICUs facilitating glucose control. Several programs have been developed and overall have been shown to be safe since the mid-1980s [19–22]. Commonly, the software is an open-loop algorithm that produces bedside recommendations about insulin titration based on different controller models as an alternative to 'written instruction with bedside calculation' [23].

The simplest type of software is the conversion of a paper-based algorithm into a software program. This system can reduce errors, but the predictive capabilities are generally limited by its simplicity [24]. The proportional-integral-derivative model (PID) [25] and the Glucommander algorithms [26] are more complex, characterized by a dynamic multiplier responsive to insulin sensitivity as judged by glucose variations for a given insulin dose, like the glucose regulation for intensive care patients algorithm (GRIP) [27].

Model Predictive Control (MPC) underlines the most recent algorithms, incorporating the administration of dextrose, insulin sensitivity, age, diagnosis of diabetes, and many other parameters for a more effective intervention, although with a greater complexity at startup [28].

An automated computer-based environment can reduce the error rate of paper-based protocols, but large-scale randomized controlled trials aiming to assess the impact of these systems on the outcome of critically ill patients are lacking. In relation to the clinical environment and specific patient needs, the defaults for the lower and upper BG targets and the initial insulin infusion rate can be changed at the beginning of the treatment. Usually these programs store BG values and dosing recommendations in a database for the review of algorithm efficacy. ICU patients, whose intensive insulin infusions were managed using software-guided programs, achieved tighter glycemic control and equal or fewer hypoglycemic episodes generally with a comparable frequency of glucose controls than paper protocols. The use of automated algorithms is promising, but requires further evidence. In the meantime their diffusion is growing.

In protocols for intravenous insulin, it is common for the patient not to take intermittent meals of carbohydrates due to difficulties to titrate up the insulin dose. In these cases, some authors have suggested administering insulin subcutaneously according to a predetermined insulin-carbohydrates ratio (1 unit every 5–10 g of carbohydrates), and some computer-based protocol models like MPC can integrate this component of the treatment.

Transition from Intravenous Insulin Infusion to Subcutaneous Insulin Treatment

Restoration of subcutaneous insulin therapy can be programmed in the postcritical phase. It is necessary to calculate the amount of insulin that the patient has received in the last 24 h to get the daily insulin requirement. This requirement (prudently reduced by 20%) should be administered for 50% as basal insulin and 50% as prandial insulin. The first subcutaneous insulin injection should be administered 2–3 h before suspending the infusion insulin.

Point of Care for the Determination of Blood Glucose

The measurement of BG concentrations in the ICU is performed intermittently in the majority of ICU, using either point-of-care (POC) glucose meters or BG analyzers.

The reference technique to accurately measure glucose levels is mass spectrometry, but alternative and less labor-intensive approaches have been developed. All glucose sensor devices are based on enzymatic reactions in which glucose is converted into a suitable product by hexokinase (central laboratory analyzers), glucose oxidase, or glucose-1-dehydrogenase. The main advantage of glucose oxidase is its specificity to glucose; however, high oxygen tensions, which are possible in mechanically ventilated patients, could result in falsely lower BG levels in glucose oxidase systems. Reducing agents, such as ascorbic acid (vitamin C) and acetaminophen (paracetamol), tend to induce underestimation of BG levels. In hemodynamically stable patients, POC measurements correlate with laboratory references values [29]; in contrast, in critically ill patients, POC fingerstick blood-glucose shows a variance compared with laboratory reference. In conditions with poor peripheral tissue perfusion as in shock, a systematic literature analysis showed that the accuracy of blood-glucose measurements with arterial blood gas analyzers was significantly higher than that of measurements with glucose meters using capillary blood, and tended to be higher than that of measurements with glucose meters using arterial blood [30].

Blood gas analyzers are a type of bench laboratory analyzers with the capability of measuring pH, pO_2, and pCO_2 often combined with oximetry. They utilize whole blood, and the glucose measurement is typically performed with a glucose electrode that utilizes glucose oxidase. Compared with hand-held POC meters, blood gas analyzers are close to laboratory standards levels. They are generally considered to be as accurate as central laboratory devices.

Accuracy of BG measurements using arterial blood gas analyzers might vary among devices, but generally BG monitoring with arterial blood gas analyzers tends to be more accurate than monitoring by glucose meters with arterial blood.

Arterial blood samples should be used rather than capillary blood samples for BG measurements in adult critically ill patients. In the hypoglycemic range, BG monitoring is less accurate than monitoring in the nonhypoglycemic range. Unstable hemodynamics and insulin infusion might increase the risk of error in BG monitoring with a glucose meter.

Central Laboratory Devices

In the majority of central laboratories, the measurement of glucose is performed with an analyzer performing multiple assays, with a lower limit of 2 mg/dl, upper limit as high as 750 mg/dl, a coefficient of variation <2%, an analytical bias of inaccuracy of <2.25, and a total error <6.0% [31].

Handled Glucose Point of Care

There are a number of POC glucose meters that target the hospital market [32]. However, the accuracy standard that is currently applied to POC meters for the home market is the only regulatory hurdle needed for hospital use. The International Organization for Standardization guideline (ISO 15197) states that 95% of readings fall within ±15% of the reference for glucose levels ≥100 mg/dl and within ±15 mg/dl of the reference for glucose levels <100 mg/dl (reference No. ISO/FDIS 15197, 2013). Although these meters are marketed specifically for use in the hospital environment, it is unclear if the technologies or accuracy profiles are actually any different or better than what these companies are marketing to the home glucose market. The inaccuracy of the POC meters has been well documented, and their possible role in iatrogenic hypoglycemia should not be ignored.

Real-Time Continuous Glucose Monitoring

Real-time continuous glucose monitoring (RTCGM) offers interesting possibilities. Automatic measurement of large numbers of BG values, even outside normal hours, alarms that warn whenever 'outlier' values are reached, or the ability to predict the imminent risk of rapid shifts toward hyper- or hypoglycemia could permit real glycemic optimization in safety. This prospect has probably less impact in the ICU, where more invasive techniques can be used for tight BG monitoring [33]. Even so, the scant data published to date from some randomized studies in ICUs indicates a lower incidence of hypoglycemia when RTCGM is used in adults under mechanical ventilation [34], and in adult [35] or pediatric patients [36], after cardiac surgery.

Before widespread use of real-time monitoring systems can be recommended in hospital, however, some questions about the accuracy of the data need to be answered. Accuracy is obviously a pressing need for almost all the current applications of RTCGM, especially in the ICU, where patients are particularly frail. In addition to the aspects normally taken into consideration for outpatients, the inpatient often presents a series of extra variables which can substantially affect the quality of measurements in interstitial fluid. These include hypotension, edema, anemia, hypothermia, pH changes, renal or hepatic insufficiency, and the use of inotropic drugs. Although various studies have given encouraging results, with high percentages of values falling within Clarke's A+B range [37–40], we still need further evidence before authorizing large-scale use of these tools. Appropriate, reliable use also implies targeted training for healthcare staff, which is not always possible outside centers of excellence.

These considerations, for example, underlie the negative position taken by the Endocrine Society in 2011 [41], whose recommendation 1.1 states: 'We recommend against the use of RTCGM alone for glucose management in the intensive care unit or operating room until further studies provide sufficient evidence for its accuracy and safety in those settings'.

This is a field, however, where technology is quickly moving ahead fast and in the near future further progress will very likely improve the reliability of the sensors. As a result, the whole question will be up for reconsideration, and these tools are likely to be used more widely in hospital.

References

1 Van den Berghe G, Wouters P, Weekers F, Verwaest C, Bruyninckx F, Schetz M, Vlasselaers D, Ferdinande P, Lauwers P, Bouillon R: Intensive insulin therapy in critically ill patients. N Engl J Med 2001; 345:1359–1367.

2 Van den Berghe G: How does blood glucose control with insulin save lives in intensive care? J Clin Invest 2004;114:1187–1195.

3 Umpierrez GE, Isaacs SD, Bazargan N, You X, Thaler LM, Kitabchi AE: Hyperglycemia: an independent marker of in-hospital mortality in patients with undiagnosed diabetes. J Clin Endocrinol Metab 2002; 87:978–982.

4 Taylor JH, Beilman GJ: Hyperglycemia in the intensive care unit: no longer just a marker of illness severity. Surg Infect (Larchmt) 2005;6:233–245.

5 Egi M, Bellomo R, Stachowski E, French CJ, Hart GK, Taori G, Hegarty C, Bailey M: Hypoglycemia and outcome in critically ill patients. Mayo Clin Proc 2010;85:217–224.

6 Egi M, Bellomo R, Stachowski E, French CJ, Hart G: Variability of blood glucose concentration and short-term mortality in critically ill patients. Anesthesiology 2006;105:244–252.

7 Krinsley JS, Egi M, Kiss A, Devendra AN, Schuetz P, Maurer PM, Schultz MJ, van Hooijdonk RT, Kiyoshi M, Mackenzie IM, Annane D, Stow P, Nasraway SA, Holewinski S, Holzinger U, Preiser JC, Vincent JL, Bellomo R: Diabetic status and the relation of the three domains of glycemic control to mortality in critically ill patients: an international multicenter cohort study. Crit Care 2013;17:R37.

8 NICE-SUGAR Study Investigators, Finfer S, Chittock DR, et al: Intensive versus conventional glucose control in critically ill patients. N Engl J Med 2009; 360:1283–1297.
9 Inzucchi SE, Siegel MD: Glucose control in the ICU – how tight is too tight? N Engl J Med 2009;360: 1346–1349.
10 Griesdale DE, de Souza RJ, van Dam RM, Heyland DK, Cook DJ, Malhotra A, Dhaliwal R, Henderson WR, Chittock DR, Finfer S, Talmor D: Intensive insulin therapy and mortality among critically ill patients: a meta-analysis including NICE-SUGAR study data. CMAJ 2009;180:821–827.
11 Umpierrez GE, Hellman R, Korytkowski MT, Kosiborod M, Maynard GA, Montori VM, Seley JJ, Van den Berghe G: Management of hyperglycemia in hospitalized patients in non-critical care setting: an endocrine society clinical practice guideline. J Clin Endocrinol Metab 2012;97:16–38.
12 Moghissi ES, Korytkowski MT, DiNardo M, Einhorn D, Hellman R, Hirsch IB, Inzucchi SE, Ismail-Beigi F, Kirkman MS, Umpierrez GE; American Association of Clinical Endocrinologists, American Diabetes Association: American Association of Clinical Endocrinologists and American Diabetes Association consensus statement on inpatient glycemic control. Diabetes Care 2009;32:1119–1131.
13 Dungan KM, Braithwaite SS, Preiser J: Stress hyperglycemia. Lancet 2009;373:1798.
14 Christensen S, Thomsen RW, Johansen MB, Pedersen L, Jensen R, Larsen KM, Larsson A, Tønnesen E, Sørensen HT: Preadmission statin use and one-year mortality among patients in intensive care – a cohort study. Crit Care 2010;14:R29.
15 Duncan AI, Koch CG, Xu M, Manlapaz M, Batdorf B, Pitas G, Starr N: Recent metformin ingestion does not increase in-hospital morbidity or mortality after cardiac surgery. Anesth Analg 2007;104:42–50.
16 Krinsley JS: Effect of an intensive glucose management protocol on the mortality of critically ill adult patients. Mayo Clin Proc 2004;79:992–1000.
17 Zimmerman CR, Mlynarek ME, Jordan JA, et al: An insulin infusion protocol in critically ill cardiothoracic surgery patients. Ann Pharmacother 2004;38: 1123–1129.
18 Goldberg PA, Siegel MD, Sherwin RS, et al: Implementation of a safe and effective insulin infusion protocol in a medical intensive care unit. Diabetes Care 2004;27:461–467.
19 Kanji S, Singh A, Tierney M, et al: Standardization of intravenous insulin therapy improves the efficiency and safety of blood glucose control in critically ill adults. Intensive Care Med 2004;30:804–810.
20 Boord JB, Sharifi M, Greevy RA, et al: Computer-based insulin infusion protocol improves glycemia control over manual protocol. J Am Med Inform Assoc 2007;14:278–287.
21 Cavalcanti AB, Silva E, Pereira AJ, et al: A randomized controlled trial comparing a computer-assisted insulin infusion protocol with a strict and a conventional protocol for glucose control in critically ill patients. J Crit Care 2009;24:371–378.
22 Braithwaite SS, Edkins R, Macgregor KL, et al: Performance of a dose-defining insulin infusion protocol among trauma service intensive care unit admissions. Diabetes Technol Ther 2006;8:476–488.
23 The Society of Thoracic Surgeons practice guideline series: blood glucose management during adult cardiac surgery. Ann Thorac Surg 2009;87:663–669.
24 Steil GM, Deiss D, Shih J, Buckingham B, Weinzimer S, Agus MS: Intensive care unit insulin delivery algorithms: why so many? How to Choose? J Diabetes Sci Technol 2009;3:125–140.
25 Rood E, Bosman RJ, van der Spoel JI, Taylor P, Zandstra DF: Use of a computerized guideline for glucose regulation in the intensive care unit improved both guideline adherence and glucose regulation. J Am Med Inform Assoc 2005;12:172–180.
26 Wintergerst KA, Deiss D, Buckingham B, Cantwell M, Kache S, Agarwal S, Wilson DM, Steil G: Glucose control in pediatric intensive care unit patients using an insulin-glucose algorithm. Diabetes Technol Ther 2007;9:211–222.
27 Davidson PC, Steed RD, Bode BW: Glucommander: a computer-directed intravenous insulin system shown to be safe, simple, and effective in 120,618 h of operation. Diabetes Care 2005;28:2418–2423.
28 Cordingley JJ, Vlasselaers D, Dormand NC, Wouters PJ, Squire SD, Chassin LJ, Wilinska ME, Morgan CJ, Hovorka R, Van den Berghe G: Intensive insulin therapy: enhanced Model Predictive Control algorithm versus standard care. Intensive Care Med 2009;35:123–128.
29 Ray JG, Hamielec C, Mastracci T: Pilot study of the accuracy of bedside glucometry in the intensive care unit. Crit Care Med 2001;29:2205–2207.
30 Inoue S, Egi M, Kotani J, Morita K: Accuracy of blood-glucose measurements using glucose meters and arterial blood gas analyzers in critically ill adult patients: systematic review. Crit Care 2013;17:R48.
31 Ricós C, Alvarez V, Cava F, García-Lario JV, Hernández A, Jiménez CV, Minchinela J, Perich C, Simón M: Current databases on biological variation: pros, cons and progress. Scand J Clin Lab Invest 1999;59: 491–500.
32 Gijzen K, Moolenaar DL, Weusten JJ, Pluim HJ, Demir AY: Is there a suitable point-of-care glucose meter for tight glycemic control? Evaluation of one home-use and four hospital-use meters in an intensive care unit. Clin Chem Lab Med 2012;50:1985–1992.
33 Thabit H, Hovorka R: Glucose control in non-critically ill inpatients with diabetes: towards closed-loop. Diabetes Obes Metab 2014;16:500–509.

34 Holzinger U, Warszawska J, Kitzberger R, Wewalka M, Miehsler W, Herkner H, Madl C: Real-time continuous glucose monitoring in critically ill patients: a prospective randomized trial. Diabetes Care 2010; 33:467–472.
35 Kopecky P, Mraz M, Blaha J, Lindner J, Svacina S, Hovorka R, Haluzik M: The use of continuous glucose monitoring combined with computer-based eMPC algorithm for tight glucose control in cardiosurgical ICU. Biomed Res Int 2013;2013:186439.
36 Agus MS, Steil GM, Wypij D, Costello JM, Laussen PC, Langer M, Alexander JL, Scoppettuolo LA, Pigula FA, Charpie R: Tight glycemic control versus standard care after pediatric cardiac surgery. N Engl J Med 2012;367:1208–1219.
37 Corstjens AM, Ligtenberg JJ, van der Horst IC, Spanjersberg R, Lind JS, Tulleken JE, Meertens JH, Zijlstra JG: Accuracy and feasibility of point-of-care and continuous blood glucose analysis in critically ill ICU patients. Crit Care 2006;10:R135.
38 Holzinger U, Warszawska J, Kitzberger R, Herkner H, Metnitz PG, Madl C: Impact of shock requiring norepinephrine on the accuracy and reliability of subcutaneous continuous glucose monitoring. Intensive Care Med 2009;35:1383–1389.
39 Rabiee A, Andreasik V, Abu-Hamdah R, Galiatsatos P, Khouri Z, Gibson BR, Andersen DK, Elahi D: Numerical and clinical accuracy of a continuous glucose monitoring system during intravenous insulin therapy in the surgical and burn intensive care units. J Diabetes Sci Technol 2009;3:951–959.
40 Yamashita K, Okabayashi T, Yokoyama T, Yatabe T, Maeda H, Manabe M, Hanazaki K: Accuracy and reliability of continuous blood glucose monitor in post-surgical patients. Acta Anaesthesiol Scand 2009;53:66–71.
41 Klonoff DC, Buckingham B, Christiansen JS, Montori VM, Tamborlane WV, Vigersky RA, Wolpert H; Endocrine Society: Continuous glucose monitoring: an Endocrine Society Clinical Practice Guideline. J Clin Endocrinol Metab 2011;96:2968–2979.

Dr. Giorgio Grassi
S.C.D.U. Endocrinologia, Diabetologia e Metabolismo
A.O. Città della Salute e della Scienza, Corso Bramante 88
IT–10126 Torino (Italy)
E-Mail giorgio.grassi@gmail.com

Bruttomesso D, Grassi G (eds): Technological Advances in the Treatment of Type 1 Diabetes.
Front Diabetes. Basel, Karger, 2015, vol 24, pp 31–46 (DOI: 10.1159/000363468)

Management of Hyperglycemia in Hospitalized Patients: Noncritical Care Setting

Ariana R. Pichardo-Lowden

Penn State University College of Medicine, Milton S. Hershey Medical Center, Hershey, Pa., USA

Abstract

Hyperglycemia is a common in-hospital problem and is associated with poor clinical outcomes. A critical review of pertinent studies and peer-reviewed publications related to inpatient glycemia was conducted. Diabetes mellitus is a problem of worldwide proportion that leads to frequent hospitalization. Hyperglycemia is often found in inpatient settings and is associated with increased risk of morbidity and mortality, surgical interventions, in-hospital infections and surgical site infections, higher admission rates to intensive care units (ICUs), increased hospital length of stay, and increased postdischarge care needs. In some studies, improved inpatient glycemia showed a positive impact in clinical outcomes. Attainment of adequate glycemic control requires addressing various clinical scenarios. The approach to hyperglycemia should abide by the principles of provision of adequate insulin regimens that consider the individual clinical situation of patients and aim for safe glucose targets. The control of hyperglycemia in the nonintensive care setting is a relevant clinical problem that requires effective and prudent strategies. This chapter provides an overview of scenarios encountered in general medical and surgical units, offers a practical approach to management of dysglycemia, lists factors contributing to hyperglycemia and hypoglycemia, reviews the recommended targets for treatment, and presents a strategy for transition to outpatient care. The research evidence available suggests that hyperglycemia is associated with poor clinical outcomes in critically and noncritically ill patients. Additionally, tight glycemic control increases the risk for hypoglycemia and mortality, and less stringent glucose targets may result in lower rates of hypoglycemia. Therefore, judicious glucose control, as opposed to stringent near-normal control proposed in previous clinical guidelines and statements, is probably sufficient to prevent poor clinical outcomes related to hyperglycemia in the ICU. The data available in non-ICU settings is less robust; however, good glucose management remains important in hospitalized patients across clinical units and an attentive attitude toward care of inpatient hyperglycemia should prevail among providers.

Overview of the Evidence of Hyperglycemia and Hypoglycemia in the Hospital

Approximately 346 million people have diabetes mellitus around the world [1], and the proportion of people over 65 years of age diagnosed with diabetes is expected to increase [2]. Patients with diabetes mellitus are frequently hospitalized and undergo surgical procedures at a greater rate than patients without diabetes [3]. Inpatient hyperglycemia is frequently encountered in intensive care units (ICUs) and general medical and surgical wards. An analysis of over 49 million point-of-care (POC) blood glucose measurements from hospitals in the USA showed a mean POC blood glucose equal to 167 mg/dl for ICU and 166 mg/dl for non-ICU patients. The prevalence of hyperglycemia (>180 mg/dl) in both settings was estimated to be approximately 32% and the prevalence of hypoglycemia (<70 mg/dl) was 6.3% for ICU patients and 5.7% for non-ICU patients [4].

Hyperglycemia in the hospital is associated with worse clinical outcomes regardless of the reason for admission to intensive [5–7] and nonintensive medical and surgical care units [5–9]. Elevations of mean glucose levels in medical and surgical ICU populations are associated with increased risk of hospital mortality and clinical complications. This association seems to be present independently of severity of illness, care units, or a diagnosis of diabetes. Furthermore, perioperative complications including surgical site infections, longer hospital length of stay (LOS), and postdischarge needs are increased in hospitalized medical and surgical patients with hyperglycemia [5, 6, 9, 10]. Although the existing data for nonintensive care populations is less robust than that data derived from critical care settings, there is growing evidence from retrospective cohorts, observational studies, and randomized trials that demonstrated a negative impact of poor glycemic control in non-ICU settings [10–12]. As data is limited in non-ICU settings, recommendations are based on extrapolation from ICU findings and other clinical settings, expert opinion, and existing guidelines.

In a prospective cohort study [13], hyperglycemia at the time of admission to the hospital was independently associated with adverse outcomes and prolonged hospital LOS in noncritically ill patients with community-acquired pneumonia. Patients with an admission blood glucose level >198 mg/dl (>11 mmol/l) had a significantly increased adjusted risk of death and in-hospital complications, which was more pronounced in those without a prior diagnosis of diabetes. A retrospective study of patients with exacerbation of chronic obstructive pulmonary disease and hyperglycemia showed that increased blood glucose concentration was associated with longer hospital LOS and death in comparison with patients who had lower blood glucose concentrations, regardless of age, sex, and history of diabetes. In this study, multivariate analysis, showed that predicted forced expiratory volume in 1 s was not a determinant of adverse outcome. Further, blood glucose independently predicted adverse clinical outcomes, whereas the severity of chronic obstructive pulmonary disease did not [14]. In a review of 2,030 medical records, newly discovered hyperglycemia was significantly associated with a higher in-hospital mortality rate (16%) in comparison with patients who had a prior history of diabetes (3%) and subjects with normoglycemia (1.7%). Patients with new hyperglycemia had a longer hospital LOS, were less likely to be discharged to home, required transfer to a nursing home or a transitional care unit more frequently, and had higher admission rates to an ICU. Non-ICU mortality was 0.8, 1.7, and 10% ($p < 0.01$) for patients with normoglycemia, known diabetes, and new hyperglycemia, respectively [10].

In surgical populations, the deleterious effects of hyperglycemia and the benefits of glucose control are distinctly relevant to surgical cardiac patients. The methodology of many studies available to date is limited by their observational and retrospective design; however, the evidence convincingly demonstrates that hyperglycemia is harmful to both critically ill and noncritically ill surgical patients. Peri-, pre- and intraoperative and postoperative hyperglycemia is associated with increased morbidity, decreased survival, and increased utilization resource [6, 15]. Data derive from surgical population including cohorts of patients who underwent mastectomy, operations for hepatobiliary and pancreatic cancer, colorectal procedures, orthopedic spinal surgery, infrainguinal vascular surgery, and total joint arthroplasty. In all of these studies, elevation of blood glucose values was associated with increased risk of surgical site infections [15].

Another relevant group of hospitalized patients are those with hospital or stress-related hyperglycemia, which refers to transient elevations in blood glucose that occur during acute illness in patients without diabetes prior to admission, or to exacerbation of hyperglycemia in subjects with diabetes mellitus. A study found that newly discovered hyperglycemia in the hospital in subjects without diabetes was found to increase risk of mortality, LOS, and need for long-term placement after hospitalization compared to patients with known diabetes [10]. Such associations should alert clinicians to the need for monitoring individuals at risk and adequately addressing and treating hyperglycemia in such patients. Medications such as octreotide, glucocorticoids, vasopressors, immunosuppressant agents, and administration of enteral or parenteral nutrition are frequent contributors to hyperglycemia in hospitalized patients [6]. Patients receiving these therapies benefit from having their blood glucose monitored and appropriate intervention offered when required [16]. It is important to recognize that in some studies, hospitalized patients with hyperglycemia without a preadmission diagnosis of diabetes have been found to have prediabetes or diabetes in as many as 42–60% of cases [17, 18]. Therefore, establishing a diagnosis prior to hospital discharge should be a priority when possible, given the potential consequences of undiagnosed diabetes. Patients with persistent hyperglycemia in the hospital should have a glycohemoglobin level drawn if not done in the preceding 3 months to identify or exclude a diagnosis of diabetes or prediabetes. Patients with glycohemoglobin levels ≥5.7% can be considered high risk and those with levels ≥6.5% are confirmed to have diabetes. There are limitations to the use of glycohemoglobin for the diagnosis of diabetes in hospitalized populations, which include the presence of hemoglobinopathies, blood transfusions, iron deficiency anemia, and high-dose salicylate use. Therefore, results need to be interpreted with caution.

Control of hyperglycemia showed positive effect in hospital outcomes. The Leuvren study, the first randomized controlled trial of intensive glucose control in ICU patients, showed reduction in morbidity and mortality in a surgical cohort [7]. Benefits of morbidity reduction were demonstrated in a subsequent trial by the same investigators; however, the benefit of mortality reduction derived from intensive glycemic management could not be replicated in a medical ICU population [19]. Other randomized controlled trials and cohort studies subsequently suggested that intensive treatment of hyperglycemia improved clinical outcomes. Later on, additional investigations continued to reveal the benefits of controlling hyperglycemia in ICU and non-ICU settings. However, a number of studies in critically ill populations failed to demonstrate mortality reduction derived from intensive glucose control, and some tied intensive glycemic control in the ICU to an increased mortality risk [20, 21]. The results of the Normoglycemia in Intensive Care Evaluation-Survival Using Glucose Algorithm Regulation (NICE-SUGAR) study and its subsequent post hoc analysis associated tight glycemic control to increased frequency of moderate and severe hypoglycemia and an increased risk of mortality [20, 22]. A systematic review and meta-analysis of 19 eligible studies, including 10 observational studies and 9 randomized controlled trials including non-ICU medical and surgical patients, suggested that intensive glycemic control was not associated with a significant effect on the risk of death, myocardial infarction, or stroke, but there was a trend toward increased risk of hypoglycemia. Intensive control of glycemia was associated with decreased risk of hospital-acquired infection primarily in surgical populations [12]. In another study in a non-cohort the number of days with hypoglycemia and the severity of hypoglycemic episodes correlated with a significantly increased risk of mortality and longer hospital stay [23].

The American Association of Clinical Endocrinologists (AACE), American Diabetes Association (ADA) [6], Endocrine Society [16], and other leading international diabetes societies [24] have issued guidelines for treatment of inpatient hyperglycemia in light of the existing evidence. Current guidelines advocate for achievable and safe glycemic targets and emphasize that the relaxation of glycemic targets should not derail efforts in controlling hyperglycemia in the hospital. It is currently recommended that the ICU glucose target be 140–180 mg/dl and non-ICU goals be premeal glucose <140 mg/dl and random glucose <180 mg/dl. Clinicians may consider glycemic goals below or above these cut-points depending on the clinical scenario, taking into the account patient's life expectancy, risk for hypoglycemia, and presence of comorbid conditions. It is important to promptly reassess insulin regimens if blood glucose is <100 mg/dl and immediately adjust if blood glucose is <70 mg/dl. Patients with stress hyperglycemia and hyperglycemia induced by medications or by parenteral or enteral nutrition (EN) lasting more than 24 h need to be treated to attain the same glucose goals as those patients with known diabetes [6, 16].

Perioperative management of hyperglycemia can be complex due to the uncertainty of when it is most critical to attain glycemic control, the heterogeneity of existing results in surgical populations, limited prospective data in non-ICU surgical patients, and limited evidence in support of definitive glycemic targets, particularly outside the critical care setting. Nonetheless, it is important to recognize that hyperglycemia in the perioperative period can lead to fluid shifts, dehydration, electrolyte disturbance, ketoacidosis, hyperosmolar states, and a predisposition to infection and impaired wound healing. Prudent control of hyperglycemia, prevention, and prompt treatment of hypoglycemia, preferably relying on standardized methods, are considered standards of care. Current glycemic control guidelines can be applicable to medical and surgical patients while maintaining the vision of attaining blood glucose targets safely.

Management of Hyperglycemia in the Medical and Surgical Wards

The management of hyperglycemia in the hospital may be confounded by a variety of clinical scenarios. Insulin therapy is often tailored to address changes in patient activity and nutritional intake, exacerbation of hyperglycemia from medications used in the hospital; by administration of enteral or parenteral nutrition, and by changes in clinical status. Consistent assessment of glycemic trends, of variations in nutritional status and clinical situation, selection of adequate insulin regimens, and prompt adjustment of insulin when indicated is necessary to optimally manage hyperglycemia and to prevent hypoglycemia in hospitalized patients.

Basal insulin prevents gluconeogenesis and ketogenesis while bolus (prandial or nutritional) insulin attempts to control glucose excursions resulting from nutrient intake. Correction or supplemental insulin aims to control existing excessive hyperglycemia. The use of insulin regimens that consider these components is an effective strategy to control hyperglycemia and to maintain euglycemia in hospitalized noncritically ill patients [11, 25, 26]. Correction or supplemental insulin should be distinguished from sliding scale insulin, which refers to insulin administered as monotherapy on an 'as needed' basis in an attempt to treat hyperglycemia after it occurs. This strategy is seldom efficacious as it does not prevent hyperglycemia while allowing suboptimal control of glucose levels. An important caveat is that patients with type 1 diabetes lack endogenous insulin and are at risk of rapid development of severe hyperglycemia and diabetic ketoacidosis in the event of failure to administer insulin properly. Therefore, the use of sliding scale insulin in patients with type 1 diabetes is dangerous and always inappropriate [16]. Patients with type 1 diabetes should never be deprived from insulin treatment or treated with sliding scale insulin as monotherapy. Randomized controlled trials comparing the safety and efficacy of subcutaneous insulin regimens consisting of basal-bolus-supplemental insulin versus sliding scale insulin in non-ICU medical and surgical populations showed superior glycemic control in participants receiving scheduled insulin in contrast to those randomized to sliding scale insulin alone. Complications such as wound infections, pneumonia, respiratory failure, acute renal failure, and bacteremia were encountered more frequently in a surgical cohort receiving sliding scale insulin [11, 26].

Table 1. Example of subcutaneous basal/bolus/correction insulin protocols for noncritically ill patients with type 2 diabetes mellitus

	Basal insulin detemir, glargine, or NPH	Nutritional or prandial insulin lispro, aspart, or regular	Supplemental or correction insulin lispro, aspart, or regular
TDD – Risk of hypoglycemia: 0.2–0.4 U/kg – Most patients: 0.5 U/kg – Insulin resistant: 0.7 U/kg	– 50% of TDD detemir or glargine – As a single injection in the morning or bedtime or NPH twice a day at the same time	– 50% of TDD divided insulin amount – Equally between meals	– Follow correction insulin algorithms – Patients eating: administer before meals and at bedtime – Patients fasting: administer every 6 h if using regular insulin or every 4–6 h if using rapid-acting insulin
Daily dose adjustment – Fasting BG target: >100 and <140 mg/dl – Random or postprandial BG target: >100 and <180 mg/dl	Increase or decrease 10–20% of dose to attain glucose fasting glucose goal	Increase or decrease 10–20% of dose to attain random or postprandial glucose goal	– Increase insulin scale for glucose persistently >140 mg/dl – Decrease insulin scale if patient develops hypoglycemia (<70 mg/dl) – Amount used in 24 h may assist in determining daily insulin dose adjustment

BG = Blood glucose.

When transitioning from home to hospital, it is recommended to discontinue oral agents in most patients with type 2 diabetes and to implement insulin therapy. Patients who have been receiving insulin prior to admission may need to have their insulin dose modified to avoid hypoglycemia or exacerbation of hyperglycemia in consideration of risk factors. The initial total daily dose (TDD) of subcutaneous insulin can be determined from the preadmission insulin dose, overall glycemic control, and body weight, or from intravenous insulin requirements for patients who are transitioning from the intravenous to the subcutaneous route. An initial weight-based calculation of total daily insulin dose may be selected between 0.2 and 0.7 U/kg/day, taking into consideration patients who may be insulin naïve, at risk for hypoglycemia, or insulin resistant such as in the case of obese subjects or patients receiving high doses of glucocorticoids. The calculated dose of insulin can be split into a basal insulin component (50%) and nutritional component (50%) which is divided equally between meals as shown in table 1.

Glucose values will often dictate the subsequent insulin dose adjustment. For instance, morning hyperglycemia or hypoglycemia in most cases indicates insufficient or excessive basal insulin respectively, and postprandial hyperglycemia often suggests an inadequate dose of insulin administered for the meal prior to glucose value in ques-

Table 2. Sample of correction or supplemental insulin algorithms

Blood glucose, mg/dl	Low-dose (for patients taking 0.2–0.4 U/kg/day)		Moderate-dose (for patients taking 0.5–0.7 U/kg/day)		High-dose (for patients taking ≥0.7 U/kg/day)	
	preprandial	bedtime	preprandial	bedtime	preprandial	bedtime
150–200	1	0	2	0	3	0
201–250	2	1	4	2	6	3
251–300	3	2	6	4	9	6
301–350	4	3	8	6	12	9
351–400	5	4	10	8	15	12
>400	6	5	12	10	18	15

Table 3. Pharmacokinetic profile of subcutaneous insulin

Insulin	Onset of action	Insulin peak	Duration of action
Rapid-acting	0.2–0.4 h (5–15 min)	1–3 h	3–5 h
Aspart			
Lispro	–		
Glulisine			
Short-acting	0.5–1 h	2–3 h	6–10 h
Regular			
Intermediate-acting	2–4 h	4–10 h	10–16 h
NPH			
Long-acting	2–3 h		
Glargine		no peak	up to 24 h
Detemir			12–23 h

tion. Supplemental or correction insulin can be scheduled to correct hyperglycemia based on predetermined blood glucose goals as shown in table 2.

In the perioperative period of major or minor surgery, it is recommended that patients receive continuous intravenous insulin or subcutaneous basal insulin and bolus insulin (when applicable) to prevent and manage hyperglycemia. This recommendation is particularly important for patients with type 1 diabetes who may develop ketoacidosis when deprived of insulin. In a study, the administration of a full preadmission dose of long-acting basal insulin (detemir or glargine) when patients are NPO ('nil per os' or 'nothing per mouth') appeared to be safe [27]. A 10–20% reduction of the dose is advisable in patients with type 1 diabetes whose control is adequate in order to prevent hyperglycemia. Intermediate insulin dose, such as neutral protamine Hagedorn (NPH), may be reduced 25–50% given its pharmacokinetic action and peak after 4 h of administration [16]. The pharmacokinetic profile of insulin types is illustrated in table 3.

Management of Hyperglycemia in Special Situations

Transition from Intravenously to Subcutaneously Administered Insulin

Transition from intravenously to subcutaneously administered insulin should not result in deterioration of glycemic control. This transition requires accurate estimation of daily insulin requirement to maintain euglycemia and to prevent hypoglycemia. If the insulin hourly rate does not fluctuate widely, the approximate 24-hour insulin requirement can be estimated by multiplying the total amount of insulin required within the past 8 or 6 h by 3 or 4, respectively. Eighty percent of this amount should constitute a reasonable TDD for subcutaneous use. In a study, the administration of 80% of the TDD, in comparison with 60 and 40%, yielded a higher percentage of blood glucose values within the target range. For patients receiving dextrose solutions while simultaneously receiving insulin intravenously, using only 60% of the total dose required in 24 h can be considered [8]. Several other protocols have been proposed to guide this transition [16]. Intravenously and subcutaneously administered insulin should overlap by at least 1–2 h (if short-acting) or 2–4 h or longer (if long-acting) before discontinuation of continuous insulin infusion. In the management of patients with type 1 diabetes, this is an extremely important step for prevention of ketoacidosis.

Patients Receiving Glucocorticoids

Glucocorticoid therapy frequently worsens existing diabetes or results in hyperglycemia. Hyperglycemia from corticosteroids results from increased hepatic glucose production, impairment of glucose uptake in peripheral tissues, and promotion of protein catabolism which provides amino acids that can be used as precursors for gluconeogenesis. Glucocorticoids exaggerate postprandial glycemia due to a reduction in glucose uptake, a situation that often requires a greater amount of prandial insulin in relation to basal insulin. It is recommended that bedside POC glucose testing be initiated in patients receiving glucocorticoid therapy regardless of a history of diabetes. Testing can be discontinued in patients without diabetes if all blood glucose values are under 140 mg/dl after at least 24–48 h of testing. Insulin needs to be initiated if there is persistent hyperglycemia. When short-term pulses of high-dose corticosteroids are used or when severe hyperglycemia ensues, intravenous insulin is the most appropriate therapy. Adjustment of the insulin dose is necessary when glucocorticoid therapy is being tapered down to prevent hypoglycemia. Although different approaches have been suggested, no study has investigated the efficacy or safety of proposed insulin protocols in the management of corticosteroid-induced hyperglycemia in the hospital, or the impact of corticosteroid-induced hyperglycemia on clinical outcomes is not clearly known [16].

Patients Receiving Total Parenteral Nutrition

Use of total parenteral nutrition can result in pronounced hyperglycemia due to a high glucose load delivered to the systemic circulation bypassing the enteral systems. Hyperglycemia in patients receiving total parenteral nutrition may lead to complications and increased mortality. POC glucose testing is recommended regardless of a history of diabetes, and insulin therapy is the optimal approach when hyperglycemia persists over 12–24 h. If no hyperglycemia ensues after 24–48 h following achievement of the target caloric intake, POC glucose testing can be discontinued [16]. An insulin drip may be required to determine the daily insulin requirement which is helpful to determine the subcutaneous dose of insulin more likely to gain the glycemic control attained. The addition of regular insulin to the nutrition formula combined with subcutaneous correction insulin can be also a practical approach. Insulin doses utilized for correction using an insulin scale may help estimate additional insulin requirements which may in turn guide the adjustment of the insulin dose to be added to the nutritional formula bag. The use of scheduled subcutaneous basal insulin guaranties that an amount of insulin will be delivered in the event that parenteral nutrition is discontinued. This approach can be considered when managing patients with type 1 diabetes [8].

Patients Receiving Enteral Nutrition

The same principles of POC glucose monitoring for patients receiving total parenteral nutrition apply to patients receiving EN [16]. There are many factors contributing to the challenge of achieving glycemic targets in enterally fed patients, such as the different schedules of EN administration, variation of nutritional formulas' caloric and carbohydrate content, and unanticipated cessation of enteral feeding. A randomized study comparing subcutaneous insulin regimens in non-ICU patients receiving EN found similar glycemic control in the groups randomized to sliding scale insulin only versus glargine. However, of the patients in the sliding scale insulin group, 48% required NPH insulin to attain glycemic goal. Commonly, patients will require basal insulin during enteral feeding. Subcutaneous regimens that can be used, include once- or twice-daily glargine or detemir, NPH every 8–12 h, scheduled regular insulin every 4–6 h, and 70/30 insulin (NPH/regular). If frequent or rapid changes of caloric intake are occurring, intermediate insulin such as NPH represents a good alternative because due to its shorter duration of action, NPH insulin can be promptly adjusted in accordance with increments or reductions of enteral feeding, or even discontinued if needed. Basal insulin combined with a correction insulin scale and prandial insulin (if applicable depending on oral intake) represent an adequate approach when using continuous EN. In patients receiving bolus feedings, prandial insulin with rapid- or short-acting insulin attempts to meet the glucose excursion after nutrition formula boluses and it can be scheduled together with basal and supplemental insulin. Supplemental insulin refers to an insulin scale used in addition to prandial insulin to correct hyperglycemia.

In patients receiving nocturnal feedings (typically, 10–12 h of EN) basal insulin and correction insulin can be used. NPH insulin administered in 2 or 3 doses may constitute a better option than long-acting insulin since therapy can be timed so that the dose of insulin given immediately prior to feeding could be higher. If patients receiving nocturnal feeding are permitted to eat meals during the day, prandial insulin may be required. In the event that EN is suddenly interrupted, initiating dextrose-containing intravenous fluids, reducing the amount of basal insulin, and increasing the frequency of POC testing can be useful strategies to avoid hypoglycemia [8].

Continuous Subcutaneous Insulin Infusion (Pump Therapy)

Patients receiving continuous subcutaneous insulin infusion in the outpatient setting may continue self-management in the hospital provided that they remain physically and mentally capable to operate their pump and have infusion sets and supplies available. Hospitals should have established policies and procedures to guide the use of this technology in the acute care setting and nursing personnel should regularly document basal insulin rates and bolus doses [16]. Insulin pumps are commonly used for management of diabetes in patients with type 1 diabetes, but can also be used to manage patients with type 2 diabetes. Insulin pumps utilize rapid-acting insulin in most cases for both basal and bolus components. The basal component consists of hourly insulin rates which will vary from patient to patient. The bolus component delivers nutritional insulin following predetermined insulin to carbohydrate ratios after patients indicate the amount of carbohydrate in the meal. Correction for hyperglycemia is based on sensitivity factors which represent the reduction of plasma blood glucose expected to occur after administration of 1 unit of insulin or fraction. Its delivery is triggered by blood glucose levels above the predetermined glucose goal, and the dose is determined by the glucose level and sensitivity factor.

If there are concerns about a patient's ability to manage insulin pump, it must be discontinued. Other reasons for removing insulin pumps include surgical procedures, magnetic resonance imaging, computed tomography scans, X-rays, and any other exposure to radiation. When discontinued, subcutaneous insulin infusion therapy must be replaced by subcutaneous insulin injections or intravenous insulin, if indicated. It is also recommended to discontinue insulin pumps in critical illness, stroke, labor and delivery, initiation of or changes in glucocorticoid therapy, enteral or parenteral nutrition, perioperative period, radiation treatment, prolonged fasting states, and if there are concerns about device malfunction. Pumps should not be used for management of hyperglycemic emergencies such as hyperglycemic nonketotic hyperosmolar states or diabetic ketoacidosis.

Glucose Meters

POC glucose meters provide immediate results and are a cost-effective tool for monitoring hospitalized patients' glucose levels. Glucose meters that have demonstrated accuracy are the preferred method for guiding glycemic management in acutely ill patients. However, it is considered that the accuracy of results from glucose meters is lower than laboratory-based blood glucose results. Discrepancies among capillary, venous, and arterial plasma samples have been observed in the presence of dehydration, hypotension, hypoperfusion, low or high hemoglobin concentrations, and interfering substances such as acetaminophen, salicylate acid, uric acid, and vitamin C. Also, equipment variability, blood sample quality, patient physiology, care of the meter, and test strips can account for some degree of discrepancy among results. Glucose results that do not correlate with the patients' clinical status should be confirmed through a laboratory sample analysis [6, 16].

Continuous Glucose Monitoring

Real-time continuous glucose monitoring (CGM) via a glucose sensor continuously measures interstitial fluid glucose levels. It requires periodic calibration in order to make acute management decisions. Glucose sensing over 24 h identifies daily patterns of hyper- and hypoglycemia and the device has an alarm that will go off at preprogrammed levels. In a study, the use of CGM contributed to reductions in glycohemoglobin levels in adult ambulatory patients with type 1 diabetes receiving intensive insulin therapy. This technology may be particularly useful in patients with hypoglycemia unawareness and/or frequent hypoglycemic events; however, studies have not shown significant reduction of severe hypoglycemia in outpatient populations [28]. Patients who use CGM as outpatients may continue to use their sensors in the hospital, but it should not be a substitute for capillary blood glucose measurements which remain the mainstay of glucose monitoring in the hospital setting.

While recent studies have suggested that CGM devices may reduce the incidence of severe hypoglycemia in acute settings, the accuracy and reliability of this technology in hospitalized patients requires further investigation [29]. Some methods of testing are potentially subject to false elevations or reductions than actual values. In critical care settings, it has been suggested that the margins of error for blood glucose measurement should be within 15 mg/dl of the reference measurement for blood sugar values less than 100 mg/dl and within 15% if above 100 mg/dl. This differs from the recommendations from the International Organization for Standardization (ISO) that suggest the margin of error be within 15 mg/dl for blood sugars less than 75 mg/dl. These devices use interstitial fluid (ISF) rather than blood to measure glucose; however, our understanding of the relationship of ISF to blood in critically ill patients is limited. In ICU settings, conditions such as hypotension receiving treatment with a vasopressor and hypothermia were associated with significant discrepancies in the accuracy of sensor readings. Therefore, caution is required when interpreting results of CGM. As published, ISO criteria were not met by several commonly used glucose meters, with all readings being higher than the reference standard. This discrepancy could lead to serious overtreatment with insulin. CGM has the potential to reduce the chance of unknown hypoglycemic events that may occur between POC measurements that may otherwise be missed, which makes this method advantageous. While it seems promising, it needs to undergo rigorous testing on a larger scale in the ICU setting before it can be recommended [30].

Table 4. Potential contributors to hypoglycemia in the hospital

No prior use of insulin
Underweight (BMI <18.5)
Changes in carbohydrate or food intake
Comorbidities such as gastroparesis and adrenal insufficiency
Failure to adjust insulin based on blood glucose patterns
Significant change in clinical status
Poor coordination of blood glucose testing/insulin administration/meal delivery
Prolonged use of sliding scale insulin as monotherapy
Inadequate communication during transfer to different units
Error in transcription and insulin administration
Discontinuation or reduction of enteral or parenteral nutrition or steroids
Use of sulfonylureas, glinides, and mixed insulins

Prevention and Management of Hypoglycemia

Insulin is recognized as a high-alert medication since harm can result in errors in prescribing, transcribing, or dosing [6]. Anticipating and promptly treating hypoglycemia in the hospital should be considered a priority. There are many potentially contributing factors as listed in table 4. Table 5 presents an example of a protocol for hypoglycemia management. An association between moderate and severe hypoglycemia and an increased risk of death was established in critically ill patients. However, a causal effect of intensive glucose control cannot be inferred from the studies conducted even though a greater frequency of hypoglycemia occurred in subjects treated intensively with insulin therapy. This association was observed in patients with hypoglycemia in the absence of insulin therapy, thus suggesting that hypoglycemia could be an indicator of severity of illness [20, 22]. The findings of this study prompted revisions and change the recommendations for glycemic targets for hospitalized patients. A retrospective study including more than 4,000 admissions analyzed frequency and severity of hypoglycemia among noncritically ill patients. The rate of hypoglycemia was 7.7% of all admissions. The investigators conducted univariate and multivariate analyses and observed a significantly increased risk of inpatient mortality, LOS, and mortality 1 year after discharge in patients with hypoglycemia. Inpatient mortality increased as the number of hypoglycemic events rose and the degree of hypoglycemia became greater. Given the retrospective nature of the study, causality could not be directly inferred [23].

Preparing for Hospital Discharge

The care of patients with diabetes or hyperglycemia in the hospital presents a window of opportunity to improve glycemic control beyond hospitalization. The identification of an elevated glycohemoglobin value facilitates the recognition of poorly controlled or

Table 5. Sample of a hypoglycemia protocol

Check and record BG (hypoglycemia is BG <70 mg/dl)
Patient alert and cooperative and can take orally: – If BG <50 mg/dl, give 25 g of dextrose intravenously; if intravenous administration of dextrose may delay prompt treatment of hypoglycemia, give 15 g of carbohydrates (4-oz fruit juice/nondiet soda, 8-oz skim milk, or 3–4 glucose tablets); 15 g carbs will raise BG approx. 25–60 mg/dl – If blood glucose >50 mg/dl, give 15 g of carbohydrates – Recheck BG every 15 min until normal, then a further 3 times every 2 h – Repeat treatment if hypoglycemia persists
Patient alert but noncooperative: – If BG <50 mg/dl, give 25 g of dextrose intravenously or 1 mg glucagon intramuscularly if no intravenous access – If BG >50 mg/dl, give 12.5 g of dextrose intravenously or 1 mg glucagon intramuscularly if no intravenous access – Recheck BG every 15 min until normal, then a further 3 times every 2 h – Repeat treatment if hypoglycemia persists
Patient not alert: – Give 25 g of dextrose intravenously or 1 mg glucagon intramuscularly if no intravenous access – Recheck BG every 15 min until normal, then a further 3 times every 2 h – Repeat treatment if hypoglycemia persists
When hypoglycemia occurs remember to: – Investigate the cause – If hypoglycemia is recurrent, or related to sulfonylurea or long-acting insulin use, consider using a continuous dextrose solution – Adjust insulin regimen – Document the event and its treatment

BG = Blood glucose.

previously undiagnosed diabetes. Clinicians may optimize or change antidiabetic treatment, emphasize the importance of adherence to therapy and dietary recommendations, and channel subsequent efforts to outpatient care. It is important that adequate patient education takes place and that planned outpatient treatment regimen in the hospital be tailored to the patient's abilities, level of understanding, motivations, and financial limitations in order to improve compliance. The transition from hospital to home should emphasize safe and effective changes in an attempt to prevent emergency department visits and readmissions. Ideally, coordinating transition to the outpatient setting should occur early during hospitalization and should consider several relevant steps as outlined in table 6. Documentation of diabetes and new hyperglycemia in the discharge documents as a way of communicating with the outpatient providers is a step forward in improving long-term patient care. The plan for discharging of patients with new hyperglycemia should include clear recommendations for short- and long-term management of glycemia, and instructions for follow-up care [6, 16, 28].

Table 6. A comprehensive hospital discharge strategy for inpatient providers

Checklist for patient self-management
Be proactive/start discharge coordination early
Assess what patients can manage at home and provide 'survival skills'
How and when to monitor and take medication
Meal plan
Instructions for sick days
Hypoglycemia management
When to contact their provider
Appointment dates with primary care provider and diabetes educator and other pertinent appointments
Reinstitute preadmission antidiabetic regimen if no contraindication exists
Consider adjustment of therapy if glycohemoglobin not at goal
If patient is new to insulin, initiate at least 1 day before discharge
Consider side effects, comorbid conditions, and costs of medications when prescribing
Confirm patient has the necessary prescriptions and supplies [when applicable: insulin, syringes or pen needles, oral medications, blood glucose meter, test strips, lancets and lancing device, urine ketone strips (type 1), glucagon emergency kit (insulin treated), medical alert (bracelet or necklace) application]
Provide clear verbal and written instructions to patient and caregivers
Checklist for follow-up care
Provide timely discharge information to primary care providers
Document primary and secondary diagnoses and diagnostic findings such as HbA_{1c} value in discharge documents
Indicate dates of hospitalization, treatment provided in the hospital, and a summary of hospital course
Clearly document discharge medications and tests pending at time of discharge
Detail follow-up arrangements
Provide the name and contact information of the responsible hospital physician

Table 7. A practical checklist for management of inpatient hyperglycemia in noncritically ill patients

If patient is hyperglycemic or has diabetes mellitus, obtain glycohemoglobin if unavailable for the past 3 months
Monitor capillary blood glucose before meals and at bedtime for patients eating or every 4–6 h for patients fasting
Clearly document glucose levels and diagnosis in the medical record
Identify contributors to hyperglycemia and hypoglycemia
Discontinue the oral antidiabetic regimen and noninsulin injectables when applicable
Utilize subcutaneous or intravenous insulin order protocols for management of hyperglycemia in the hospital when applicable, preferably using a standardized approach
When using subcutaneous insulin, select a regimen to include basal (long or intermediate-acting) and prandial/supplemental (short- or rapid-acting) insulin when applicable
Aim for glucose targets between 140 and 180 mg/dl
Assess control daily and adjust insulin therapy as needed
Avoid using sliding scale insulin
Consider reducing insulin dose when patient will be fasting for tests or procedures
Suspect, prevent, identify, and manage hypoglycemia promptly
Provide diabetes education when required
Arrange for adequate continuity of care
Provide clear documentation of hyperglycemia in the hospital and discharge plans

Hospital Efforts

Diabetes leading societies advocated that hospitals implement programs in an effort to improve glycemic control in their inpatient population. It is recommended that hospitals provide administrative support for an interdisciplinary steering committee to target system approaches, establish a uniform method of collecting and evaluating POC testing data, utilize accurate glucose measuring devices, and facilitate staff education to update knowledge on diabetes and adverse events related to diabetes management [6, 16]. Attempts to address existing barriers to inpatient glycemic control should ideally recognize limitations of hospitals and their personnel that may potentially impede the optimization of care. There exist knowledge, attitude, confidence and clinical decision barriers to hospital glycemic control among inpatient providers and physicians in training [Pichardo-Lowden and Haidet, unpubl. data] which may represent potential targets for staff education and system changes. Adequate management of hyperglycemia is often neglected, and the use of sliding scale insulin regimens in many hospitals prevails despite proven inferiority and known detrimental effects of this strategy in relation to basal-bolus insulin. This inertia may, perhaps constitute one of the stronger barriers to managing inpatient hyperglycemia. Therefore, systematic changes, education of personnel, and a proactive attitude toward the problem of inpatient glycemic control is essential to improving our processes [8]. Table 7 presents a practical checklist for management of inpatient hyperglycemia in noncritically ill patients.

References

1 World Health Organization: Media Centre. 2012. http://www.who.int/mediacentre/factsheets/fs312/en/index.html.

2 Wild S, Roglic G, Green A, Sicree R, King H: Global prevalence of diabetes: estimates for the year 2000 and projections for 2030. Diabetes Care 2004;27: 1047–1053.

3 American Diabetes Association: Economic costs of diabetes in the US in 2007. Diabetes Care 2008;31: 596–615.

4 Swanson CM, Potter DJ, Kongable GL, Cook CB: Update on inpatient glycemic control in hospitals in the United States. Endocr Pract 2011;17:853–861.

5 Furnary AP, Gao G, Grunkemeier GL, Wu Y, Zerr KJ, Bookin SO, Floten HS, Starr A: Continuous insulin infusion reduces mortality in patients with diabetes undergoing coronary artery bypass grafting. J Thorac Cardiovasc Surg 2003;125:1007–1021.

6 Moghissi ES, Korytkowski MT, DiNardo M, Einhorn D, Hellman R, Hirsch IB, Inzucchi SE, Ismail-Beigi F, Kirkman MS, Umpierrez GE: American Association of Clinical Endocrinologists and American Diabetes Association consensus statement on inpatient glycemic control. Diabetes Care 2009;32:1119–1131.

7 Van den Berghe G, Wouters P, Weekers F, Verwaest C, Bruyninckx F, Schetz M, Vlasselaers D, Ferdinande P, Lauwers P, Bouillon R: Intensive insulin therapy in critically ill patients. N Engl J Med 2001;345:1359–1367.

8 Pichardo-Lowden AR, Fan CY, Gabbay RA: Management of hyperglycemia in the non-intensive care patient: featuring subcutaneous insulin protocols. Endocr Pract 2011;17:249–260.

9 Furnary AP, Zerr KJ, Grunkemeier GL, Starr A: Continuous intravenous insulin infusion reduces the incidence of deep sternal wound infection in diabetic patients after cardiac surgical procedures. Ann Thorac Surg 1999;67:352–360, discussion 60–62.

10 Umpierrez GE, Isaacs SD, Bazargan N, You X, Thaler LM, Kitabchi AE: Hyperglycemia: an independent marker of in-hospital mortality in patients with undiagnosed diabetes. J Clin Endocrinol Metab 2002;87:978–982.

11 Umpierrez GE, Smiley D, Jacobs S, Peng L, Temponi A, Mulligan P, Umpierrez D, Newton C, Olson D, Rizzo M: Randomized study of basal-bolus insulin therapy in the inpatient management of patients with type 2 diabetes undergoing general surgery (RABBIT 2 surgery). Diabetes Care 2011;34:256–261.

12 Murad MH, Coburn JA, Coto-Yglesias F, Dzyubak S, Hazem A, Lane MA, Prokop LJ, Montori VM: Glycemic control in non-critically ill hospitalized patients: a systematic review and meta-analysis. J Clin Endocrinol Metab 2012;97:49–58.

13 McAlister FA, Majumdar SR, Blitz S, Rowe BH, Romney J, Marrie TJ: The relation between hyperglycemia and outcomes in 2,471 patients admitted to the hospital with community-acquired pneumonia. Diabetes Care 2005;28:810–815.

14 Baker EH, Janaway CH, Philips BJ, Brennan AL, Baines DL, Wood DM, Jones PW: Hyperglycaemia is associated with poor outcomes in patients admitted to hospital with acute exacerbations of chronic obstructive pulmonary disease. Thorax 2006;61:284–289.

15 Pichardo-Lowden A, Gabbay RA: Management of hyperglycemia during the perioperative period. Curr Diab Rep 2011;12:12.

16 Umpierrez GE, Hellman R, Korytkowski MT, Kosiborod M, Maynard GA, Montori VM, Seley JJ, Van den Berghe G; Endocrine Society: Management of hyperglycemia in hospitalized patients in non-critical care setting: an Endocrine Society clinical practice guideline. J Clin Endocrinol Metab 2012;97:16–38.

17 Clement S, Braithwaite SS, Magee MF, Ahmann A, Smith EP, Schafer RG, Hirsch IB: Management of diabetes and hyperglycemia in hospitals. Diabetes Care 2004;27:553–591.

18 Dungan KM, Braithwaite SS, Preiser JC: Stress hyperglycaemia. Lancet 2009;373:1798–1807.

19 Van den Berghe G, Wilmer A, Hermans G, Meersseman W, Wouters PJ, Milants I, Van Wijngaerden E, Bobbaers H, Bouillon R: Intensive insulin therapy in the medical ICU. N Engl J Med 2006;354:449–461.

20 Finfer S, Chittock DR, Su SY, Blair D, Foster D, Dhingra V, Bellomo R, Cook D, Dodek P, Henderson WR, Hebert PC, Heritier S, Heyland DK, McArthur C, McDonald E, Mitchell I, Myburgh JA, Norton R, Potter J, Robinson BG, Ronco JJ: Intensive versus conventional glucose control in critically ill patients. N Engl J Med 2009;360:1283–1297.

21 Griesdale DE, de Souza RJ, van Dam RM, Heyland DK, Cook DJ, Malhotra A, Dhaliwal R, Henderson WR, Chittock DR, Finfer S, Talmor D: Intensive insulin therapy and mortality among critically ill patients: a meta-analysis including NICE-SUGAR study data. CMAJ 2009;180:821–827.

22 Finfer S, Liu B, Chittock DR, Norton R, Myburgh JA, McArthur C, Mitchell I, Foster D, Dhingra V, Henderson WR, Ronco JJ, Bellomo R, Cook D, McDonald E, Dodek P, Hebert PC, Heyland DK, Robinson BG: Hypoglycemia and risk of death in critically ill patients. N Engl J Med 2012;367:1108–1118.

23 Turchin A, Matheny ME, Shubina M, Scanlon JV, Greenwood B, Pendergrass ML: Hypoglycemia and clinical outcomes in patients with diabetes hospitalized in the general ward. Diabetes Care 2009;32:1153–1157.

24 Australian Diabetes Society. Guidelines for Routine Glucose Control in Hospital. 2012. https://www.diabetessociety.com.au/documents/ADSGuidelinesforRoutineGlucoseControlinHospitalFinal2012_000.pdf.

25 Umpierrez GE, Hor T, Smiley D, Temponi A, Umpierrez D, Ceron M, Munoz C, Newton C, Peng L, Baldwin D: Comparison of inpatient insulin regimens with detemir plus aspart versus neutral protamine Hagedorn plus regular in medical patients with type 2 diabetes. J Clin Endocrinol Metab 2009;94:564–569.

26 Umpierrez GE, Smiley D, Zisman A, Prieto LM, Palacio A, Ceron M, Puig A, Mejia R: Randomized study of basal-bolus insulin therapy in the inpatient management of patients with type 2 diabetes (RABBIT 2 trial). Diabetes Care 2007;30:2181–2186.

27 Mucha GT, Merkel S, Thomas W, Bantle JP: Fasting and insulin glargine in individuals with type 1 diabetes. Diabetes Care 2004;27:1209–1210.

28 Standards of medical care in diabetes – 2014. Diabetes Care 2014;37(Suppl 1):S14–S80.

29 Umpierrez GE, Hellman R, Korytkowski MT, et al: Management of hyperglycemia in hospitalized patients in non-critical care setting: an Endocrine Society clinical practice guideline. J Clin Endocrinol Metab 2012;97:16–38.

30 Klonoff DC, Buckingham B, Christiansen JS, et al: Continuous glucose monitoring: an Endocrine Society Clinical Practice Guideline. J Clin Endocrinol Metab 2011;96:2968–2979.

Ariana R. Pichardo-Lowden, MD
Penn State Hershey Endocrinology, Diabetes and Metabolism
500 University Drive
Hershey, PA 17033 (USA)
E-Mail apichardolowden@hmc.psu.edu

Bruttomesso D, Grassi G (eds): Technological Advances in the Treatment of Type 1 Diabetes.
Front Diabetes. Basel, Karger, 2015, vol 24, pp 47–62 (DOI: 10.1159/000363474)

Self-Monitoring in Diabetes: When and How Much?

Basilio Pintaudi · Antonio Nicolucci

Department of Clinical Pharmacology and Epidemiology, Fondazione Mario Negri Sud, Santa Maria Imbaro, Italy

Abstract

Self-monitoring of blood glucose (SMBG) is an integral component of diabetes care for patients with type 1 diabetes mellitus (T1DM). It is an essential tool for the improvement of glycemic control and to increase patient empowerment and adherence to treatment. The standard recommended frequency of SMBG in T1DM is 3–4 times daily, even though many patients might require more frequent monitoring in special conditions. The frequency of testing should be agreed upon by the patients and their healthcare teams. As a general rule, more blood glucose tests are needed as the therapy becomes more intensive. People using insulin pump therapy should perform SMBG at least 4–6 times daily, and especially during establishment of pump therapy. To confirm hypoglycemia, patients must perform SMBG and repeat it every 15 min until euglycemia. Patients undergoing frequent asymptomatic hypoglycemia should perform SMBG more often. During intercurrent illness, patients need to monitor their blood glucose levels at least every 4 h, or every 2 h when blood glucose levels keep rising, to avoid diabetic ketoacidosis. With physical activity, patients should perform SMBG before, during, and after exercise. While driving, SMBG should be performed before leaving and at 2-hour intervals during long journeys. The issue of SMBG in women with T1DM deserves specific attention, especially during the menstrual period, preconception time, pregnancy (at least 7 tests/day), and breastfeeding.

Between 1964 and 1967, a new method for measuring glucose, Dextrostix, was introduced. Based on finger puncture with a lancet or with an injection needle, these strips extemporaneously determined capillary blood glucose, and provided an alternative for the sticks that determined urinary glucose. The test was performed by putting a thick drop of blood on the stick, washing it under water for the elimination of other blood constituents, and then comparing it, after 1 min of reaction, with a color scale ranging from light yellow to darker colors, depending on the amount of glucose contained. This method was able to measure blood glucose levels ranging from 0 to more than 250 mg/dl. However, because determination of the colors in the gray to blue zone was inaccurate with this subjective visual method, the test was replaced in 1967 with a reflectometer, an objective self-reading tool on a portable, rechargeable battery that measured light reflected from the color strip and converted it into glucose blood concentration. Today, more precise measurement technologies have been developed and improved upon, and it is now possible to accurately check blood glucose levels.

Self-monitoring of blood glucose (SMBG) has certainly represented a significant step forward in the treatment of type 1 diabetes mellitus (T1DM), although its benefits were not immediately accepted. Controlled trials of SMBG in T1DM were performed in the 1980s and 1990s [1–8]. Most of these studies failed to demonstrate significantly lower glycated hemoglobin (HbA_{1c}) levels in the group performing SMBG [1–6]. These studies were small, however, with less than 20 patients per group in most cases. A systematic review also failed to provide evidence to support the clinical effectiveness of SMBG in improving glycemic control [9].

Despite the lack of solid scientific evidence, there were a number of reasons to consider SMBG as an integral component of diabetes care for individuals with T1DM. First, when SMBG was tested as a component of specific training programs, this led to a sustained improvement of glycemic control [10–12]. Similarly, in the Diabetes Control and Complications Trial (DCCT) [13] and the Stockholm Diabetes Intervention Study [14], SMBG was a key component of the protocol for the intensive insulin treatment, and these protocols were associated with better clinical outcomes. Second, the use of SMBG has become essential with the development of intensive conventional insulin treatment protocols. To tailor the dosage of insulin to current needs over the day, it is essential to follow the course of blood glucose levels by SMBG. Third, SMBG allows prompt determination of hypoglycemia or hyperglycemia that not only can improve patients' safety, but can also motivate them to make appropriate changes in diet, exercise, and insulin administration [15, 16]. In the presence of too low or too high blood glucose tests results, if properly educated and trained, patients will adjust their behavior accordingly (i.e. insulin administration, diet). To the extent these adjustments are successful, blood glucose values are likely to be in the normal range more often. Finally, by enhancing patient education on the impact of nutrition, activity, and medication choices, SMBG can increase patient empowerment and adherence to treatment, which in turn can lead to better glycemic control. It is now widely accepted that the improvement of blood glucose leads to good metabolic control, lower risk of long-term complications, lower healthcare costs, and improved quality of life [13, 17, 18]. Therefore, a combination of several arguments led the medical community to consider SMBG as an essential component of diabetes care in T1DM.

It is thus necessary to provide clear recommendations on how to use SMBG to help physicians, diabetes educators, and patients establish the correct behavior to attain and maintain daily glycemic control. The American Diabetes Association (ADA) initially addressed the issue of SMBG in a consensus conference in 1987 [19], without specific guidance regarding its frequency; afterwards, guidelines on the recommended frequency and timing of SMBG were made [20–23]. These guidelines had substantial variations in their recommendations, which can be attributed to the poor methodological quality of most of the existing clinical studies in which the patients were often unaware of actions to be undertaken in response to SMBG results.

For this reason, a global consensus conference of recognized diabetes experts was held to clarify the role of SMBG as a tool to help optimize glycemic control while minimizing hypoglycemia and maintaining quality of life [24]. This international panel of experts established that guidelines for the use of SMBG in glycemic control should contain more specific recommendations regarding frequency, timing, and integration of SMBG into the management strategy. They recommended the frequency of SMBG testing be dependent on the degree of glycemic control, the risk of hypoglycemia, the need for short-term adjustment of treatment, and special situations (before and during pregnancy, intercurrent illness, hypoglycemia unawareness, etc.). SMBG at different times of the day was recommended to provide an overall view of fasting, preprandial, and postprandial glycemic control. In order to optimize therapy, it is recommended to monitor blood glucose 3–4 times daily, even though many patients might require more frequent monitoring (particularly in cases of hyperglycemia or frequent hypoglycemia), including both pre- and postprandial (and occasionally even at 2:00–3:00 a.m.) values.

More recent clinical practice recommendations encourage the use of daily SMBG [25–27]. SMBG is considered beneficial, when supported by education, for all patients with T1DM [25]. This statement is supported by a recent systematic review showing that SMBG is associated with improvements in diabetes control, although further robust research was recommended to identify the optimum frequency of SMBG in T1DM [26]. SMBG should be a key component of self-management in T1DM when used as an integration tool along with patient education.

Even though the present recommendations are clear, adherence to SMBG is suboptimal as the number of patients who never practice SMBG is significant, also in countries in which glucometer strips are provided free of charge [28]. Data from the DCCT/Epidemiology of Diabetes Interventions and Complications (EDIC) studies show that up to 64% of patients with T1DM do not regularly self-monitor their blood glucose levels [29].

A recent study assessed the frequency of and the reasons for SMBG in relation with clinical, behavioral, and demographic characteristics [30]. In this cross-sectional Danish-British multicenter survey evaluating 1,076 consecutive patients with T1DM, SMBG was performed daily by 39% and less than weekly by 24%. Sixty-seven percent reported performing routine testing, while the remaining 33% only when hypo- or hyperglycemia was suspected. The authors also found that lower HbA_{1c} was associated with more frequent testing.

The same result was found in a study of a pediatric population of 132 adolescents with T1DM, recruited from Children's Hospital of Pittsburgh, who were interviewed annually for 5 consecutive years after routine clinical evaluations [31]. Adolescents monitoring blood glucose more frequently were younger, belonged to families of a higher social status, were on insulin pumps, and had higher self-efficacy. Among children and adolescents with T1DM, it appeared that older age [32, 33] and longer duration of diabetes were associated with less frequent testing [34]. Other demographic variables that have been linked to more frequent SMBG include female sex [35], having married biological parents compared to single, separated or divorced parents [36], being white, and having a higher education level [35].

Another significant aspect that is causing worldwide restrictions on the number of strips being prescribed and on the lack of choice of glucometers is a patient's financial situation. Although costs are of increasing importance, they should not become the leading criteria. Healthcare professionals are encouraged to evaluate the frequency of testing based on patients' needs. According to this, in August 2012, the Diabetes UK Care recommendations on SMBG for adults with T1DM were published [37], establishing key points for SMBG and clarifying the circumstances of when more frequent testing is required. Although testing more than 10 times/day has been shown to provide no added benefit with respect to lowering HbA_{1c} [38], testing above the recommended frequency levels is advised in special situations.

Starting/Changing Therapy

The timing of T1DM diagnosis represents the first crucial chance for the patient to acquire the skills necessary for the execution and interpretation of data deriving from SMBG. At this time the diabetes team has the task of playing an essential educational role. The prescription of insulin therapy by the physician is a medical procedure that inevitably exposes the patient to the risk of hypoglycemia. In addition, patients must adapt insulin therapy to their lifestyle and eating habits. All of this involves the possible occurrence of blood glucose fluctuations ranging from episodes of hypoglycemia, both diurnal and nocturnal, to unexpected hyperglycemia. People with T1DM trained in the use of SMBG experience fewer acute complications and are able to use SMBG to predict future episodes of mild, moderate, or severe hypoglycemia [39]. It is therefore necessary to inform the patient of the opportunity to perform a number of glycemic controls in order to avoid sudden glucose excursions. Although the time when the disease is diagnosed is highly challenging from a psychological point of view, the patient should understand that measuring blood glucose within the time specified by the healthcare professional is the only way to optimize blood sugar.

The latest ADA recommendations [27] suggest SMBG at least prior to meals and snacks, and occasionally postprandially. For many patients, this will require testing

Table 1. Specific recommendation for T1DM patients on when and how frequent to perform glucose self-monitoring

When	How much
Normal daily life	At least prior to meals and snacks, occasionally postprandially, at bedtime [27]
Person injecting 1–2 times/day	At least 2 times a day [37]
Person who alters insulin doses at mealtimes	At least 4 times a day [37]
Hypoglycemia	To confirm hypoglycemia, every 15 min after treating low blood glucose until the euglycemia [27]
Driving	Before driving and at 2-hour intervals during long journeys [37] Before driving and at regular intervals for journeys of 1 h or longer in drivers who are at risk for developing hypoglycemia [52]
Intercurrent illness	Every 4 h as a minimum; at 2-hour intervals if the glucose levels keep rising [25] Every hour in case of DKA episodes [44]
Physical activity	1 h before and 30 min before exercise, during, and afterwards [56]
Insulin pump	At least 4–6 times daily [37]
Pregnancy	At least 7 tests per day (fasting, 1 h after every meal and before going to bed) [66]

6–8 times daily, although individual needs may be greater. The frequency of testing should be agreed upon between the patient and his/her healthcare team. As a general rule, more blood glucose tests are needed as the therapy becomes more intensive. Patients injecting 1 or 2 times per day should be taught to undertake SMBG at least twice a day, including fasting, preprandial, and postprandial to identify trends (table 1). Twice a day is the minimum required and patients who need to change insulin doses at mealtime should be encouraged to monitor glucose at least 4 times a day [37].

In order to properly and independently manage the frequency of blood glucose measurements, it is essential that the patient receives the necessary education. Diabetes educators play multiple roles, have many responsibilities, and are involved in the continuum of SMBG, self-care, and patient behavior. The educator's role ranges from teaching the simple skills of performing a test, to how to interpret results and solve problems, and to modify behaviors and therapy based on the information acquired. The diabetes educator also helps patients choose appropriate and accurate blood glucose monitoring systems. SMBG is most effective when it is a continuous key of the diabetes management process [40].

To answer the question, 'Can the SMBG that every T1DM patient already uses be applied in a better way?', Skeie et al. [41] designed the 'MEASURE' (Metabolic Effects of Accurate Blood Sugar Results and Education in Type 1 Diabetes) trial. They evaluated the effect of a simple, structured, realistic SMBG intervention on the metabolic control in patients with T1DM and long-standing experience in performing SMBG. The intervention was based on monthly contacts with a nurse, use of a blood glucose diary, a 'fasting blood glucose map', and hypoglycemia registration. This approach was able to significantly improve metabolic control in the experimental group as compared to the control group (mean HbA_{1c} difference of 0.6).

Structured assessment of self-monitoring skills, the quality and use made of the results obtained, and the equipment used should be performed annually, or more frequently according to need, and reinforced when appropriate [37]. For example, in cases of insulin rate changes, blood glucose levels may vary widely, both to hypo- or hyperglycemia, sometimes even unawareness, making it necessary to perform SMBG more frequently.

Hypoglycemia

Patients perform SMBG more frequently during hypoglycemia, defined as a blood glucose value <70 mg/dl [27]. Of concern, sometimes apparently unjustifiable episodes of morning hyperglycemia may be a rebound of nocturnal hypoglycemia, making it advisable to perform seriated nocturnal controls. Patients might be unaware of hypoglycemia due to impaired counterregulatory responses, with a sixfold risk increase of confusion, coma, and seizure [42]. As a consequence, patients undergoing frequent asymptomatic hypoglycemia should perform SMBG more often (table 1).

Intercurrent Illness

Illness and infections, as well as other forms of stress, can raise blood glucose levels. It is possible to help prevent the more serious effects of illness on diabetes, keeping blood glucose levels down. For this reason, it is necessary to increase the frequency of SMBG. Patients should be advised that they need to monitor their blood glucose levels at least every 4 h, or every 2 h when blood glucose levels continue to rising (table 1) [25, 43]. Children and young people with T1DM and their families should be offered clear information and protocols ('sick day rules') for the management of T1DM during intercurrent illness.

The most serious consequence is the possibility to develop diabetic ketoacidosis (DKA). Children and young people with T1DM should have short-acting insulin or rapid-acting insulin analogues and blood and/or urine ketone testing strips available for use during intercurrent illness. Testing for ketones should be done once or twice a day, or more, depending on the presence of ketonuria [25, 43].

There is no specific number of SMBG tests recommended in case of DKA. The British Society for Paediatric Endocrinology and Diabetes [44] recommends hourly capillary blood glucose measurements in its guidelines for the management of DKA.

Ziegler et al. [45] studied the correlation between frequency of SMBG, HbA_{1c} levels, and acute complications in children and adolescents with T1DM. Data on 26,723 children and adolescents aged 0–18 years, collected during 1995 and 2006, were derived from the Diabetes-Patienten-Verlaufsdaten (DPV)-Wiss-database, a standardized, prospective, computer-based documentation of diabetes care and clinical outcomes. In this study, the incidence of DKA was significantly and inversely related to SMBG frequency; the DKA rate decreased by 0.38 events/100 person-years for each additional glucose measurement.

Driving

Recurrent severe hypoglycemia in patients with diabetes is strongly associated with the risk of a crash while driving [46, 47]. Over half of the patients with T1DM in a US study reported at least one hypoglycemia-related driving mishap over a 12-month period [48], while in the UK approximately 27 hypoglycemia-related driving accidents are reported every month to the Driver and Vehicle Licensing Agency (DVLA) [46]. To help ensure road safety, recent changes were made to European Union driving regulations for patients with diabetes, such as revoking the driving license in case of more than one episode of severe hypoglycemia within 12 months [49]. In addition to these recommendations, a diabetic driver in the UK will need to carry out more testing to meet DVLA rules [50]. Since 2011 the DVLA requires drivers with a group 1 license (cars, motorcycles) who are on insulin therapy to test blood glucose levels before driving and every 2 h during a long journey; on the other hand, group 2 drivers (lorries/passenger carrying vehicles) must monitor blood glucose at least twice daily, whenever relevant to driving, and every 2 h using a glucose meter with a memory function.

It seems self-evident that safe driving requires regular monitoring [51]. Since cognitive impairment may persist for up to 30 min following the treatment of hypoglycemia, driving should not be resumed until 40 min of euglycemia. The ADA position statement on diabetes and driving [52] suggests that special care should be taken to prevent hypoglycemia while operating any vehicle in drivers with T1DM who are at risk for developing hypoglycemia and that they should be taught to always check their blood glucose before getting behind the wheel and at regular intervals while driving for periods of 1 h or longer (table 1).

Driving is an even more dangerous activity for adolescents due to the possibility of extreme blood glucose excursion. Unfortunately, this are not much data concerning driving safety and adolescents with T1DM. A survey of 72 parents of adolescent drivers aged 16–19 years with T1DM showed that over half (56%) of them reported moderate to extreme worry about how diabetes impacted their adolescent's driving, while only 21% thought their adolescents had similar concerns [53] as nondiabetic adolescents. Almost a third of their parents thought their adolescents did not need to treat low blood glucose until it fell below 70 mg/dl, while 13% thought they could safely drive with blood glucose below 65 mg/dl. Furthermore, 31 and 14% of parents, respectively, reported their adolescents had been involved in a crash or were stopped by the police over the past years due to episodes of both hypo- and hyperglycemia. Adolescents reportedly took steps to prevent hypo- and hyperglycemia while driving, but more aggressively avoided hypoglycemia.

Physical Activity

The importance of regular physical activity for individuals withT1DM is widely recognized. However, it is fundamental to exercise without causing large fluctuations in blood sugar (hyper-/hypoglycemia) or ketosis episodes. Available guidelines for physical activity for T1DM were developed by the ADA in collaboration with the American College of Sports Medicine (ACSM) [54]. Guidelines on practical applications of sports in athletes with diabetes have also been published by the International Diabetes Athletes Association (IDAA) [55], now called the Diabetes Exercise Sports Association (DESA), and these were taken from the Italian National Association of Athletes Diabetics (ANIAD). The majority of the guidelines for T1DM on management during exercise are not supported by evidence-based findings, but are due to personal experiences or clinical practice.

The ability to adjust the therapeutic regimen (insulin and nutritional therapy) to achieve high performance and safe participation in sports activities has recently been recognized as an important strategy in the management of T1DM. In particular, the important role that the patient has to collect data of SMBG in response to exercise and using them to improve performance and increase safety is now fully accepted. Blood sugar should be in a good range prior to exercise, as well as during and even after it [56], and this can only be achieved by prudent monitoring of blood sugar. To avoid wide swings, it is advisable to check blood sugar 1 h before and 30 min before an activity (table 1), as this will give a downward or upward glycemic trend and time enough to adjust it, if needed. For the possibility of having hypoglycemia during exercise, especially when starting a new activity, it is absolutely recommended to interrupt it and perform appropriate glucose checks. If during a sports activity the patient faces hypoglycemia, it is important to check blood sugar not only in the time immediately following the end of the activity, but until at least 24 h after its end. In fact, hypoglycemic episodes generally occur several hours after the end of the activity and even up to 24 h later.

Insulin Pump

Insulin pump therapy, or continuous subcutaneous insulin infusion, was introduced more than 30 years ago [57] as a procedure to improve glycemic control in patients with T1DM by mimicking the normal insulin-delivery patterns. A portable pump infuses rapid-acting insulin at a slow basal rate, 24 h a day, through a fine cannula implanted in the subcutaneous tissue, with patient-activated insulin boluses administered at mealtimes. With insulin pumps in current use, it is important to calculate the appropriate insulin dose at mealtime, as estimated on the basis of carbohydrate intake, preprandial and target blood glucose levels, insulin sensitivity, and a calculation of the insulin remaining since the previous bolus [58]. Insulin pump therapy can improve glycemic control in patients with T1DM because it can reduce the within-day and between-day glycemic variability that is seen with insulin injections [59]. It is important for the patient to be motivated to use the insulin pump. The necessary activities include frequent SMBG (4–6 times daily), carbohydrate counting, adjustment of the insulin dose according to the estimated amount of carbohydrate intake, and working with the pump team to learn pump procedures [60]. Diabetes UK recommendations [37] suggest that people using insulin pump therapy should monitor their blood glucose levels at least 4–6 times daily (table 1), or even more, especially during the establishment of pump therapy or during intercurrent illness.

Women

The issue of SMBG in women with T1DM deserves specific attention. Beginning with adolescence, women with T1DM need to be adequately informed that maintaining optimal blood glucose levels can be affected by a number of physiological events. With the support of their healthcare team, they must be able to deal calmly with blood sugar imbalances that can occur during the menstrual period, pregnancy, and breast feeding, and learn how important the preconception time is.

Menstrual Cycle

It has been recognized that postovulatory exacerbation of hyperglycemia contributes to the instability of diabetes in many women of reproductive age [61]. It has been suggested that increasing plasma levels of progesterone and estrogen may induce insulin resistance and consequently lead to increased hyperglycemia during the luteal phase of the menstrual cycle. Since menstrual cycles may vary in length and the fact that it takes patients several days to achieve a steady state with regard to insulin dosage adjustment, it is difficult to design an insulin regimen that maintains euglycemia throughout the menstrual cycle. This is why women with T1DM should practice more intensive monitoring of blood glucose.

Preconception

Major congenital malformations remain the leading cause of mortality and serious morbidity in infants of mothers with T1DM. Clinical trials of preconception care to achieve stringent blood glucose control in the preconception period and during the first trimester of pregnancy have demonstrated striking reductions in rates of malformations compared with infants of diabetic women who did not participate in preconception care [62, 63]. Preconception care programs are multidisciplinary and are designed to train patients in diabetes self-management with diet, intensified insulin therapy, and SMBG. Individualized targets for SMBG should be agreed upon with diabetic women who are planning to become pregnant, taking into account the risk of hypoglycemia. Planned pregnancies greatly facilitate preconception diabetes care. Unfortunately, nearly two thirds of pregnancies in women with diabetes are unplanned, leading to a persistent excess of malformations in infants of diabetic mothers [27].

Pregnancy
If pregnancy is confirmed, SMBG should be a key component of diabetes therapy during pregnancy and should be included in the management plan. Daily SMBG both before and after meals, at bedtime, and occasionally at 2:00–4:00 a.m. will provide optimal results (table 1) [63].

The value of postprandial testing in pregnancy is supported by controlled trials [64, 65]. Postprandial capillary glucose measured 1 h after starting a meal on average best approximates postprandial peak glucose measured continuously, even though due to individual differences it may be useful for each patient to determine her own postprandial peak testing time. Frequent sampling is optimal in pregnancy due to the increased potential for rapid-onset hypoglycemia in the absence of food or during exercise, and the exacerbated hyperglycemic responses to food ingestion, psychological stress, and intercurrent illness. Use of alternate site testing in the dynamic state of pregnancy with rapid changes in blood glucose may give different results than fingerstick testing, so fingerstick SMBG represents the best option in pregnancy [63]. During pregnancy, the National Institute for Health and Care Excellence (NICE) recommends to test fasting blood glucose levels and blood glucose levels 1 h after every meal and at bedtime [66]. To enable insulin adjustment, preprandial testing is necessary, and at least 7 tests per day are therefore needed. Extra testing is likely to be needed with the increased incidence of hypoglycemia caused by starving to achieve tighter diabetes control.

Breastfeeding
Immediately after delivery, the insulin requirement declines to approximately 60% of the prepregnancy dose, and remains 10% lower during breastfeeding [67, 68]. Women with T1DM should reduce their insulin administration immediately after birth and monitor their blood glucose levels carefully to establish the appropriate insulin dose to achieve adequate glycemic control. They should be informed that they are at increased risk of hypoglycemia in the postnatal period, especially when breastfeeding, and they should be advised to have a meal or snack available before or during feeds [66] and to check their blood sugar before meals and at bedtime.

Lifestyle

T1DM lifestyle determines how frequently a person with T1DM needs to test. There are a number of factors related to personal habits or activities that may require an increase in the frequency of SMBG, despite the lack of specific recommendations. A first issue is represented by alcohol intake. The association between alcohol and hypoglycemia has been known for some time. The main pathogenetic mechanism is undoubtedly represented by the inhibition of gluconeogenesis. In hypoglycemia induced by alcohol, it is obviously easier to find insusceptible individuals and/or those suffering from postprandial hypoglycemia. Another circumstance is represented by travel, especially if associated with a change in time zone. In such cases the patient should know the correct timing to administer insulin dose (especially if the patient is in a multiple daily injection regimen) and the subsequent need of SMBG tests. Another situation requiring more frequent testing is when the patient changes his/her work/job. The change of working activity, especially if nocturnal, involves a proactive self-management, particularly to avoid hypoglycemia. Performing a different type of work, with a different working timetable, can cause blood sugar imbalances that must be promptly identified and corrected. For all of the circumstances mentioned above, it is important that the patient performs a greater number of SMBG tests and understands how to act autonomously to optimize glycemia.

Recent Technological Advancements in Self-Monitoring Blood Glucose

Health professionals working in the field of diabetes have a wide choice of blood glucose meters to give patients, with different options for monitoring and recording blood glucose results. All the meters have to meet the International Organization for Standardization (ISO) criteria. The continuous advances in technology have allowed modern blood glucose meters to be precise and well manageable for the patient. The autocoding provides that test strips calibrate themselves, which means the patient gets accurate results without the extra work of entering a code into the meter, thus reducing possible errors. The devices provide the patient clear instructions starting when they are automatically turned on once a strip is inserted. The large display also allows visually impaired persons to see clearly [69] and produces a high level of contrast and low levels of reflection. A common source of testing errors is simply not drawing enough blood in the sample. The modern meters are effective with smaller samples, giving more reliable results, with less pain. Significant technological improvements have been made in the field of lancing fingertips or alternative sites for obtaining a blood sample to address key customer needs, including better performance (regarding pain, wound healing, and long-term sensitivity), reduced costs, and higher integration with other components of blood glucose monitoring (e.g. integration of the lancing device with the glucose monitor) [70].

Technological advancement in treatment of T1DM suggests that mobile diabetes management systems may represent a strategy to improve the quality of diabetes care. Goldberg et al. [71] designed and tested a Web-based diabetes program consisting of interactive disease management tools and safe messaging. Patients could upload their glucose measurements to a shared electronic medical record using a wired interface to their home computer. Participants cited the dependence on their personal computer for uploads as a significant barrier to usability. For this reason the same Web-based system was extended to mobile phones, using a mobile phone application called Health Reach Mobile, designed to help patients with diabetes understand day-to-day trends in their blood glucose and communicate with care providers between office visits. It provided feedback on the phone itself, minimizing the need for a computer or direct clinician involvement [72]. The authors also tested mobile wireless glucose meter uploads and graphical and tabular approaches to mobile phone-based feedback on glycemic control.

Mobile technology may be usefully applied to help adolescents with T1DM. Young patients admitted that they did not test as much as they were supposed to, causing great anxiety in their parents who worried about the long-term complications associated with the disease [73, 74].

Cell phones can create an active link between adolescents and both parents and healthcare providers. For this reason HealthPia Inc. (Palisades Park, N.J., USA) has developed a prototype system that integrates a glucose monitoring system onto a conventional cell phone. The HealthPia GlucoPack™ Diabetes Monitoring System has a small blood glucose monitoring device integrated into the battery pack of a cell phone. The device consists of a strip sensor, analog circuit, microcontroller unit, communication interface, and phone input/output. When the strip is inserted, data are sent to the specific phone input/output protocols. The information is sent both to the phone display and to a secure server through a cellular signal. Glucometer data are transmitted to a server that, through a website, allows patients, parents, and clinicians to view these blood glucose values in a number of formats over a safe Internet connection [75]. Adolescents reported positive feelings about this technology [76].

Another recent instrument that represents an important technological advancement in SMBG is the iBGStar™ (Sanofi-Aventis) meter, which uses dynamic electrochemical technology for blood sample analysis. It can be used alone or linked to an iPhone or iPod touch Apple to view, manage, and easily communicate patient information on diabetes [77].

Conclusions

SMBG requires that patients prick their fingers with a lancet device to obtain a small blood sample. The blood is applied to a reagent strip or blood glucose test strip, and glucose concentration is determined by inserting the strip into a reflectance photometer or an electrochemical sensor. Results, based on an automated reading, are available from the photometer within 5–30 s and can be stored in the glucose meter's electronic memory or recorded in the patient's logbook. It is interesting and surprising that something so simple can offer the T1DM patient the ability to manage alone many situations that everyday life presents.

A recent study investigating the patient's perspective of SMBG showed that due to a variety of factors, there is a wide variety in the performance of SMBG [78], including the patients' perception, his/her goals, and personal and contextual factors. Patients did not always perceive SMBG as a positive tool, which would have enabled them to achieve good glycemic control. They mentioned many experiences which support a negative perception of SMBG, making it more difficult to self-monitor. They also felt that healthcare providers were predominantly focused on good glycemic control. The greatest skill of the physician should be to arm the patient's self-management and, specifically for SMBG, teach them the true meaning of 'when' and 'how much'. New technology advances might be of great help in improving the acceptability of the monitoring systems and the compliance with recommended testing frequency.

References

1 Worth R, Home PD, Johnston DG, Anderson J, Ashworth L, Burrin JM, Appleton D, Binder C, Alberti KG: Intensive attention improves glycaemic control in insulin-dependent diabetes without further advantage from home blood glucose monitoring: results of a controlled trial. Br Med J 1982;285:1233–1240.

2 Miller PF, Stratton C, Tripp JH: Blood testing compared with urine testing in the long term control of diabetes. Arch Dis Child 1983;58:294–297.

3 Mann NP, Noronha JL, Johnston DI: A prospective study to evaluate the benefits of long-term self-monitoring of blood glucose in diabetic children. Diabetes Care 1984;7:322–326.

4 Daneman D, Siminerio L, Transue D, Betschart J, Drash A, Becker D: The role of self-monitoring of blood glucose in the routine management of children with insulin-dependent diabetes mellitus. Diabetes Care 1985;8:1–4.

5 Terent A, Hagfall O, Cederholm U: The effect of education and self-monitoring of blood glucose on glycosylated hemoglobin in type I diabetes. A controlled 18-month trial in a representative population. Acta Med Scand 1985;217:47–53.

6 Gordon D, Semple CG, Paterson KR: Do different frequencies of self-monitoring of blood glucose influence control in type 1 diabetic patients? Diabet Med 1991;8:679–682.

7 Starostina EG, Antsiferov M, Galstyan GR, Trautner C, Jorgens V, Bott U, Mühlhauser I, Berger M, Dedov II: Effectiveness and cost-benefit analysis of intensive treatment and teaching programmes for type 1 (insulin-dependent) diabetes mellitus in Moscow – blood glucose versus urine glucose self-monitoring. Diabetologia 1994;37:170–176.

8 Carney RM, Schechter K, Homa M, Levandoski L, White N, Santiago J: The effects of blood glucose testing versus urine sugar testing on the metabolic control of insulin-dependent diabetic children. Diabetes Care 1983;6:378–380.

9 Coster S, Gulliford MC, Seed PT, Powrie JK, Swaminathan R: Monitoring of blood glucose control in diabetes mellitus: a systematic review. Health Technol Assess 2000;4:1–93.

10 Mühlhauser I, Bruckner M, Berger D, Cheta V, Jorgens C, Ionescu-Tîrgovişte V, Scholz I, Mincu I: Evaluation of an intensified insulin treatment and teaching programme as routine management of type 1 (insulin-dependent) diabetes. The Bucharest-Düsseldorf Study. Diabetologia 1987;30:681–690.

11 Pieber TR, Brunner GA, Schnedl WJ, Schattenberg S, Kaufmann P, Krejs GJ: Evaluation of a structured outpatient group education program for intensive insulin therapy. Diabetes Care 1995;18:625–630.

12 DAFNE Study Group: Training in flexible, intensive insulin management to enable dietary freedom in people with type 1 diabetes: Dose Adjustment for Normal Eating (DAFNE) randomised controlled trial. Br Med J 2002;325:746.

13 The effect of intensive treatment of diabetes on the development and progression of long-term complications in insulin-dependent diabetes. The Diabetes Control and Complications Trial Research Group. N Engl J Med 1993;329:977–986.

14 Reichard P, Nilsson BY, Rosenqvist U: The effect of long-term intensified insulin treatment on the development of microvascular complications of diabetes mellitus. N Engl J Med 1993;329:304–309.

15 Owens D, Barnett AH, Pickup J, Kerr D, Bushby P, Hicks D, Gadsby R, Frier B: Blood glucose self-monitoring in type 1 and type 2 diabetes: reaching a multidisciplinary consensus. Diabetes Prim Care 2004;6: 8–16.

16 Schütt M, Kern W, Krause U, Busch P, Dapp A, Grziwotz R, Mayer I, Rosenbauer J, Wagner C, Zimmermann A, Kerner W, Holl RW; DPV Initiative: Is the frequency of self-monitoring of blood glucose related to long-term metabolic control? Multicenter analysis including 24,500 patients from 191 centers in Germany and Austria. Exp Clin Endocrinol Diabetes 2006;114:384–388.

17 The Writing Team for the Diabetes Control and Complications Trial/Epidemiology of Diabetes Interventions and Complications Research Group: Sustained effect of intensive treatment of type 1 diabetes mellitus on development and progression of diabetic nephropathy: the Epidemiology of Diabetes Interventions and Complications (EDIC) study. JAMA 2003;290:2159–2167.

18 The Writing Team for the Diabetes Control and Complications Trial Epidemiology of Diabetes Interventions and Complications Research Group: Effect of intensive therapy on the microvascular complications of type 1 diabetes mellitus. JAMA 2002; 287:2563–2569.

19 Consensus statement on self-monitoring of blood glucose. Diabetes Care 1987;10:95–99.

20 American Diabetes Association: Standards of medical care in diabetes. Diabetes Care 2004;27(Suppl 1): S15–S35.

21 American Association of Clinical Endocrinologists and the American College of Endocrinology: Medical guidelines for the management of diabetes mellitus: the AACE system of intensive diabetes self-management – 2002 update. Endocr Pract 2002;8: 40–82.

22 Canadian Diabetes Association: Canadian Diabetes Association 2003 clinical practice guidelines for the prevention and management of diabetes in Canada. Can J Diabetes 2003;27(Suppl 2):S1–S152.

23 Burgers JS, Bailey JV, Klazinga NS, Van Der Bij AK, Grol R, Feder G; AGREE Collaboration: Inside guidelines: comparative analysis of recommendations and evidence in diabetes guidelines from 13 countries. Diabetes Care 2002;25:1933–1939.

24 Bergenstal RM, Gavin JR III; Global Consensus Conference on Glucose Monitoring Panel: The role of self-monitoring of blood glucose in the care of people with diabetes: report of a global consensus conference. Am J Med 2005;118:1S–6S.

25 NICE: Type 1 Diabetes: Diagnosis and Management of Type 1 Diabetes in Adults. Clinical Guideline 15. London, NICE, 2004.

26 Optimal therapy report. Systematic review of use of blood glucose test strips for the management of diabetes mellitus. Can Agency Drugs Technol Health 2009;3:e0101.

27 American Diabetes Association. Standards of Medical Care in Diabetes – 2013. Diabetes Care 2013; 36(Suppl 1):S11–S66.

28 Evans JM, Newton RW, Ruta DA, MacDonald TM, Stevenson RJ, Morris AD: Frequency of blood glucose monitoring in relation to glycaemic control: observational study with diabetes database. BMJ 1999; 319:83–86.

29 DCCT/EDIC Research Group: Modern-day clinical course of type 1 diabetes mellitus after 30 years' duration: the Diabetes Control and Complications Trial/Epidemiology of Diabetes Interventions and Complications and Pittsburgh Epidemiology of Diabetes Complications experience (1983–2005). Arch Intern Med 2009;169:1307–1316.

30 Hansen MV, Pedersen-Bjergaard U, Heller SR, Wallace TM, Rasmussen AK, Jørgensen HV, Pramming S, Thorsteinsson B: Frequency and motives of blood glucose self-monitoring in type 1 diabetes. Diabetes Res Clin Pract 2009;85:183–188.

31 Helgeson VS, Honcharuk E, Becker D, Escobar O, Siminerio L: A focus on blood glucose monitoring: relation to glycemic control and determinants of frequency. Pediatr Diabetes 2011;12:25–30.

32 Haller MJ, Stalvey MS, Silverstein JH: Predictors of control of diabetes: monitoring may be the key. J Pediatr 2004;144:660–661.

33 Evans JM, Newton RW, Ruta DA, MacDonald TM, Stevenson RJ, Morris AD: Frequency of blood glucose monitoring in relation to glycaemic control: observational study with diabetes database. BMJ 1999; 319:83–86.

34 Dorchy H, Roggemans MP, Willems D: Glycated hemoglobin and related factors in diabetic children and adolescents under 18 years of age: a Belgian experience. Diabetes Care 1997;20:3–6.

35 Karter AJ, Ackerson LM, Darbinian JA, D'Agostino RB, Ferrara A, Liu J, Selby JV: Self-monitoring of blood glucose levels and glycemic control. The Northern California Kaiser Permanente Diabetes registry. Am J Med 2001;111:1–9.

36 Urbach SL, LaFranchi S, Lambert L, Lapidus JA, Daneman D, Becker TM: Predictors of glucose control in children and adolescents with type 1 diabetes mellitus. Pediatr Diabetes 2005;6:69–74.

37 Self-monitoring of blood glucose (SMBG) for adults with type 1 diabetes. Diabetes. UK care recommendation. 2012. http://www.diabetes.org.uk/upload/Position statements/SMBGType1positionstatement.pdf (accessed January 29, 2013).

38 Davidson PC, Bode BW, Steed RD, Hebblewhite HR: A cause-and-effect-based mathematical curvilinear model that predicts the effects of self-monitoring of blood glucose frequency on hemoglobin A_{1c} and is suitable for statistical correlations. J Diabetes Sci Technol 2007;1:850–856.

39 Janssen M, Snoek F, Jongh R, Casteleijn S, Deville W, Heine RJ: Biological and behavioural determinants of the frequency of mild, biochemical hypoglycaemia in patients with type 1 diabetes on multiple insulin injection therapy. Diabetes Metab Res Rev 2000;16:157–163.

40 The American Association of Diabetes Educators position statement: self-monitoring of blood glucose. http://www.diabeteseducator.org/export/sites/aade/_resources/pdf/research/Self-Monitoring_of_Blood_Glucose.pdf (accessed January 29, 2013).

41 Skeie S, Kristensen GB, Carlsen S, Sandberg S: Self-monitoring of blood glucose in type 1 diabetes patients with insufficient metabolic control: focused self-monitoring of blood glucose intervention can lower glycated hemoglobin A_{1C}. J Diabetes Sci Technol 2009;3:83–88.

42 Geddes J, Schopman JE, Zammitt NN, Frier BM: Prevalence of impaired awareness of hypoglycaemia in adults with type 1 diabetes. Diabet Med 2008;25:501–504.

43 Rosindale S: Ensuring good management of diabetes in intercurrent illness. Nursing Times 2004;22:34–36.

44 Savage MW, Dhatariya KK, Kilvert A, Rayman G, Rees JA, Courtney CH, Hilton L, Dyer PH, Hamersley MS; Joint British Diabetes Societies: Joint British Diabetes Societies guideline for the management of diabetic ketoacidosis. Diabet Med 2011;28:508–515.

45 Ziegler R, Heidtmann B, Hilgard D, Hofer S, Rosenbauer J, Holl R; DPV-Wiss-Initiative: Frequency of SMBG correlates with HbA_{1c} and acute complications in children and adolescents with type 1 diabetes. Pediatr Diabetes 2011;12:11–17.

46 Shaw K: Driving and diabetes: new licensing standards by European Union directive. Pract Diabetes Int 2011;28:375–376.

47 Cox DJ, Gonder-Frederick LA, Kovatchev BP, Julian DM, Clarke WL: Progressive hypoglycemia's impact on driving simulation performance. Occurrence, awareness and correction. Diabetes Care 2011;23:163–170.

48 Cox DJ, Ford D, Gonder-Frederick L, Clarke W, Mazze R, Weinger K, Ritterband L: Driving mishaps among individuals with type 1 diabetes. Diabetes Care 2009;32:2177–2180.

49 Department for Transport: Proposals to amend driving license standards for vision, diabetes and epilepsy: annex III to directive 91/439/EEC. Annex A impact assessment for proposals to amend driving license standards for diabetes. http://www.dft.gov.uk/dvla/consultations.aspx (accessed October 6, 2012).

50 DVLA: At a glance guide to the current medical standards of fitness to drive. 2012. www.dft.gov.uk/dvla/medical/ataglance.aspx (accessed January 1, 2013).

51 Frier BM: Hypoglycaemia and driving performance. Diabetes Care 2000;23:148–149.

52 American Diabetes Association: Diabetes and driving. Diabetes Care 2012;35(Suppl 1):S81–S86.

53 Cox DJ, Gonder-Frederick LA, Shepard JA, Campbell LK, Vajda KA: Driving safety: concerns and experiences of parents of adolescent drivers with type 1 diabetes. Pediatr Diabetes 2012;13:506–509.

54 American College of Sports Medicine and American Diabetes Association joint position statement. Diabetes mellitus and exercise. Med Sci Sports Exerc 1997;29:i–vi.

55 International Diabetes Athletes Association. http://www.insulindependence.org/ (accessed January 1, 2013).

56 Colberg SR: Use of clinical practice recommendations for exercise by individuals with type 1 diabetes. Diabetes Educ 2000;26:265–271.

57 Pickup JC, Keen H, Parsons JA, Alberti KG: Continuous subcutaneous insulin infusion: an approach to achieving normoglycaemia. BMJ 1978;1:204–207.

58 Pickup J, Pender S, Kidd J, Yemane N: Running an insulin pump service; in Pickup JC (ed): Insulin Pump Therapy and Continuous Glucose Monitoring. Oxford, Oxford University Press, 2009, pp 23–37.

59 Pickup JC, Kidd J, Burmiston S, Yemane N: Determinants of glycaemic control in type 1 diabetes during intensified therapy with multiple daily insulin injections or continuous subcutaneous insulin infusion: importance of blood glucose variability. Diabetes Metab Res Rev 2006;22:232–237.

60 Pickup JC: Insulin-pump therapy for type 1 diabetes mellitus. N Engl J Med 2012;366:1616–1624.

61 Widom B, Diamond M, Simonson D: Alterations in glucose metabolism during menstrual cycle in women with IDDM. Diabetes Care 1992;15:213–220.

62 Kitzmiller JL, Block JM, Brown FM, Catalano PM, Conway DL, Coustan DR, Gunderson EP, Herman WH, Hoffman LD, Inturrisi M, Jovanovic LB, Kjos SI, Knopp RH, Montoro MN, Ogata ES, Paramsothy P, Reader DM, Rosenn BM, Thomas AM, Kirkman MS: Managing preexisting diabetes for pregnancy: summary of evidence and consensus recommendations for care. Diabetes Care 2008;31:1060–1079.

63 American Diabetes Association: Preconception care of women with diabetes. Diabetes Care 2004; 27(Suppl 1):S76–S78.

64 de Veciana M, Major CA, Morgan MA, Asrat T, Toohey JS, Lien JM, Evans AT: Postprandial versus preprandial blood glucose monitoring in women with gestational diabetes mellitus requiring insulin therapy. N Engl J Med 1995;333:1237–1241.

65 Manderson JG, Patterson CC, Hadden DR, Traub AI, Ennis C, McCance DR, et al: Preprandial versus postprandial blood glucose monitoring in type 1 diabetic pregnancy: a randomized controlled clinical trial. Am J Obst Gynecol 2003;189:507–512.

66 NICE: Diabetes in pregnancy. Management of diabetes and its complications from preconception to the postnatal period. Clinical guideline 63. http://publications.nice.org.uk/diabetes-in-pregnancy-cg63/guidance (accessed January 1, 2013).

67 Riviello C, Mello G, Jovanovic LG: Breastfeeding and the basal insulin requirement in type 1 diabetic women. Endocr Pract 2009;15:187–193.

68 Stage E, Norgard H, Damm P, Mathiesen E: Long-term breast-feeding in women with type 1 diabetes. Diabetes Care 2006;29:771–774.

69 Morgan V, Blubaugh BBA, Uslan MM: Accessibility attributes of blood glucose meter and home blood pressure monitor displays for visually impaired persons. J Diabetes Sci Technol 2012;6:246–251.

70 Heinemann L, Boecker D: Lancing: Quo Vadis? J Diabetes Sci Technol 2011;5:966–981.

71 Goldberg HI, Ralston JD, Hirsch IB, Hoath JI, Ahmed KI: Using an Internet comanagement module to improve the quality of chronic disease care. Jt Comm J Qual Saf 2003;29:443–451.

72 Harris LT, Tufano J, Le T, Rees C, Lewis GA, Evert AB, Flowers J, Collins C, Hoath J, Hirsch IB, Goldberg HI, Ralston JD: Designing mobile support for glycemic control in patients with diabetes. J Biomed Inform 2010;43:S37–S40.

73 Carroll AE, Marrero DG: The role of significant others in adolescent diabetes: a qualitative study. Diabetes Educ 2006;32:243–252.

74 Carroll AE, Marrero DG: What adolescents with type I diabetes and their parents want from testing technology: a qualitative study. Comput Inform Nurs 2007;25:23–29.

75 Carroll AE, Marrero DG, Downs SM: The HealthPia GlucoPack Diabetes Phone: a usability study. Diabetes Technol Ther 2007;9:158–164.

76 Carroll AE, DiMeglio LA, Stein S, Marrero DG: Using a cell phone-based glucose monitoring system for adolescent diabetes management. Diabetes Educ 2011;37:59.

77 Pfützner A, Mitri M, Musholt PB, Sachsenheimer D, Borchert M, Yap A, Forst T: Clinical assessment of the accuracy of blood glucose measurement devices. Curr Med Res Opin 2012;28:525–531.

78 Hortensius J, Kars MC, Wierenga WS, Kleefstra N: Perspectives of patients with type 1 or insulin-treated type 2 diabetes on self-monitoring of blood glucose: a qualitative study. BMC Public Health 2012; 12:167.

Dr. Antonio Nicolucci
Laboratory of Clinical Epidemiology of Diabetes and Chronic Diseases
Mario Negri Sud Foundation, Via Nazionale 8/a
IT–66030 Santa Maria Imbaro (Italy)
E-Mail nicolucci@negrisud.it

Bruttomesso D, Grassi G (eds): Technological Advances in the Treatment of Type 1 Diabetes.
Front Diabetes. Basel, Karger, 2015, vol 24, pp 63–80 (DOI: 10.1159/000363475)

Interfering Factors in Quality of Glucose Measurement

Richard Hellman

Heart of America Diabetes Research Foundation and Kansas City School of Medicine, University of Missouri, Kansas City, Mo., USA

Abstract

The use of point-of-care (POC) glucose meters has revolutionized the measurement of blood glucose, but the new technologies have also introduced challenges due to interfering factors which may affect the accuracy of the measurements. Although new regulatory standards have just been proposed, both the ISO 15197 revised standard and the two new FDA standards, none of these standards solve some of the current problems faced by the clinicians and patients. Among the most serious problems are clinical 'outliers', where the POC glucose measurement is misleading, leading to clinical errors and patient harm. In addition to the above issues, this chapter looks at the special problems of using POC glucose measurement in inpatient units and particularly in critical care settings, the impact of glucose meter accuracy in clinical decisions and the pitfalls that may occur, the distinction between total analytical error and the total error (which is usually significantly larger and more important clinically), and the problems in pediatric care which add to the complexity of ascertaining the true glucose values of the patient. We provide recommendations for changes in both regulatory bodies, both for premarket approval and postmarket monitoring of both POC glucose devices and glucose reagent strips.

The development of point-of-care (POC) glucose meters has revolutionized the measurement of blood glucose both for in- and outpatients, greatly adding to the tools available for the care of diabetes and resulting in improved clinical outcomes. But with the new technology have come challenges, for the new meters have interfering factors that need to be understood and dealt with by those who use and rely upon the information derived from POC glucose meters.

The invention of the first widely used POC blood glucose measurement tool, the Dextrostix, was in 1963 [1], followed 7 years later by the Ames Reflectance Meter. The use of POC glucose meters has continued to increase every year. In 2008, more than 44 million tests were performed daily worldwide. POC glucose testing resulted in USD 8.8 billion in annual revenue in 2008 [2]. The glucose meters and strips have been continually improved upon and now, 50 years later, both patients and clinicians have a wide variety of devices and strips to choose from, with very diverse technologies, each with strengths and weaknesses, many of which are poorly understood by the purchaser or the user. In this review, I will focus on the POC glucose meters and their strips, and discuss the relevant aspects of the newer technologies of these instruments and the many examples of factors interfering with the quality of glucose measurement. Although the POC glucose meters are greatly improved, serious problems remain with accuracy and reliability, especially in, but not limited to, critical care situations. Patients, clinicians, and purchasers all need to be aware of the shortcomings of these devices and of factors that can lead to catastrophic errors in care.

The Scope of the Problem

Urgent information about the true blood glucose of the patient is often needed, and this information may be crucial not only for the surgeon, anesthesiologist, or intensivist, but also for the person with diabetes who is driving a motor vehicle, the parent of a child with diabetes, or the emergency room physician examining an unconscious patient. All these persons need real-time knowledge of the actual blood glucose value, and POC glucose meters are increasingly used as the reference to decide what to do next. Even patients who use continuous glucose monitoring systems (CGMS) will compare their CGMS results to the results of their POC glucose meter in order to validate the values of their CGMS instrument and check the accuracy of their clinical decisions. In patients using CGMS, validation by POC glucose meter may be very important since the interstitial glucose measured by CGMS may lag significantly behind the true blood glucose level of the patient in some clinical circumstances.

There is little question that glucose levels from a central hospital laboratory cannot replace POC glucose testing. Even in inpatient settings, a central hospital laboratory, although it can perform glucose measurements with a high degree of accuracy and precision, is often impractical in emergent clinical situations since glucose levels may change rapidly in critical care patients. When the rate of change of glucose levels is greater than 2–3 mg/dl/min, a delay of 20 min in reporting the glucose level from the central laboratory may lead to a clinically significant error in decision-making. And, if the true glucose is in the hypoglycemic range, the delayed central laboratory glucose level frequently leads to confusion and to a clinical error. Also, a significant delay in processing the central laboratory glucose should be avoided since a delay in running the sample may allow glycolysis to proceed, falsely lowering the result by up to 5–7%/h [3], which is a preanalytic error. Clearly, real-time POC glucose measurement in is optimal, and for that reason, accurate POC instrumentation is needed. Our task is thus to improve POC glucose measurement, to understand the limitations of the present instrumentation, and to know when to use other methods of POC glucose measurement.

It is surprising how often people assume that the POC glucose meters currently in use are accurate and precise enough to always allow a sound clinical decision. Furthermore, many believe that accuracy is not significantly different from meter to meter, or strip lot to strip lot. Also, it is commonly believed that the data output from the meter truly reflects what the meter measured. Yet, all of those assumptions may be incorrect. In fact, POC glucose meters vary widely in their accuracy across the clinical range of glucose values, and many meters are very uneven in their relative accuracy in different parts of the range. There are many circumstances in which some, or, less often, all of the meters now in use are quite inaccurate. Fortunately, we now know a great deal about the circumstances in which inaccurate results are more likely to be present. We have also learned about 'outliers', the measured glucose levels from the POC glucose meters which are so inaccurate as to lead both the clinician and the patient into clinical decisions that may cause serious injury or even death.

The Regulatory Agencies and Their Standards

Many of the POC glucose meters currently in use have only had to meet the 2003 standard of the International Organization for Standardization (ISO) which stated that the meter's performance must have at least 95% of the glucose measurements within ±20% of a blood glucose reference standard when the glucose is ≥75 mg/dl, and ±15 mg/dl when the glucose level is <75 mg/dl. This standard (ISO 15197) was widely criticized by many as being too lax [4]. For example, the standard allowed up to 5% of the results to be as serious an error as the instrument can report, yet such errors, which theoretically could occur as much as 1 out of every 20 readings, could result in very misleading information, resulting in what are called clinical outliers, potentially leading to patient harm.

In January 2013, the ISO 15197 standard was revised. The revised standard [5] however, will not become mandatory until 2015. The new criteria are: (1) 95% of the measured glucose values must be within ±0.83 mmol/l (±15 mg/dl) of the reference measurement if glucose is <5.55 mmol/l (<100 mg/dl), or within ±15% if glucose is ≥5.55 mmol/l (≥100 mg/dl), and (2) 99% of the individual measured glucose values shall fall within zones A and B of the consensus error grid for type 1 diabetes patients.

The two criteria listed above are also relevant for the reagent lots (meter strips) tested in the application for approval. Criterion 1 is applied to each reagent lot individually. Criterion 2 is applied only to the overall performance of all the reagent lots tested in the application for approval. In addition, the revised ISO 15197 standard mandates limits to the degree that variations in hematocrit (and other interfering substances) can affect the accuracy of the glucose measurement.

In the USA, the FDA has recently proposed two new standards to replace their present standards, which require a meter's performance to be within ±20% of a blood glucose reference standard for 95% of the values ≥100 mg/dl and an allowable error of ≤12 mg/dl for all values <100 mg/dl. The new proposed FDA standards are only advisory, but they expect these to be mandatory by the end of 2015. In their comments, the FDA stated that the new 2013 ISO 15197 standards were inadequate and therefore new, more extensive standards are needed. These standards, however, are only for new meters not yet marketed.

The most stringent FDA standards are regarding the test systems for prescription POC meter use, for devices used by medical professionals, in hospitals, clinics, doctors' offices, nursing homes and other clinical settings. The advisory standards for accuracy under these devices are that 99% of the values must be within ±10% of the glucose levels ≥3.85 mmol/l (≥70 mg/dl), and within ±0.385 mmol/l (±7 mg/dl) for glucose levels <3.85 (<70 mg/dl). Moreover, 100% of values must be within ±20% of the reference values for samples ≥3.85 mmol/l (≥70 mg/dl) or within ±15 mg/dl for values <3.85 mmol/l (<70 mg/dl) [6].

They also recommend testing for a considerable number of interfering substances as well as hematocrit. They recommend a minimum hematocrit range of 10–65%. Other recommendations included checking for variations due to oxygen tension, temperature, humidity, and altitude changes, as well as resistance to shock and vibration.

However, the new FDA recommendations for the larger group, the POC glucose meters and strips that will be used by patients and the public, were somewhat less stringent. They set limits of 95% for all self-monitoring of blood glucose results needing to be ±15% across the entire claimed measuring range of the device, and 99% of all self-monitoring of blood glucose test results needing to be within ±20% of the glucose reference standard across the entire claimed measuring range of the device [7]. Surprisingly, they allowed the claimed measuring range to be as narrow as 50–400 mg/dl, allowing meters to be used by the public which cannot distinguish between a glucose level of 49 and 20 mg/dl. Likewise, these devices may be acceptable to the FDA even if they cannot distinguish between a glucose level of 401 mg/dl and one of 600 mg/dl. The hematocrit range that is acceptable to the FDA for these POC glucose meters designed for the lay public is 20–60%, again significantly narrower than the range approved for medical personnel (10–65%).

Yet even the proposed FDA standard for general use and the revised ISO 15197 standard allow some of the reported values to be large enough as to be clinical outliers. Moreover, both organizations only discuss analytical error and not total error, which, as we will explain later, is really what is relevant to the user of these devices, and almost certainly will be larger – often considerably larger – than the total analytical error (TAE) which the regulatory agencies are considering. When the clinician must know how far the glucose measurement result is from the true glucose of the patient, the most relevant value is the total error, not just the TAE. The total error is the sum of the TAE, the pre- and postanalytic error, and what the normal biologic variation is.

For the most part, however, the regulatory agencies rely on information submitted by the manufacturer, and do not retest the devices in their laboratories. Many of the manufacturers of the POC glucose meters currently available have not had their factories inspected nor their data directly verified by any regulatory agency, and if the approval was some time ago, the meters and their strips almost certainly have not been retested [8]. Also, some manufacturers will submit their applications with the claim that their technology is so similar to other previously approved meters that there should be a relatively low bar for acceptance as long as their submitted results meet the ISO or FDA standard. In 2010, however, when Freckmann et al. [8] reviewed 27 meters that had been approved in Europe from 18 companies, careful analytic testing showed that 41% of the meters tested did not meet even the minimal standards of the ISO. Also, and most importantly, many of the meters were accurate and precise only in a portion of the clinical range. Particularly disturbing was the finding that in the hypoglycemic range a number of the meters were much more inaccurate, a finding recently verified by Rebel et al. [9]. Accuracy during the hypoglycemic range is particularly crucial since in this set the patient is very vulnerable to injury and delayed treatment often leads to harm.

In 2009, Kristensen et al. [10] tested nine meters for the accuracy of their strips within certain hematocrit ranges. They found that, in contrast to the claims of five of the manufacturing companies, their strips showed relatively large variations within these ranges. Other authors [8, 9] have also found that their analytical retesting of previously approved meters have resulted in poorer performance of the meters than the manufacturers claim.

The data indicate that there is a need for an independent agency or agencies to test and retest these meters and their strips, both initially, when the POC glucose meter comes on the market, and afterwards. This information, which is crucial to the end-user, is simply not available at present. There is, however, a Scandinavian organization supported by Sweden, Norway, and Denmark [Scandinavian Evaluation of Laboratory Equipment for Primary Healthcare (SKUP)] which independently evaluates diabetes diagnostic and therapeutic equipment before it enters the marketplace.

Outliers

Outliers [4] in POC glucose measurement are defined as glucose levels that are far enough from the true glucose level to lead to potential errors in the care of the patient. Outliers can lead to catastrophic errors. In 2009, the FDA [11] reported serious problems due to interfering substances in POC glucose meters that used a glucose 1-dehydrogenase enzyme to convert glucose to gluconolactone using the coenzyme pyrroloquioline quinone (PQQ), often referred to as the glucose dehydrogenase (GDH)-PQQ methodology. The PQQ coenzyme method offers an advantage in being less sensitive to ambient oxygen and electrochemical interference than other GDH methods. But, unfortunately, this method is very prone to interference with nonglucose sugars, such as maltose, galactose, mannose, xylose, and ribose, which are reported as glucose.

In 2009, the FDA discussed reports of 13 deaths that had occurred when meters with the GDH-PQQ methodology were used in patients on peritoneal dialysis. In each case, the health providers overdosed the patient with insulin because the POC glucose meter indicated erroneously that the patient was hyperglycemic, reporting maltose present in patients' blood as glucose. Maltose was present in blood because the peritoneal fluid contained icodextrin, which is broken down to maltose. In reality, these patients were having severe hypoglycemia at the very moment they were receiving what later proved to be lethal doses of insulin. Other substances used in patient care that also contain maltose include some intravenous gamma globulin solutions such as Octagam 5, gammaimmune 5%, and drugs such as Orencia (abatacept). These too must be considered as potential interfering substances for glucose measurement if a GDH-PQQ type glucose meter is in use. The impact of health foods with large amounts of these nonglucose sugars on the accuracy of GDH-PQQ type meters has not yet been studied.

A clinical outlier which leads to a catastrophic error in care can occur due to a falsely low reported glucose level as well. Blank et al. [12] reported that in diabetic ketoacidosis (DKA), the true blood glucose may be 300 mg/dl or more higher than the reported glucose from a POC glucose meter. They speculate that this is due to dehydration as well as other undefined factors which are noted in the blood of a patient with DKA. Similar examples of falsely low outlier results with POC glucose meters are frequent in critical care in hyperosmolar states.

In a 2001 article, Boyd and Bruns [13] used a computer simulation to analyze and model the impact of TAE on clinical decision. They concluded that a TAE of 5%, a much smaller error rate than what was allowable in the ISO or FDA standards, would result in an 8–23% clinical error rate in choosing insulin doses from a glucose level-based insulin algorithm. If the TAE was 10%, however, their modeling showed that the resultant clinical error rate was 16–45%. If the TAE was 15%, the range of clinical error was even higher with a very significant incidence of large errors. These larger errors were in the range of errors that would likely be clinically very significant. As they pointed out, TAE, which is obtained under the most optimal conditions, such as carefully chosen glucose meters and strips as well as tests performed by highly trained laboratory personnel, underestimates the total amount of error that may be present in ordinary daily life.

Why Outliers Are Dangerous

Outliers can mislead both the patient and the provider and cause harm to the patient. A falsely high glucose level delays recognition and treatment of hypoglycemia that already exists. Worse yet, it may encourage treatment that will worsen the hypoglycemia, such as shown with the GDH-PQQ experience in patients on peritoneal dialysis.

On the other hand, a falsely low glucose level will lead to delay in the diagnosis of serious hyperglycemia and decrease the intensity of treatment. An example of this is a patient with hyperglycemia and DKA in which the POC glucose meter may initially

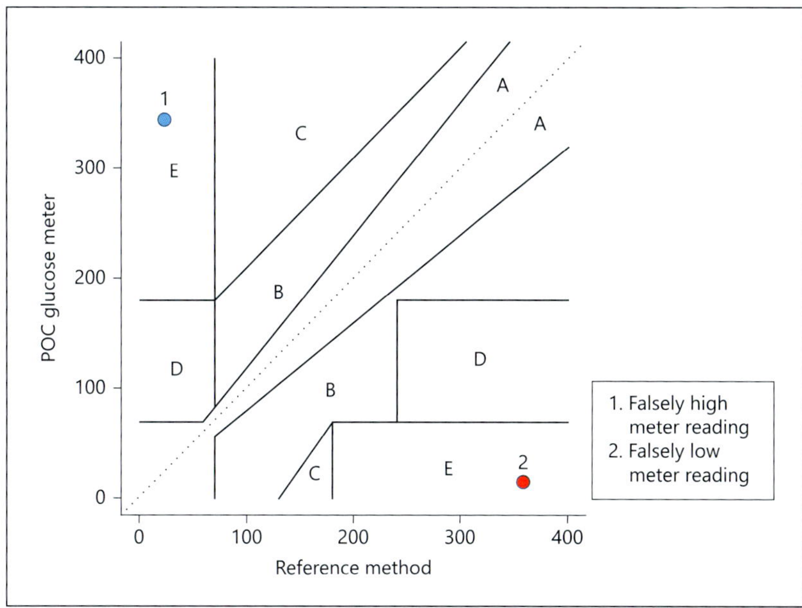

Fig. 1. Why outliers are dangerous: Clarke error grid.

give a reading that is as much as 300 mg/dl lower than the true blood glucose, leading the unwary clinician to delay treatment or diagnosis of the DKA present in the patient until much later, increasing the risk of harm to the patient.

In figure 1, a Clarke error grid shows two points, 1 and 2, that illustrate the two examples noted above. Note that point 1 shows a true hypoglycemic value in zone E that the POC meter read as elevated as in the problem with GDH-PQQ meters. In the second example, point 2 shows an elevated glucose level that is 300 mg/dl higher than the POC meter reported value, as in DKA. The use of the Clarke error grid is one method to display the clinical importance of the variance, or true error of the measured glucose value by POC glucose meters.

Basic Technologies and Interfering Factors of the Point-of-Care Glucose Meters in Common Use

Current POC glucose meters usually use either a glucose oxidase (GO) or a GDH enzyme method to measure glucose. With the GO method, the enzyme converts the glucose molecule to gluconic acid and hydrogen peroxide. The amount of hydrogen peroxide produced is proportional to the glucose concentration in the sample of blood. It is the change in hydrogen peroxide concentration that is measured either by a color change in an indicator (photometric method) or in the newer meters, by measuring electron capture (amperometric method).

While the GO methods are extremely specific and do not react with other sugars, the method is often influenced by the blood oxygen concentration [14–16], which is not a concern for the GDH method. The GO meters are influenced by hypoxia, oxygen administration, and altitude. When there are high levels of dissolved oxygen in the sample, the change in oxygen tension leads to a falsely reduced blood glucose level reported by the GO meter, and conversely, when the patient is hypoxic, or the tissue sample comes from a hypoxic region, then the glucose reported will be falsely increased. These variations are usually small but in the very ill patient, with a PaO_2 <40 or >100 mm Hg, the errors may be over 15% [9, 16]. GO test strips using a ferrocene method for electron capture are more susceptible to changes in PaO_2 than the GO test strips using MBTH (peroxide/meta[3-methyl 2 benzothiazoline hydrazine] *N*-sulfonyl benzene sulfonic acid). In a study by Tang et al. [15], the ferrocene-containing strips he studied resulted in 20–31.6% of the values being outside the set limits due to the oxygen interference, which was significantly poorer than those using MBTH methodology.

The GO methodology interferences are not limited only to oxygen tension, but can also include drugs, such as ascorbic acid which causes both GO and GDH devices and strips to read falsely lower, and acetaminophen, which in therapeutic concentrations may falsely lower GO meter results but increase GDH-type POC glucose meter results.

Other factors include anemia, which affects nearly all glucose meters similarly. The mechanism is as follows: anemia causes lower amounts of red cells/volume of blood. The current POC glucose meters measure the total glucose from the sample, but are designed to assume a normal hematocrit when reporting the whole blood glucose value. Since glucose levels are much lower in red cells than in plasma, anemia will lead to a falsely elevated POC glucose value except in the meters that are designed to compensate for a significant change in hematocrit. A meter, such as the Hemocue, which first lyses the red cells, is less affected by hematocrit change. Some of the newer meters directly measure hematocrit in order to calculate an adjusted glucose level and make it closer to the true value.

Likewise, in most meters (both the GO and GDH types), polycythemia will cause a falsely lower glucose value reported by the POC glucose meter. The water composition of whole blood can also be affected by conditions such as severe hypertriglyceridemia or paraproteinemia, both of which will lower the water concentration in the blood sample, also leading to a 'pseudo-hypoglycemia' result [9, 14].

Source of Sample

Among the variables to consider is the source of the sample, whether arterial, capillary, or venous. POC glucose meters are usually thought of as using capillary blood, but a whole blood sample can be obtained from either arterial, capillary, or venous sources. In general, the concentrations of glucose in arterial blood at a normal PaO_2 will be 5 mg/dl higher than in capillary blood and 10 mg/dl higher than in venous blood, but the comparisons of POC glucose meters using these different sources are

Table 1. Effect of interfering substances on glucose measurement

Interfering substance	Type of meter	
	GO	GDH
Maltose	none	↑↑ (GDH-PQQ type) ↑ (most other GDH methods)
Xylose or galactose (health foods, etc.)	none	↑↑ (GDH-PQQ type) ↑ (most other GDH methods)
Ascorbic acid	small	↑
Acetaminophen	↓	↑
Dopamine	none	↓
Mannitol	↑	none

complex, incomplete, and sometimes contradictory, as shown in a recent review by Dungan et al. [14].

There is, however, considerable agreement among experts that the difference between plasma and whole blood (specimen matrix) is usually the most important variable to be considered when the choice for glucose measurement is made and should be carefully considered. In situations where the water content or lipid and protein concentrations or cellular components of whole blood are seriously disordered, if whole blood is to be used, a reliable and accurate method or methods to account for the effects of those factors on the quality of blood glucose measurement must be present in order to make the whole blood glucose measurements reliable enough to use in clinical decision-making.

One study provided data to show that the site of the capillary blood may at times be more important than the specimen matrix and must be considered [17]. The different sites used in obtaining capillary blood specimens may introduce considerable unwanted variation in the glucose measurements and should be considered, especially if results are discordant with each other. An example of some of these factors can be seen in table 1. In table 2, the effects of other kinds of preanalytic errors are noted on the reported glucose levels from each of the types of meters.

From the clinical standpoint, we are most interested in what the true glucose is at the moment the measurement is made. As stated earlier, the measured blood glucose is not only affected by the TAE of the meter, but also by preanalytic factors, i.e. errors made before the specimen is measured. As seen in table 2, there are many factors which are due to handling and storage of the meter and the strips and the conditions in which the instrument is used that may cause an increase in the total error.

Other factors may also occur postanalytically, such as the reporting tool of the meter giving a false result because of either software problems or mechanical failure [4]. Some manufacturers have programmed their devices to give no result if the strip is

Table 2. Effect of preanalytic errors on glucose measurement

Preanalytic error	Type of meter	
	GO	GDH
Exposure of strips to elevated temperature[a]	↓	↓
Exposure of strips to decreased temperature[a]	↑	↑
Exposure of strips to humidity, vibration, dirt[a]	↑ or ↓	↑ or ↓
Out-of-date strips[a]	↑ or ↓	↑ or ↓
Failure to calibrate strips	↑ or ↓	↑ or ↓
Failure to wash hands	↑↑	↑↑
Failure to dry hands	↓	↓
Inadequate drop size	↓	↓

[a] May destroy strip.

outdated, or the electrical system of a meter may fail and give a discordant result or none at all. On March 25, 2013, Reuters and other international news agencies reported that LifeScan was voluntarily recalling nearly 2 million glucose meters because they malfunctioned at high glucose levels. At levels at or above 1,024 mg/dl, the meters either reported no results or shut down. Just 3 weeks later, on April 15, 2013, Reuters and other agencies reported that Abbott was recalling meters of the FreeStyle InsuLinx® type because at glucose levels of 1,024 mg/dl or higher, the meters read much lower numbers, often in the hypoglycemic range. These are just two examples of POC glucose meters creating a postanalytic error, 'outlier' results of great magnitude.

There are numerous ways in which postanalytic errors may occur. For example, a patient reading the meter display results might not recognize that the units used for display are not the ones they are used to seeing, e.g. mmol/l versus mg/dl, or cannot read the numbers correctly, as can occur when people of limited visual acuity look at a small or poorly lit display screen, resulting in postanalytic error. It is the total sum of all the errors, i.e. the total error, that should be considered clinically. The total error is the sum of the analytic error of the measuring instrument, the preanalytic error, the postanalytic error, and normal biologic variation.

Some of the most important and common preanalytic errors are due to the handling and use of the instrument, or user error. Hand washing, an essential feature for all of the strips used at present, is a key step, but unfortunately many users omit this step leading to preanalytic errors as high as 35% or more. The cause of the error is due to the food or other interfering substances which are still left on the unwashed finger before the sample was obtained, but are subsequently measured by the meter. Falsely elevated glucose levels are common in this circumstance.

On the other hand, failure to dry the finger before obtaining the sample is also very common. This error will lead to dilution of the sample and a falsely low glucose result, an occurrence common in, but not limited to, the pediatric population. Hand washing and drying is frequently and routinely omitted by adults who are unaware of the errors they are introducing in their results.

In pediatric populations, however, the data is very strong. In a study by Perwien et al. [18] in 2000, in children ages 7–14 years, only 19.1% washed their hands before testing themselves for blood glucose, and only 14.6% of the children dried their finger after hand washing prior to glucose testing. Additionally 29.4% of children failed to cap the bottle of the strip container, leading to an increased risk of degrading the strips due to exposure to temperature and excessive humidity variation.

Children are particularly at risk for postanalytic issues in the accuracy of reporting of their glucose levels because of their desire to mislead those in authority regarding their level of compliance. In a study by Wilson and Endres [19], 42% of the children aged 12–18 years fabricated test results and 18% failed to report the results. There is also a relationship between high depression scores and the providing of misleading glucose results in children [20].

But again, the problem of falsification of glucose results is hardly restricted to children. A much earlier study by Mazze et al. [21] showed the high frequency of adults who transcribed incorrect, but consistently lower, blood glucose levels when showing their glucose records to physicians and healthcare providers. The results the adults wrote down were very different from those results found in the memory of their glucose meters. The postanalytic problem of misrepresentation of their glucose values is a universal one it seems, and is often a significant source of poor clinical decisions and clinical outliers.

Problems in Inpatient Care Settings

Perhaps the most critical areas in which any significant errors of POC glucose meters may lead to an adverse event in clinical care is in the inpatient setting, particularly in critical care [22]. However, it is not the prevention of hypoglycemia that is most crucial in inpatient settings. On the contrary, it is poorly controlled hyperglycemia that leads to the largest amount of in-hospital morbidity and mortality. The role of hyperglycemia in causing both increased morbidity and mortality is well-established in inpatient settings [23, 24], where good glucose control and real-time reporting are critically important [24].

It is not surprising that in contrast to the wide acceptance of POC glucose meters in the outpatient setting, many authors have questioned the wisdom of using POC glucose meters for blood glucose measurements in the operating room suite or in the intensive care unit (ICU). In *Clinical Chemistry* in 2009, Scott et al. [22] wrote a key article questioning the uncritical use of POC glucose meters in critical inpatient care. In critical care, due not only to DKA, but also in nonketotic hyperglycemic states, severe hypotension, hypoxia, and shock states, there are multiple factors, ranging from low tissue O_2 levels, acidosis, and poor blood flow to the accumulation of other intracellular substances, which decrease the accuracy of the POC glucose measurements [9, 22]. Rice et al. [25] and Pitkin and Rice [26] discussed the cardiovascular changes in the operating room which lead to rapid and deleterious changes in regional blood flows, thus decreasing the accuracy of fingerstick blood glucose measurements. In a recent review by Kanji et al. [27], both peripheral edema and vasopressor therapy had a particularly adverse effect on POC glucose monitoring and led to significant discordance of POC glucose results with the central laboratory values. In these studies, when compared to arterial sampling, capillary sampling was significantly less accurate, particularly in the critical hypoglycemic range. In the presence of hypotension <70 mm Hg, the variance of the capillary POC readings and the central laboratory were sufficiently large enough to lead to 'outliers' that affected clinical decision-making and it was worsened by hypotension with an arterial pressure <70 mm Hg. Other studies, such as Hoedemaekers et al. [28] in 2008, also confirm Kanji's findings.

These multiple factors most often lead to POC glucose levels that are falsely elevated, masking true hypoglycemia. Other factors, however, may also do the same, most notably anemia, which is common in critically ill patients, and which may occur rapidly, and be large in degree. In the NICE-SUGAR study, Cembrowski [29] observed differences in sensitivity to fluctuations in hematocrit in 5 of the 7 test strip lots used at his institution and thought that falsely elevated glucose levels may have delayed recognition of true hypoglycemia in the study subjects, delaying treatment and contributing to adverse outcomes. Although there are newer POC glucose meters which use a new technique called dynamic electrochemistry [30, 31] that are supposedly less sensitive to variations in hematocrit, these techniques may also be susceptible to other interferences as well.

There are other data as well that report problems in critical care. A study by Stork et al. [32], for example, showed the limitations using POC glucose meters in the hypoglycemic range, and two studies in neonates also showed the inadequacy of POC glucose meters in the neonatal ICU setting [33, 34].

It is for these reasons that Van den Berghe et al. [35] advocate the use of blood gas multichannel analyzers as the POC instrument in their ICUs. The wet chemistry method of the blood gas analyzers resembles the central laboratory methods in the level of accuracy, and arterial lines are used by Dr. Van den Berghe rather than capillary blood. Some newer meters have been proposed as more appropriate for inpatient use because of their improved accuracy and resistance to hematocrit variation [36–39], but all of these may be less accurate in the critical care setting in the presence of severe hypotension and use of vasopressors. Some authorities recommend that although POC glucose meters can be used safely in a carefully tested and validated environment in hospital settings, in operating rooms and in critical care, the arterial blood gas multichannel analyzer at the point of care may be a better choice for glucose measurement. More research needs to be done in this area since not all studies indicate poor results with capillary samples in critical care settings. A large study by Karon et al. [40] in cardiac surgery showed relatively good results when using capillary blood samples with intensive insulin therapy, but most authors agree that we should use POC glucose meters in the hospital setting only after the inherent vulnerabilities of this system are minimized.

Recommended Strategies in the Hospital Environment

Given that the POC glucose meters have an important role in the hospital care of patients with abnormal glucose levels, how then can we minimize their current shortcomings? Data show that training and education of those who use the POC glucose meters improves performance [41]. Skeie et al. [42] showed that both laboratory technicians and patients can be successfully trained to increase their proficiency with the use of POC glucose meters. These researchers also performed a small randomized study with insulin-requiring diabetic patients which showed that improving the technique of their self-blood glucose monitoring led to a small, nonsignificant, improvement in HbA_{1c} levels [42].

In contrast, the use of POC meters in hospitals is often done by the most poorly trained staff, even though proper technique is key to optimal results. Education of those who use and interpret the results, in both inpatient and outpatient areas, is crucial. Such educational programs should be designed also to increase the likelihood that the clinician will seek a central glucose check when either the clinical setting (shock, hypotension, or severe hyperglycemia) or the clinical conditions (patient on peritoneal dialysis or comatose with an elevated glucose level by POC glucose meter) suggests the possibility of an inaccurate POC glucose meter result (a clinical 'outlier').

Both the choice of glucose meter for the hospital setting and the choice of an educational plan for teaching about interfering factors in glucose measurement and the particular vulnerabilities of the individual meter used in the hospital are critical decisions. These decisions should be the responsibility either of those who are in charge of the clinical care of patients with abnormal glucose levels or the physician-in-chief of the hospital. There are studies that show the value of having the director of clinical pathology having a comprehensive quality control program [43, 44] for the POC glucose meters. Additionally, if a significant number of patients who are cared for in the ICU of the institution are found to have discordant results when the POC measurements are compared to glucose levels run by the central laboratory, the use of a POC blood-gas multichannel analyzer to deliver POC glucose results from arterial samples should be strongly considered instead of the POC glucose meters.

Recommendations in the General Setting

If possible, the choice of the glucose meter should be made not by the payer, who far too often focuses primarily on cost, but instead an informed decision should be made based primarily on the clinical performance of the meter. A key factor should be the total analytical accuracy of the meter, and ideally, the meter being considered should be tested against reference glucose standards. Unfortunately, unlike plasma or serum glucose, for which there are international standards, there is no international standard for whole-blood glucose because of the analytical complexity and variability of whole blood [8]. Unfortunately, there is also no agreement as to which instrumentation should be a reference standard for measurement of whole blood; if there were, at the very least all glucose meters could be tested against the accuracy of simultaneous ice-chilled plasma samples simultaneously drawn from the same patient and tested by the same reference laboratory instrument. Even agreement in this area would greatly simplify the process of comparison.

In contrast, without such standards, available data show that a random choosing of several glucose meters from different manufacturers can lead to differences of 60–75 mg/dl when obtaining samples from the same patient at the same time [14]. This is an unacceptable situation that frequently leads to confusion.

We also need to consider the usefulness of the POC glucose meter under consideration for the individual patient. Can the patient with neuropathy use the proposed choice of meter or does the patient need one with larger or more prominent buttons? Can the patient with diminished vision see the meter screen under usual conditions? Is there a hands-on instructor-led program for the patient, and is there an opportunity for the patient to be retested on their proficiency within two weeks? The work of Mykityshyn et al. [45] showed that older patients often do poorly in self-learning the use of a new glucose monitor, and if written material alone was used, their retention was poor and they often could not remember what they were told two weeks before. A better education program for the use of POC glucose meters for elderly patients should include a two-week follow-up in which their skills are retested. Children, on the other hand, learn best when the teaching method is appropriate for their age, education level, and culture, and the method includes follow-up supervision, re-education, and shared responsibility [46]. There are some innovative methods that are being used to improve adherence for the younger patients [47].

It is even more important today that clinicians be alert to the wide variety of interfering factors that can affect the reliability of POC glucose measurements by their patient. With payers often under pressure to cut costs, it is not uncommon in the USA for patients to be sent a POC meter they have never seen or used before to replace the meter and strips they were accustomed to. A forced change to a newer glucose meter may result in an improvement, but more often leads to a decrease in the accuracy of their glucose monitoring. Also, improper handling, storage or transport at any point in the delivery chain, from the manufacturer to the warehouse or from the clinic to patients' homes, may have an adverse effect on the accuracy and precision of measurements.

Unfortunately, there are also no good studies on the lifespan of meters. We have no data on whether some meters degrade in functioning quickly and which meters are much more sensitive to environmental influences. We also have almost no information on the usual lot-to-lot variation of strips or cartridges made by the different manufacturers, and as the number of new meters continues to increase, we have far too little data on the newer, less well-tested instruments. We also are keenly aware that patients who use their POC glucose meter for validation of the CGMS reading are also at risk of increased errors if their CGMS is validated against a less accurate POC glucose meter. It is also important to consider strip handling. Many of our patients are unaware of the fact, as pointed out by Kristensen et al. [10], that the temperature at which the strips are stored may affect the results as well, as strips stored at cold temperatures, at 10°C, will read falsely elevated glucose levels for up to 15 min, while those stored at 39.5°C will give falsely low values. Extremes of temperature may destroy the strips entirely.

Current Trends

Fortunately, we are beginning to see a change in the behavior of the more responsible members of the industry. There is much more discussion regarding the relative accuracy of the meters and the engineering of some of the more recent meters is becoming more sophisticated and aimed at dealing with some of the shortcomings delineated in this review. Although there is strong resistance from the competing companies in the use of an industry standard interface so that any glucose reading of the meters in common use can be downloaded without the need for the proprietary software, attempts are starting to be made to allow a common instrument to download many POC glucose meters without their proprietary company software. While privacy issues must be addressed, as the patient's information must be kept secure, increasing the ease of access of the clinical team to a person's current and recent blood glucose data increases the ability of the health provider to intelligently guide the patient and improve their glycemic control.

Recommendations for Change

The regulatory bodies need to consider tightening the acceptable minimal standard of accuracy [2, 4, 14, 48, 49] and precision for all glucose meters. Strip lots should also be randomly tested by an independent, scientifically based, regulatory entity for efficacy, and the results should be made available to the public in a timely manner. Every meter should be tested in such a way that the accuracy standards can be achieved not

Table 3. Proposed standards for TAE

	Glucose levels	
	≥75 mg/dl	<75 mg/dl
95% of values	≤10%	≤10 mg/dl
99% of values	≤15%	≤12 mg/dl
99.9% of values	≤20%	≤15 mg/dl

only by highly trained hospital personnel, but also by patients in everyday settings. Moreover, the payers should recognize that their role is not to select the meter without clinical input, but to work closely with the experts to choose a more accurate and user-friendly POC glucose meter. It is important that the patients can have meters that are useful for them, more accurate than many of those at present, and more reliable. They also need an opportunity to continue to learn and receive help on how to use their POC glucose meter properly. It is hoped that the new emphasis on encouraging manufacturers to focus more on the accuracy and ease of use of the meters will hasten transformation of the field into more useful and relevant instrumentation than sometimes is the case today.

Clearly the time has come for a change in standards of accuracy of POC glucose meters. Currently, there are a number of new meters using more advanced technology that can achieve a TAE of less than 4–5% [31–33]. In 2010, at the 70th Annual Scientific Sessions of the American Diabetes Association [50], I recommended a new standard for total allowable error (table 3). It was feasible in 2010 to reach the standards of accuracy I proposed then. It is certainly even more widely feasible today. Note that part of the recommendations is not just to lower the range of acceptable values overall, but to make 'outliers' very rare. If our goal is to achieve safety so that it is very rare that a patient is harmed by a very inaccurate result from a POC glucose meter, it is reasonable to include a higher standard for outliers as well.

References

1 Tonyushkina K, Nichols JH: Glucose meters: a review of technical challenges to obtaining accurate results. J Diabetes Sci Technol 2009;3:971–980.

2 Scott MG: Glucose meters: need for greater accuracy (lab perspective). Presentation at the American Diabetes Association/American Association for Clinical Chemistry Symposium, 'Point-of-Care Devices for Glucose and HbA1C: Are They Up to the Task?'. American Diabetes Association's 70th Scientific Sessions, Orlando, 2010.

3 Arabadjief D, Nichols JH: Assessing glucose meter accuracy. Curr Med Res Opin 2006;22:2167–2174.

4 Krouwer JS, Cembrowski GS: A review of standards and statistics used to describe blood glucose monitor performance. J Diabetes Sci Technol 2010;4:75–83.

5 ISO 15197:2013(E). In vitro Diagnostic Test Systems – Requirements For Blood-Glucose Monitoring Systems for Self-Testing in Managing Diabetes Mellitus. Geneva, ISO, 2013.

6 Blood Glucose Monitoring Test Systems for Prescription Point-of-Care Use – Draft Guidance for Industry and Food and Drug Administration Staff. Washington, US Department of Health and Human Services, Food and Drug Administration, Center for Devices and Radiological Health, Office of In Vitro Diagnostic Device Evaluation and Radiological Health, Division of Chemistry and Toxicology Devices, 2014.
7 Self-Monitoring Blood Glucose Test Systems for Over-the-Counter Use – Draft Guidance for Industry and Food and Drug Administration Staff. Washington, US Department of Health and Human Services, Food and Drug Administration, Center for Devices and Radiological Health, Office of In Vitro Diagnostic Device Evaluation and Radiological Health, Division of Chemistry and Toxicology Devices, 2014.
8 Freckmann G, Baumstark A, Jendrike N, Zschornack E, Kocher S, Tshiananga J, Heister F, Haug C: System accuracy evaluation of 27 blood glucose monitoring systems according to DIN EN ISO 15197. Diabetes Technol Ther 2010;12:221–231.
9 Rebel A, Rice MA, Fahy BG: The accuracy of point-of-care glucose measurements. J Diabetes Sci Technol 2012;6:396–411.
10 Kristensen GB, Monsen G, Skeie S, Sandberg S: Standardized evaluation of nine instruments for self-monitoring of blood glucose. Diabetes Technol Ther 2008;10:467–477.
11 US Food and Drug Administration: Public health notification: potentially fatal errors with GDH-PQQ glucose monitoring technology. 2009. http://www.fda.gov/medicaldevices/safety/alertsandnotices/publichealthnotifications/ucm176992.htm.
12 Blank FS, Miller M, Nichols J, Smithline H, Crabb G, Pekow P: Blood glucose measurement in patients with suspected diabetic ketoacidosis: a comparison of Abbott MediSense PCx point-of-care meter values to reference laboratory values. J Emerg Nurs 2009; 35:93–96.
13 Boyd JC, Bruns DE: Quality specifications for glucose meters: assessment by simulation modeling of errors in insulin dose. Clin Chem 2001;47:209–214.
14 Dungan K, Chapman J, Braithwaite SS, Buse J: Glucose measurements: confounding issues in setting targets for inpatient management. Diabetes Care 2007;30:403–409.
15 Tang Z, Louie RF, Lee JH, Lee DM, Miller EE, Kost GJ: Oxygen effects on glucose meter measurements with glucose dehydrogenase- and oxidase-based test strips for point-of-care testing. Crit Care Med 2001; 29:1062–1070.
16 Tang Z, Louie RF, Payes M, Chang KJ, Kost GJ: Oxygen effects on glucose measurements with a reference analyzer and three handheld meters. Diabetes Technol Ther 2000;2:349–362.
17 Stahl M, Brandslud I: Measurement of glucose content in plasma from capillary blood in diagnosis of diabetes mellitus. Scan J Clin Lab Invest 2003;63:431–440.
18 Perwien AR, Johnson SB, Dymtrow D, Silverstein J: Blood glucose monitoring skills in children with type 1 diabetes. Clin Pediatr 2000;39:351–357.
19 Wilson DP, Endres RK: Compliance with blood glucose monitoring in children with type 1 diabetes mellitus. J Pediatr 1986;108:1022–1024.
20 Hellman R: Glucose meter accuracy and the impact on the care of diabetes in childhood and adolescence. Pediatr Endocrinol Rev 2011;8:200–207.
21 Mazze RS, Shamoon H, Pasmantier R, Lucido D, Murphy J, Hartmann K, Kuykendall V, Lopatin W: Reliability of blood glucose monitoring by patients with diabetes mellitus. Am J Med 1984;77:211–217.
22 Scott MG, Bruns DE, Boyd JC, Sacks DB: Tight glucose control in the intensive care unit: are glucose meters up to the task? Clin Chem 2009;55:18–20.
23 Umpierrez GE, Hellman R, Korytkowski MT, Kosiborod M, Maynard GA, Montori VM, Seley JJ, Van den Berghe G: Management of hyperglycemia in hospitalized patients in non-critical care setting: an Endocrine Society clinical practice guideline. J Clin Endocrinol Metab 2012;97:16–38.
24 Van den Berghe G, Wouters P, Weekers F, Verwaest C, Bruyninckx F, Schetz M, Vlasselaers D, Ferdinande P, Lauwers P, Bouillon R: Intensive insulin therapy in critically ill patients. N Engl J Med 2001; 345:1359–1367.
25 Rice MJ, Pitkin AD, Coursin DB: Glucose measurement in the operating room: more complicated than it seems. Anesth Analg 2010;110:1056–1065.
26 Pitkin AD, Rice MJ: Challenges to glycemic measurement in the perioperative and critically ill patient: a review. J Diabetes Sci Technol 2009;3:1270–1281.
27 Kanji S, Buffie J, Hutton B, Bunting PS, Singh A, McDonald K, Fergusson D, McIntyre LA, Hebert PC: Reliability of point-of-care testing for glucose measurement in critically ill adults. Crit Care Med 2005; 33:2778–2785.
28 Hoedemaekers CW, Klein Gunnewiek JM, Prinsen MA, Willems JL, Van der Hoeven JG: Accuracy of bedside glucose measurement from three glucometers in critically ill patients. Crit Care Med 2008;36: 3062–3066.
29 Cembrowski GS, Tran DV, Slater-Maclean L, Chin D, Gibney RTN, Jacka M: Could susceptibility to low hematocrit interference have compromised the results of the NICE-SUGAR trial? Clin Chem 2010;56: 1193–1195.
30 Mushholt PB, Schipper C. Thomé N, Ramljak S, Schmidt M, Forst T, Pfützner A: Dynamic electrochemistry corrects for hematocrit interference on blood glucose determinations with patient self-measurement devices. J Diabetes Sci Technol 2011;5: 1167–1175.

31 Rice MJ: Dynamic electrochemistry: a step in the right direction. J Diabetes Sci Technol 2011;5:1176–1178.
32 Stork AD, Kemperman H, Erkelens DW, Veneman TF: Comparison of the accuracy of the HemoCue glucose analyzer with the Yellow Springs Instrument glucose oxidase analyzer, particularly in hypoglycemia. Eur J Endocrinol 2005;153:275–281.
33 Rosenthal M, Ugele B, Lipowsky G, Küster H: The Accutrend sensor glucose analyzer may not be adequate in bedside testing for neonatal hypoglycemia. Eur J Pediatr 2006;63:99–107.
34 Bellini C, Serra G, Risso D, Mazzella M, Bonioli E: Reliability assessment of glucose measurement by HemoCue analyzer in a neonatal intensive care unit. Clin Chem Lab Med 2007;45:1549–1554.
35 Van den Berghe G, Bouillon R, Mesotten D: Glucose control in critically ill patients. N Engl J Med 2009; 361:89.
36 Weitgasse R, Hofmann M, Gappmayer B, Garstenauer C: New, small, fast-acting blood glucose meters: an analytical laboratory evaluation. Swiss Med Wkly 2007;137:536–540.
37 Bewley B, O'Rahilly S, Tassell R, DuBois J, Donald E: Evaluation of the analytical specificity and clinical application of a new-generation hospital-based glucose meter in a dialysis setting. Point of Care 2009;8:61–67.
38 Holtzinger C, Szelag E, DuBois JA, Shirey TL, Presti S: Evaluation of a new POCT bedside glucose meter and strip with hematocrit and interference corrections. Point of Care 2008;7:1–6.
39 Castano Lopez MA, Fernandez de Liger Serrano JL, Robles Rodriguez JL, Marquez Marquez T: Validation of a glucose meter at an intensive care unit. Endocrinol Nutr 2012;59:28–34.
40 Karon BS, Gandhi GY, Nuttall GA, Bryant SC, Schaff HV, McMahon MM, Santrach PJ: Accuracy of Roche Accu-Chek inform whole blood capillary, arterial, and venous glycose values in patients receiving intensive intravenous insulin therapy after cardiac surgery. Am J Clin Pathol 2007;127:919–926.
41 Kristensen GB, Nerhus K, Thue G, Sandberg S: Standardized evaluation of instruments for self-monitoring of blood glucose by patients and a technologist. Clin Chem 2004;50:1068–1071.
42 Skeie S, Kristensen GBB, Carlsen S, Sandberg S: Self-monitoring of blood glucose in type 1 diabetes patients with insufficient metabolic control: focused self-monitoring of blood glucose intervention can lower glycated hemoglobin A_{1c}. J Diabetes Sci Technol 2009;3:83–88.
43 Lewandrowski K, Cheek R, Nathan DM, Godine JE, Hurxthal K, Eschenbach K, Laposata M: Implementation of capillary blood glucose monitoring in a teaching hospital and determination of program requirements to maintain quality testing. Am J Med 1992;93:419–426.
44 Zarbo RH, Jones BA, Friedberg RC, Valenstein PN, Renner SW, Schifman RB, Walsh MK, Howanitz PJ: Q-tracks: a College of American Pathologists program of continuous laboratory monitoring and longitudinal tracking. Arch Pathol Lab Med 2002;126: 1036–1044.
45 Mykityshyn AL, Fisk AD, Rogers WA: Learning to use a home medical device: mediating age-related differences with training. Hum Factors 2002;44:354–364.
46 Anderson B, Ho J, Brackett J, Finkelstein D, Laffel L: Parental involvement in diabetes management tasks: relationships to blood glucose monitoring adherence and metabolic control in young adolescents with insulin-dependent diabetes mellitus. J Pediatr 1997; 130:257–265.
47 Klingensmith GJ, Aisenberg J, Kaufman F, Halvorson M, Cruz E, Riordan ME, Varma C, Pardo S, Viggiani MT, Wallace JF, Schachner HC, Bailey T: Evaluation of a combined blood glucose monitoring and gaming system (Didget) for motivation in children, adolescents, and young adults with type 1 diabetes. Pediatr Diabetes 2013;14:350–357.
48 Kristensen GBB, Nerhus K, Thue G, Sandberg S: Results and feasibility of an external quality assessment scheme for self-monitoring of blood glucose. Clin Chem 2006;52:1311–1317.
49 Heinemann L: Measurement quality of blood glucose meters: is there a need for an institution with an unbiased view? J Diabetes Sci Technol 2007;1:178–180.
50 Hellman R: Glucose meters: need for greater accuracy (clinician perspective). Presentation at the American Diabetes Association/American Association for Clinical Chemistry Symposium, 'Point-of-Care Devices for Glucose and HbA1C: Are They Up to the Task?'. American Diabetes Association's 70th Scientific Sessions, Orlando, 2010.

Richard Hellman, MD, FACP, FACE
Heart of America Diabetes Research Foundation
2790 Clay Edwards Dr, Ste 1250
North Kansas City, MO 64116-3260 (USA)
E-Mail rhellman@nkcendo.com

Bruttomesso D, Grassi G (eds): Technological Advances in the Treatment of Type 1 Diabetes.
Front Diabetes. Basel, Karger, 2015, vol 24, pp 81–98 (DOI: 10.1159/000363479)

Continuous Glucose Monitoring: Professional and Real Time

Howard Zisser · Jennifer E. Lane · Joseph P. Shivers
Sansum Diabetes Research Institute, Santa Barbara, Calif., USA

Abstract
Continuous glucose monitors are a valuable tool to obtain tight glycemic control in people with diabetes. Since 1999 when the first continuous glucose monitor became commercially available, continuous glucose monitors have continued to evolve, becoming more accurate and user-friendly. Novel uses have also been discovered, including tracking glucose during sleep and finding trends in glucose levels that may lead to diet or exercise changes. While continuous glucose monitors are continually advancing in accuracy and reliability, their 'hassle factor' and invasiveness have investigators seeking alternative routes of glucose measurement. New models of continuous glucose monitors are being pursued including implantable, intraperitoneal, and fluorescence-based glucose sensors, as well as noninvasive models that are used on the surface of the skin. Regardless of system type, the ultimate goal is to find the continuous glucose monitor that is best-suited for use in systems that automate insulin delivery partially (e.g. low glucose suspend) or entirely (e.g. 'fully closed-loop' artificial pancreas).

Technical Description

A continuous glucose monitor is a device that measures the concentration of glucose in the subcutaneous (interstitial) fluid, automatically and periodically. Compared to self-monitoring with a glucose meter, continuous glucose monitoring (CGM) measurements can give patients and healthcare providers a better understanding of glycemic trends and patterns. This is because CGM provides much more data than self-monitoring and can be quite accurate in portraying the direction and speed of glucose changes. However, individual glucose measurements tend to be less accurate with

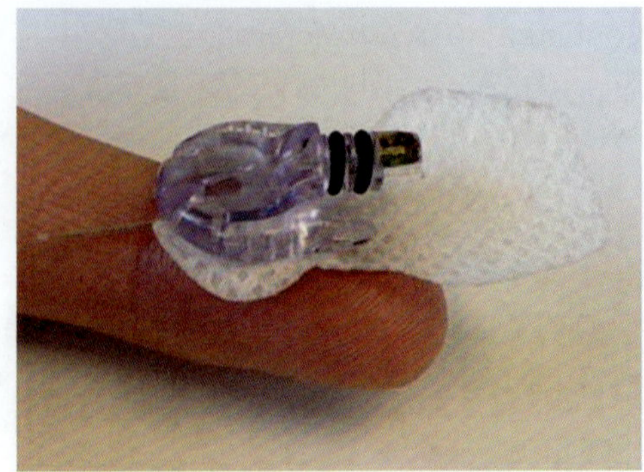

Fig. 1. Medtronic Sof-Sensor.

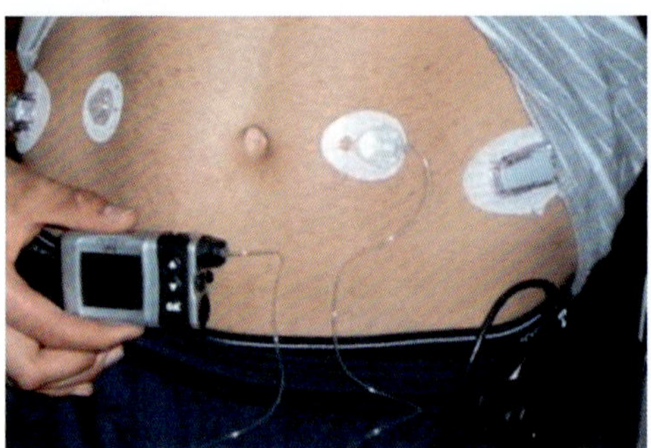

Fig. 2. Dexcom transmitter (farthest right) connected to the sensor that is inserted into the skin. The transmitter sends information to the receiver that is clipped on the belt.

CGM than with a blood glucose meter. Thus, the FDA has approved continuous glucose monitors only as adjuncts to blood glucose meters, not as sources of information sufficient for adjusting insulin therapy.

The CGM system consists of a sensor, a transmitter, and a receiver. The sensor consists of a wire catheter 5–14 mm long and 20–25 gauge thick (fig. 1). This sensor is inserted underneath the skin for several days at a time. Like an insulin pump catheter, the sensor operates best when placed in a fleshy area such as the abdomen, upper arm, buttocks, or back. The sensor is coated in glucose oxidase which oxidizes glucose to gluconolactone and reduces oxygen to hydrogen peroxide (H_2O_2) [1]. In turn, the breakdown of hydrogen peroxide produces an electrical current on an electrode surface in the sensor that measures this electrical current.

Professional versus Real-Time Systems

In a 'real-time' CGM system, the glucose sensor is connected to a transmitter that is worn outside the body and taped to the skin (fig. 2). This transmitter wirelessly sends measurements of current to a receiver that converts the 'raw' measurement of electrical current into an estimate of glucose concentration. In some CGM systems, this receiver is a standalone handheld device; in others, the receiver's functions are performed by an insulin pump. The receiver displays glycemic data numerically and pictorially so that patients can monitor their glucose trends in real time, perform blood glucose measurements, and/or modify their behavior and therapy accordingly. The receiver can also beep, buzz, or vibrate to inform the patient of potentially dangerous glucose values and trends. Additionally, the receiver stores information for weeks at a time. This information can be downloaded and reviewed, enabling retrospective pattern analysis by the patient and his/her healthcare provider.

In a 'professional' CGM system, data are stored for retrospective analysis but are not displayed in real time. Some continuous glucose monitors can be switched from real-time to a 'blinded' professional mode (which effectively involves turning off the receiver's data display and alert functions). Other continuous glucose monitors, designed exclusively for professional use, have a digital recorder instead of a transmitter, with no receiver at all. The chief advantage of professional CGM is that it gives clinically useful insights into the typical glycemic pattern of a patient who does not use real-time CGM, whereas access to real-time data would likely change the patient's behavior. However, by not displaying glucose values or sounding alerts about hypo- and hyperglycemic excursions, professional CGM also deprives the patient of information that could be life-saving [2].

History of Continuous Glucose Monitoring

Medtronic

The first continuous glucose monitor was the MiniMed (Medtronic, Northridge, Calif., USA) Continuous Glucose Monitoring System (CGMS), which became commercially available in 1999 (fig. 3). This retrospective continuous glucose monitor stored readings every 5 min and could be worn for up to 3 days [1]. The system had a high accuracy rating, with 96.6% of paired sensor-BGSM readings falling in zones A and B of the Clarke error grid. However, a relatively high amount of sensor error was experienced [3]. The company's second continuous glucose monitor was the MiniMed CGMS Gold, which became commercially available in 2003. The Gold was a retrospective continuous glucose monitor that stored readings every 5 min and could hold up to 14 days' worth of readings. Medtronic's first real-time continuous glucose monitor, the MiniMed Guardian RT-System, was approved in 2005. This was the first Medtronic continuous glucose monitor that allowed people to see their glucose measurements on the receiver without downloading the data to a computer. The Guardian RT-System monitor had a range of up to 6 feet from the sensor, and it introduced a feature whereby the user could enter events such as insulin administration, meals, or exercise [4].

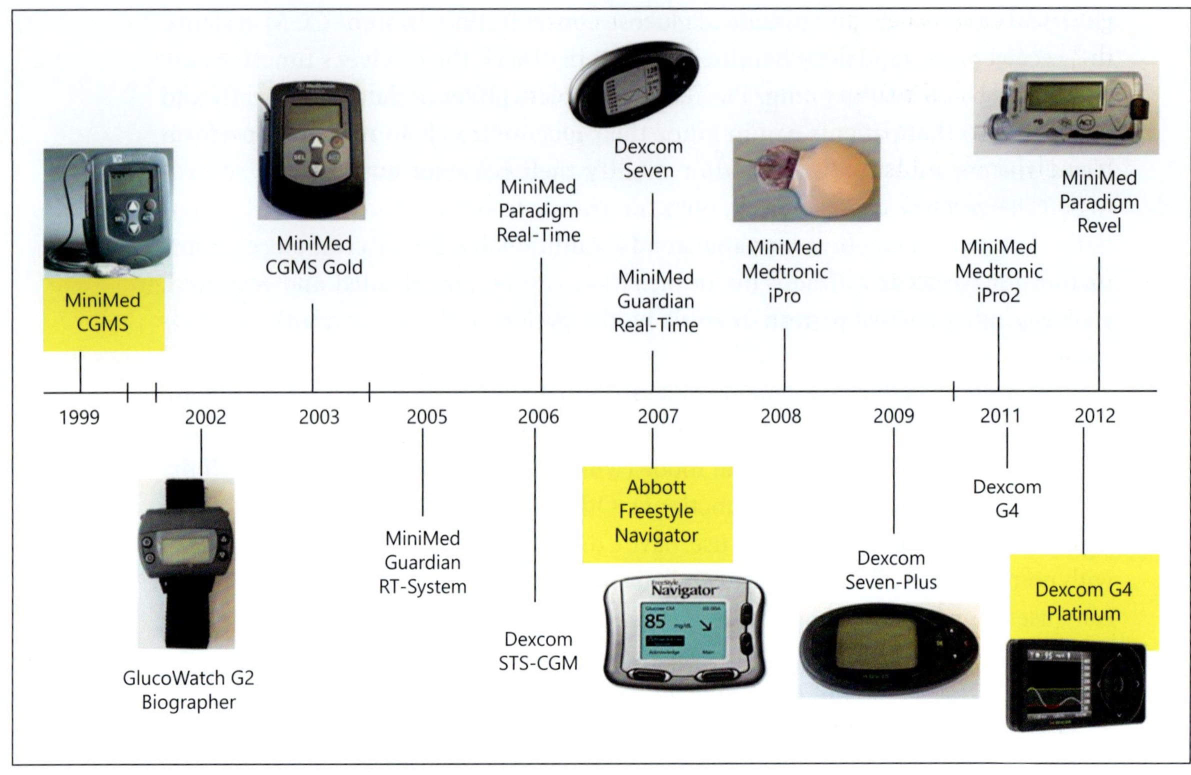

Fig. 3. Timeline of continuous glucose monitors.

In 2006 and 2007, Medtronic put out two real-time continuous glucose monitors, the MiniMed Guardian Real-Time Continuous Glucose Monitor and the MiniMed Paradigm Real-Time Continuous Glucose Monitor. These two continuous glucose monitors, which are similar in design and use the same algorithm, differ in function. The Paradigm Real-Time is a continuous glucose monitor and insulin pump integrated together in one device, while the Guardian is a real-time continuous glucose monitor alone. The Paradigm Real-Time was the first FDA-approved integrated insulin pump and continuous glucose monitor. This system was later adapted into the MiniMed Paradigm Veo, a system that integrated a low glucose suspend feature. If the user's glucose drops below the set hypoglycemia threshold and does not respond to the pump's alarms, the pump automatically suspends insulin delivery for up to 2 h. Medtronic also further developed the technology for retrospective continuous glucose monitors.

In 2008 Medtronic released an easy-to-use retrospective continuous glucose monitor called the iPro. This continuous glucose monitor is inserted into the subcutaneous area and can be left on for up to 3 days, after which the user can download software called Solutions to a personal computer and download the iPro wirelessly with a wireless link called ComLink. Once the iPro has been downloaded, the user can analyze glucose trends using reports including sensor summary, sensor modal day, and sensor daily detail [5].

In 2011 the iPro2 was released. This second generation iPro had several advantages over the first iPro. The iPro2 could be worn for up to 6 days, was more user friendly, compatible with more meters, and used a Web-based application for download that provided the user with suggestions based on their glucose trends.

Medtronic's newest integrated pump and continuous glucose monitor in the USA, the MiniMed Paradigm Real-Time Revel System, was released in 2010. It is similar to the Veo, but lacks the low glucose suspend feature, which has not yet been approved by the FDA. Since the release of Revel, Medtronic has released the new Enlite sensor, which received CE Marking in Europe in 2011 and is under regulatory review in the USA. In clinical trials the Enlite sensor had a mean absolute relative difference (MARD) of 13.86%, based on 6,404 plasma-sensor glucose paired points [6]. This is an improvement compared to NexSensor, which was found to have a MARD of 17.1% using abdomen site data, and Sof-Sensor, which was found to have a MARD of 19.7% [7].

Cygnus

The first continuous glucose monitor with which the user could follow glucose measurements in real time on a receiver was the GlucoWatch 2 Biographer (Cygnus Inc., Redwood, Calif., USA). Although it was the first of its kind and a historical device in diabetes technology, users reported a high degree of inaccurate readings and false alarms, along with irritation at the insertion site. Clinical studies reported that this continuous glucose monitor did not actually improve glycemic control [8].

Dexcom

Dexcom (San Diego, Calif., USA), another CGM company that only produces continuous glucose monitors, has produced 5 different versions of continuous glucose monitors starting in 2006. Their first was the Dexcom STS-CGM System, which monitors in real time. The STS-CGM system showed a MARD of 21.2% when 6,767 paired sensor-self monitoring of blood glucose (SMBG) data points, collected during in-clinic days, were compared [9]. Their second real-time continuous glucose monitor, released in 2007, was the Dexcom Seven, which could be worn for up to 7 days. Comparing the Dexcom Seven CGM measurements with venous blood glucose measurements (n = 2,318) using a YSI Glucose Analyzer (YSI Life Sciences; Yellow Springs, Ohio, USA), the MARD was determined to be 16.7% [10]. After the Seven came the Seven-Plus, released in 2009. With its updated software, the Seven-Plus was found to be more accurate than the Seven with a MARD of 13.0% [11]. The Seven-Plus also introduced trend arrows. These new trend arrows were displayed on the patient's receiver as a safety feature that would indicate which direction the patient's blood glucose was headed and at what rate. Other improvements of the Seven-Plus were the option of putting in event markers such as dinner, exercise, etc.

In 2011, Dexcom partnered with Animas to release a CGM/pump system, the Animas Vibe, in Europe. The Animas Vibe featured a color screen and a CGM system, referred to as the G4, with changes to the CGM transmitter, sensor design, membrane, and algorithm. Dexcom then added more updates to the sensor membrane and sensor algorithms before releasing the G4 as a stand-alone CGM product, the G4 Platinum, in Europe and the USA in 2012.

Abbott

In 2007, Abbott (Alameda, Calif., USA) released its first continuous glucose monitor, the Freestyle Navigator. When compared against the Dexcom Seven-Plus and Medtronic Guardian, this continuous glucose monitor was shown to have the best overall accuracy, with a MARD of all paired points of 11.8 as compared to 16.5% (Seven-Plus) and 20.3% (Guardian) [12]. However, in 2011 Abbott withdrew the Freestyle Navigator from the market in the USA. In a press release on the Abbott website in 2011, this discontinuation was claimed to be due to the company's inability to provide a consistent supply of the product and replacement components [13]. In 2012, Abbott released the Navigator 2.0, which is commercially available in a few European countries.

Negatives and Positive of Current Continuous Glucose Monitoring

CGM provides detailed information that patients can use to address (or prevent) glucose excursions. It can also be a valuable educational tool by revealing how glucose levels change in response to food, insulin, physical activity, stress, illness, etc. On the other hand, CGM also has several downsides that must be anticipated and managed by patients and healthcare providers using the technology.

Negatives

One set of CGM's disadvantages can be broadly classified as 'hassle factor'. Inserting a glucose sensor requires the skin to be punctured with an inserter needle, a process that many patients find painful. The sensor and transmitter (or recorder) must then be worn both day and night, with the receiver kept nearby and its alarms – some of them cautionary, redundant, or outright false – addressed by the patient. These non-stop requirements can pose a variety of inconveniences, physical discomforts, and psychological burdens. According to their labels, sensors are to be replaced every 3–7 days. Sometimes sensors continue to operate beyond this timeline, but other times they malfunction unexpectedly, requiring troubleshooting and/or premature replacement. Even when functioning optimally, continuous glucose monitors must be calibrated with blood glucose measurements roughly twice a day [14, 15]. As noted above, patients are also supposed to measure their blood glucose every time they modify their insulin therapy even if they are using real-time CGM (though many patients choose to interpret this guideline loosely).

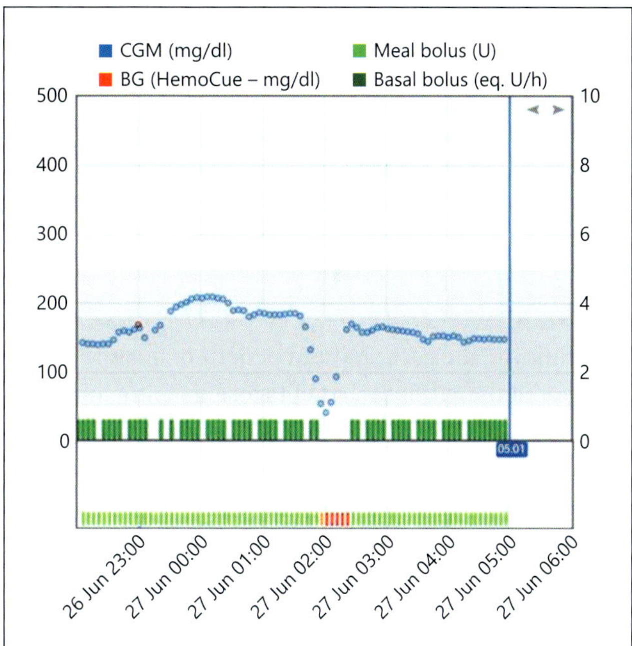

Fig. 4. At approximately 2:00 a.m. the subject rolled onto their sensor putting pressure on the area and causing a compression artifact.

Other drawbacks to CGM involve sensor accuracy. For a start, glycemic excursions in the interstitial fluid occur slightly after those seen in the blood, due to the time required for fluid transport within the space. Thus, when glucose levels are changing rapidly, even CGM readings that are perfectly accurate will differ from blood glucose measurements taken at the same time. Of course, CGM readings are not always perfectly accurate measurements of interstitial glucose concentration. This inaccuracy is due in part to limitations of the sensor chemistry, in part to 'biofouling' and other physiological responses to the sensor insertion, and in part to the fact that CGM readings are based on calibrations with blood glucose meters, which are themselves less accurate than more accepted measurement methods such as YSI Glucose Analyzers. Errors can also arise when blood flow around the sensor is restricted (e.g. when a patient rolls over in bed so that their body weight is pressing against the sensor). The sensor may falsely indicate that hypoglycemia is occurring, and the 'compression artifact' can last as long as blood flow around the sensor is relatively restricted (fig. 4).

For many patients, the key hurdles around CGM are financial. In the USA, the up-front costs of a CGM transmitter and receiver total anywhere from USD 500 to 1,500, and the ongoing costs of sensors add several hundred dollars per month. Many US insurers reimburse for CGM in people with type 1 diabetes, but require documentation of some special circumstances to justify the added expense beyond blood glucose monitoring. Such circumstances include higher glucose values in the morning than when going to bed, extreme sensitivity to insulin, pregnancy or predicted pregnancy, history of frequent hypoglycemia, and unawareness of hypoglycemia. European reimbursement for CGM varies by jurisdiction, but generally tends to be more stringent than in the USA. Depending on their interest in CGM and their financial resources, some patients might work with their healthcare providers to use the technology only briefly or intermittently as a diagnostic, educational, and/or motivational tool, rather than a core aspect of daily diabetes management.

Positives

Determining the accuracy and benefit of a continuous glucose monitor is not definitive due to the different benefits and dangers that must be considered. While the ultimate goal of using a continuous glucose monitor is to achieve better glucose control, this cannot be measured with glycated hemoglobin (HbA_{1c}) alone. It is also important to minimize hyper- and hypoglycemic episodes. These episodes are important to monitor because studies show that falsely lowered HbA_{1c} may be due to increased prevalence of hypoglycemia. Within-target HbA_{1c} may also be a poor measure of stability because it may be an average of the hyper- and hypoglycemic spikes that are frequent [16]. Therefore, monitoring HbA_{1c} alone is an incorrect measure of glucose control.

Advancements in CGM have allowed for this problem to be rectified, as reported in 2012 in a JDRF-funded study. In this study, use of a continuous glucose monitor not only lowered HbA_{1c}, but did so without increasing the frequency of hypoglycemic episodes. While maintaining HbA_{1c} below 7.0%, time spent per day in the hypoglycemic range (<70 mg/dl) decreased from 91 min at baseline to 54 min. Upon follow-up, these results were sustained up to 1 year, proving use of CGM to be beneficial. Among children participating in the study, at the end of the year only 21% were able to maintain CGM use for 6 days or more a week. However, those who did were able to decrease their HbA_{1c} 0.9% within the first 6 months and sustain this decrease for the full 12 months of use [17].

It is also important to consider other factors that have been found to be correlated with HbA_{1c} levels. For example, when looking at HbA_{1c} to determine poor or high-quality glycemic control, one must also consider metabolic control (average glucose), glucose variability (standard deviation), hyperglycemia, hypoglycemia, and postprandial indices [16]. Due to the extensive variables, the Endocrine Society attempted to summarize the subgroups of patients living with diabetes that would most benefit from CGM. The clinical practice guideline's authors recommended CGM for adults wishing to achieve target HbA_{1c}, as well as for adults with nocturnal hypoglycemia, the dawn phenomenon, postprandial hyperglycemia, hypoglycemia unawareness, and when significant changes are made to their diabetes regimen. While CGM is also recommended as a supplemental tool for adults in hospital settings, it is not recommended as the sole glucose management tool until further studies have been conducted. In children and adolescents, CGM was recommended for those who wish to achieve target HbA_{1c} levels while still limiting the risk of hypoglycemia. However, no recommendation was made for children younger than 8 years [18].

Type 2 Diabetes

Benefits of CGM are not only for patients living with type 1 diabetes. In 2012, CGM was proven beneficial in the largest group of people living with diabetes, patients with type 2 diabetes not taking mealtime insulin. Intermittent wear in this subgroup of people was shown to lower HbA_{1c} levels when compared to standard SMBG during a 12-week period. Even when the CGM group returned to SMBG after the initial 12 weeks, their HbA_{1c} levels continued to improve until 24 weeks, and the improvement was maintained for 52 weeks [19]. This shows that intermittent CGM helps improve glycemic control for people living with type 2 diabetes.

Novel Uses

Continuous Glucose Monitoring during Sleep and Dead-in-Bed Syndrome

Continuous glucose monitors have been shown to be helpful in acute scenarios that without them may have gone unexplained. These episodes are especially prevalent during sleep hours when users are not cognizant of their blood glucose measurements. Both hypoglycemia and hyperglycemia are two occasions in which use of a continuous glucose monitor may bring explanations to these glucose fluctuations.

One novel case presents a 36-year-old man who showed hyperglycemic spikes of 350–400 between midnight and 8:00 a.m. (fig. 5a). Upon review by his doctor of the professional CGM data, these periods of dangerous nocturnal hyperglycemia spikes appeared to be repeating themselves on several occasions. Upon questioning, the subject denied being awake or eating during these times. Further investigation of his medication showed the subject was on zolpidem, a nonbenzodiazepine sedative hypnotic, approved by the FDA for treatment of insomnia. A link has recently formed between the use of zolpidem and the exhibiting of complex sleep behaviors, which include sleep eating, sleep driving, sleep cooking, and sleep conversations (including telephone calls and texting) [20]. After bringing sleep eating into question, the subject disclosed that several mornings he had found what appeared to be dirty cereal bowls in his kitchen sink. This led to the belief that the nocturnal hyperglycemia was due to sleep eating and the zolpidem was immediately discontinued. CGM tracings following the discontinuation of the zolpidem demonstrated resolution of the overnight hyperglycemia (fig. 5b). These hyperglycemic episodes, due to sleep eating, would not have been observed and rectified had it not been for his use of a continuous glucose monitor [21].

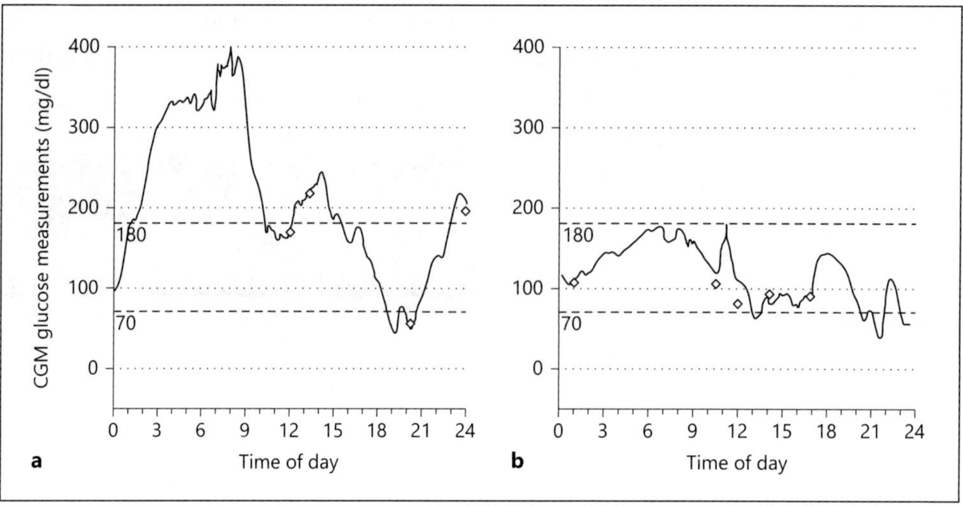

Fig. 5. a Large spike in blood glucose between 12:00 a.m. and 8:00 a.m. **b** Resolution of overnight hyperglycemia after discontinuing zolpidem.

A more severe result of profound overnight hypoglycemic episodes is 'dead-in-bed' syndrome, in which patients with type 1 diabetes die unexpectedly in their sleep. This was first documented in 2010 when a 23-year-old man wearing a continuous glucose monitor reached a low of 30 mg/dl at 3 a.m. and died, presumably from cardiac arrhythmia due to hypoglycemia between 5 and 8 a.m. [2]. While death due to nocturnal hypoglycemia is hard to verify with an autopsy, the subject's use of the continuous glucose monitor made this conclusion reasonable. As a further example, a 44-year-old man with type 1 diabetes who was found dead in his basement was originally thought to have died from hypoglycemia. Upon further inspection of his continuous glucose monitor, the man was shown to be in his target range with a blood glucose measurement of 145 mg/dl. With this information, along with the performance of an autopsy, the man was suspected to have died from a cardiovascular event due to an exacerbation of asthma [22].

In the above cases, the subject's glucose levels at the time of activity or death might never have been known without CGM. Use of a continuous glucose monitor can provide the details necessary to further inspect an unusual episode, fatal or not, or to provide insight on how to improve future continuous glucose monitors to help eradicate hyper- and hypoglycemic episodes.

Remote Monitoring

New innovations using telemedicine have also come into play to make hypoglycemic episodes less prevalent and to allow faster responses to the episodes that do occur. Telemedicine is defined as the use of information and communication technology to support medical care and decision-making. With the advancements in this type of

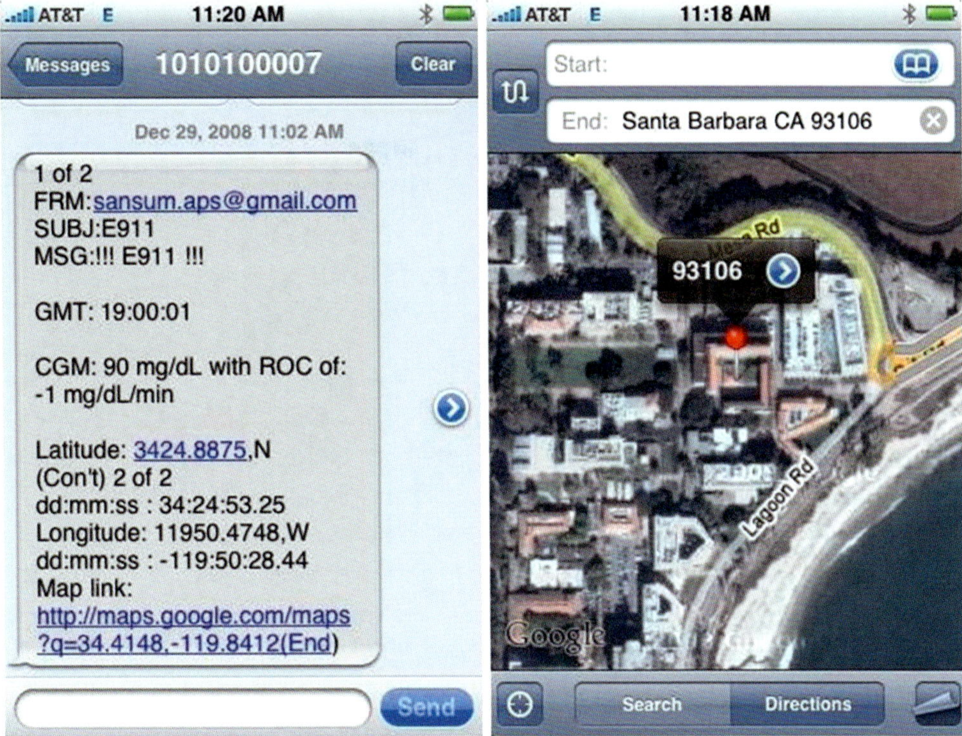

Fig. 6. Example of SMS message containing current CGM data and rate of change, GPS coordinates, and hyperlink to Google maps and Google map pinpoint location.

medicine, continuous glucose remote monitoring has made it possible to display a user's up-to-date information in real time in distant locations. This type of safety setting is beneficial for monitoring people with hypoglycemia unawareness as well as children and adolescents who are away from home or are sleeping.

In 2009, the Enhanced 911/Global Position System Wizard (E911) was proposed. This remote monitoring system allowed for the user's continuous glucose monitor to be integrated with a global positioning system (GPS). The goal of this integrated system is to detect adverse events, such as hypoglycemia, in real time, suggest a solution, and send an alert to specified contacts or emergency healthcare provider. This platform automatically sent a SMS message containing the user's current continuous glucose monitor reading along with its rate of change and the location of the user including a Google map (fig. 6). The E911 device includes alerts that can be sent to the patient to inform them of their hypoglycemia, a specified contact, a call center for the device, a physician, and/or an emergency service (e.g. 911 in the USA; fig. 7). If none of the alerts facilitate a response from the user, the E911 may suspend insulin delivery to provide further protection from hypoglycemia [23]. Integration of the E911 system with CGM would improve the risk of hypoglycemia unawareness and provide a safety net at times when hypoglycemia is not avoided.

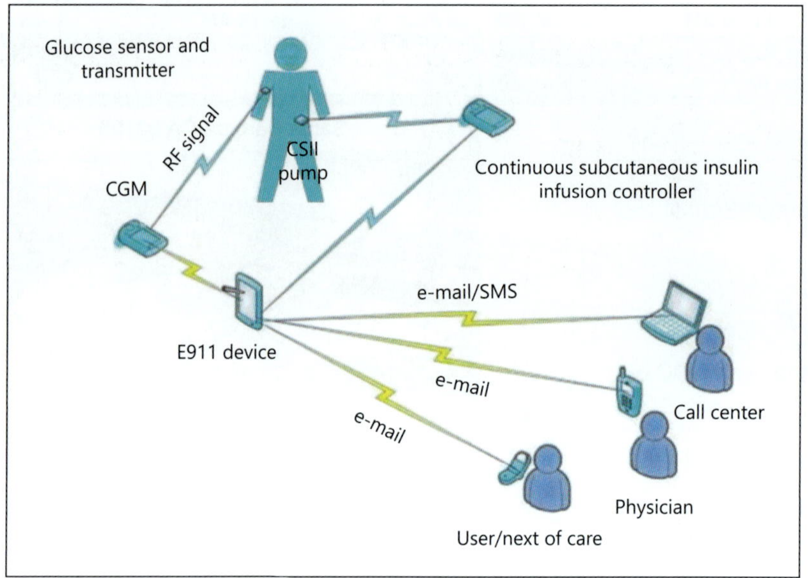

Fig. 7. Schematic of how the E911 device can broadcast an alert to the user, caregiver, physician, and call center by SMS message or e-mail. CSII = Continuous subcutaneous insulin infusion.

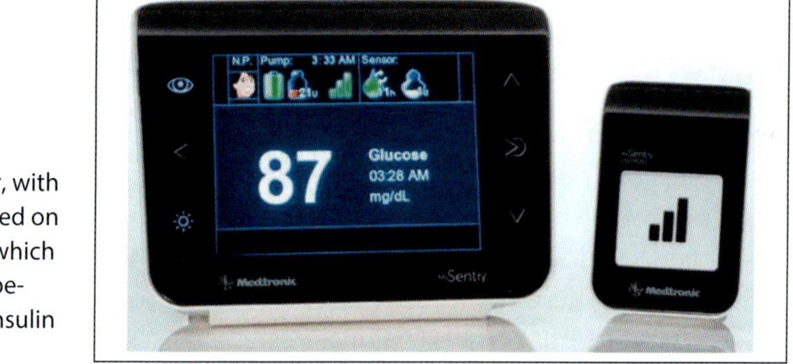

Fig. 8. mySentry monitor, with CGM information displayed on the screen, and outpost which acts as a communicator between the monitor and insulin pump.

Although GPS- and cell phone-based remote monitoring systems such as the E911 system are not yet available, hypoglycemia for children remains a risk in the home as well, for instance during sleep. In 2012, the FDA approved the first in-home remote monitoring system for commercial use, the Medtronic mySentry Remote Glucose Monitor. This system allows guardians access to their child's CGM readings via a small monitor that can be placed at their bedside (fig. 8). The system is comprised of three parts: the monitor that displays the wearer's insulin pump and CGM information, the outpost that is used to send and receive information from the wearer's insulin pump and send it to the monitor (which can be placed up to 6 feet away from the insulin pump and 50 feet away from the monitor), and the MiniMed Paradigm Real-Time Revel insulin pump that can send and receive information to the outpost. It also

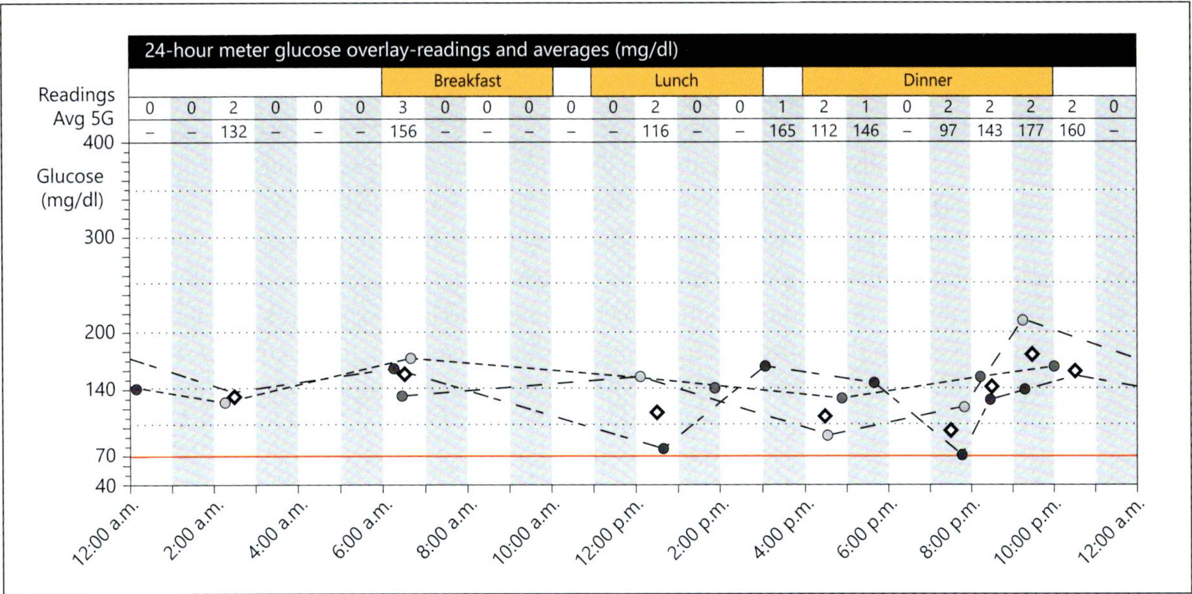

Fig. 9. CareLink modal day report showing 3 days of glucose measurements displayed on a 24-hour time scale.

displays the pump's predictive hyper- and hypoglycemia alarms so that those monitoring the wearer may be alerted when the wearer is headed out of target range. mySentry is a new innovation that acts as a preventative agent for monitoring dangerous overnight hyper- and hypoglycemia.

Analyzing Continuous Glucose Monitoring Data

Another evolving aspect of CGM is the process of data collection and analysis. Currently, each continuous glucose monitor manufacturer has its own proprietary data download software, and some third-party companies (e.g. DiaSend, Askim, Sweden) have also designed CGM data analysis programs. These software systems all share certain general functions, such as a 'modal day' display of multiple days' worth of glycemic data on a single 24-hour time scale (fig. 9), but many details are particular to each system and must be learned separately by patients and healthcare providers. To address this issue, some have advocated for continuous glucose monitor manufacturers to adopt the same universal 'title page' in their data readouts. This proposed overview page could be based on the International Diabetes Center's Ambulatory Glucose Profile (AGP) or an alternative summary graphic [24, 25].

In addition to data aggregation, some software systems offer explicit considerations about how patients and/or healthcare providers can adjust diabetes therapy. CareLink Pro 3, Medtronic Diabetes' software for healthcare providers, offers detailed analyses and therapeutic considerations of glycemic excursions in patients who have collected at least 5 days of data using an integrated pump and continuous glucose monitor [26]. The software was launched in the USA in 2010 and internationally in 2012. Whereas CareLink Pro is designed for retrospective data analysis by healthcare providers, other software is intended for real-time use by patients. The DIAdvisor, an investigational European system sponsored in part by Novo Nordisk, uses CGM data to predict glucose levels 20 min into the future and advise patients accordingly [27]. The most obvious application for such onboard predictive software will be in artificial pancreas products and their precursors. However, future stand-alone CGM systems could also conceivably become more sophisticated with regard to predictive alerts, retrospective pattern analysis, and individualized learning (all pending clinical validation and regulatory approval, naturally).

New Continuous Glucose Monitor Models

Despite the many benefits of continuous glucose monitors, the vast majority of patients with type 1 diabetes do not use the technology [28]. Some people are simply satisfied with traditional 'finger-stick' SMBG. Others are attracted to the benefits of CGM, but repelled by practical concerns, e.g. cost, time, and effort; pain of insertion; imperfect accuracy; imperfect reliability, and psychological burden. Some of these issues can be addressed by modifying current systems. However, certain drawbacks are inherent to any continuous glucose monitor that uses subcutaneous, glucose-oxidase-based sensors requiring replacement several times per month. Thus, many companies and academic institutions are studying other approaches to CGM. In this section, we discuss a few of these alternative approaches, which have the potential to improve CGM's clinical utility and facilitate new applications such as automated insulin delivery (i.e. the 'artificial pancreas').

Implantable Glucose Sensors

For many years, a major goal in continuous glucose monitor development has been to design implantable glucose sensors that can operate for long periods (i.e. 6 months or more). Long-term implantable sensors would resolve many of the hassles associated with wearing and replacing current continuous glucose monitor sensors. However, groups developing implantable sensors face several difficult technical challenges. These challenges include making the sensors small enough that they can be implanted and removed relatively easily on an ongoing basis, supplying the sensor with power, and ensuring that the sensor will still function after it has been implanted for many months (during which time the body might encapsulate the sensor, potentially closing it off from the body's fluids).

Some implantable sensors use electrochemistry similar to that of today's CGM. For example, GlySens Inc. (San Diego, Calif., USA) has conducted 6-month clinical stability testing with a glucose-oxidase-based sensor that uses catalase to break down H_2O_2 and

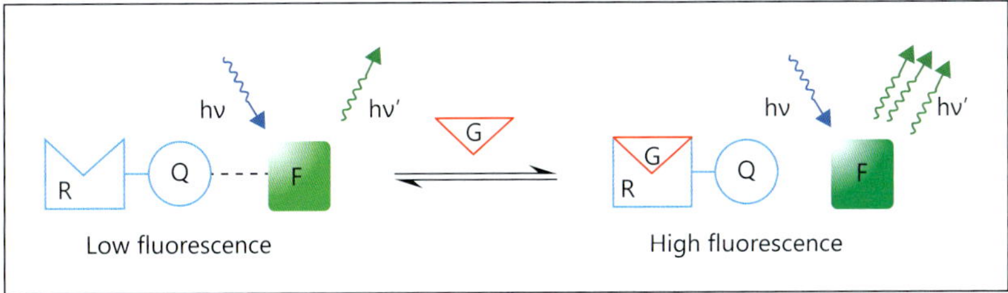

Fig. 10. In fluorescence-based glucose sensors, when glucose is present it binds to the receptor drawing away the quencher and allowing for higher fluorescence. This higher fluorescence depicts a higher glucose concentration. R = Receptor; Q = quencher; F = fluorophore; G = glucose; hν = photon energy.

thus improve sensor longevity [29]. Other implantable sensors use fluorescence. Month-long clinical data have been presented on a wrist-implanted sensor developed by Senseonics (Germantown, Md., USA) [30], and 4-month data have been reported on a subconjunctival sensor developed by EyeSense GmbH (Grossostheim, Germany) [31].

Intraperitoneal Sensors

Many implantable glucose sensors are designed for the subcutaneous space, but ultimately a more favorable location could be the abdominal (intraperitoneal) cavity. Compared to the subcutaneous space, the intraperitoneal cavity has greater and more uniform blood flow, which could increase a sensor's long-term stability and reduce intersensor variability [32]. The intraperitoneal cavity is also larger, which eases the constraints on sensor size. Additionally, preclinical research indicates that blood glucose excursions can be detected earlier in the intraperitoneal space compared to the subcutaneous space [32]. To these authors' knowledge, intraperitoneal glucose sensing has not been tested in humans.

Fluorescence-Based Sensors

Some believe that fluorescence-based glucose sensors can be more accurate and long-lasting than enzyme-based sensors, in part because fluorescent measurements do not consume biological molecules or produce chemical byproducts. At a basic level, most fluorescent sensors rely on fluorescent molecules (fluorophores) coupled to other molecules that bind glucose (e.g. lectin). When glucose molecules bind to the fluorophores in the sensor, the fluorescence signal changes in a way that can be quantified precisely (fig. 10). The changes in fluorescence can thus be used to calculate glucose concentration. One problem with fluorescence-based glucose sensors is the interference of photobleaching, the destruction of fluorophores due to light exposure. This destruction makes it hard to observe and measure the fluorescent molecules, compromising the sensors performance and accuracy.

Becton Dickinson is developing a subcutaneous fluorescence-based glucose sensor that would be worn similarly to current sensors. This sensor, which uses glucose-galactose-binding protein, has been evaluated in a 12-hour feasibility comparison to current CGM [33]; further clinical research is ongoing as of this writing [34]. Medtronic is also developing a subcutaneous fluorescence-based glucose sensor for short-term wear. The company plans to integrate this optical sensor into a CGM system that also uses an electrochemical sensor, with the stated goal of making the entire system accurate and reliable enough to support automated insulin delivery [35]. The fluorescence-sensing technology was acquired by Medtronic in 2009 from PreciSense A/S (Horsholm, Denmark) [36], which has studied the sensor in humans for up to 14 days [37]. EyeSense has also conducted clinical research on a subcutaneous fluorescence-based continuous glucose monitor sensor [38].

Noninvasive Glucose Sensors

Another longstanding goal in CGM development is to design noninvasive (or minimally invasive) glucose sensors. Many noninvasive glucose-monitoring prototypes use some form of spectroscopy. The physics underlying these methods is extremely complex, and the signal can be affected by a patient's skin attributes and disrupted if the sensor moves [39]. In 2012, a Raman spectroscopy-based continuous glucose monitor developed by C8 Medisensors (San Jose, Calif., USA) was approved for use in Europe. However, the reported data accuracy for the system, which is worn around the waist, did not appear competitive with those of current CGM systems [40].

Not all noninvasive CGM systems use spectroscopy. For example, GlucoWatch used a transdermal method called reverse iontophoresis that had limited accuracy and could cause skin irritation [39]. More recently, Echo Therapeutics (Philadelphia, Pa., USA) has conducted multiple clinical trials of a system whereby a small area of skin is permeated with a microdermabrasion device, allowing interstitial glucose concentration to be measured with a glucose-oxidase-based sensor on the skin's surface [41].

Conclusion

As new innovations come along and sensors become more accurate, the ultimate goal of 'closing the loop' and creating an artificial pancreas product – a combination continuous glucose monitor/insulin pump system that automatically controls glucose levels – begins to come in sight. Over the history of continuous glucose monitors, products have become more accurate, more user-friendly, less invasive, and safer for day-to-day use. With the development of the new alerts, suspend systems, and suggestive treatment systems, continuous glucose monitors are beginning to do more of the work that most people living with diabetes have to do several times a day on their own. This review has suggested that although there are downsides and hassles to its use, CGM is advancing towards a diabetes technology that will ultimately provide patients with a life in which their diabetes is controlled for them and not by them.

References

1 Cengiz E, Tamborlane WV: A tale of two compartments: interstitial versus blood glucose monitoring. Diabetes Technol Ther 2009;11(Suppl 1):S11–S16.

2 Tanenberg RJ, Newton CA, Drake AJ: Confirmation of hypoglycemia in the 'dead-in-bed' syndrome, as captured by a retrospective continuous glucose monitoring system. Endocr Pract 2010;16:244–248.

3 Sachedina N, Pickup JC: Performance assessment of the Medtronic-MiniMed Continuous Glucose Monitoring System and its use for measurement of glycaemic control in type 1 diabetic subjects. Diabet Med 2003;20:1012–1015.

4 Diabetes Research in Children Network (DirecNet) Study Group: The accuracy of the Guardian RT continuous glucose monitor in children with type 1 diabetes. Diabetes Technol Ther 2008;10:266–272.

5 Blevins TC: Professional continuous glucose monitoring in clinical practice. J Diabetes Sci Technol 2010;4:440–456.

6 Keenan DB, Mastrototaro JJ, Zisser H, Cooper KA, Raghavendhar G, Lee SW, Yusi J, Bailey TS, Brazg RL, Shah RV: Accuracy of the Enlite 6-day glucose sensor with guardian and Veo calibration algorithms. Diabetes Technol Ther 2012;14:225–231.

7 Peoples T, Bailey T, Ronald B, Zisser HC, Janowski B, Huang S, Talbot C, Yang Q: Accuracy performance of the Medtronic NexSensor for 6 days in an inpatient setting using abdomen and buttocks insertion sites. J Diabetes Sci Technol 2011;5:358–364.

8 Diabetes Research in Children Network (DirecNet) study Group: Youth and parent satisfaction with clinical use of the GlucoWatch G2 Biographer in the management of pediatric type 1 diabetes. Diabetes Care 2005;28:1929–1935.

9 Garg S, Zisser H, Schwartz S, Bailey T, Kaplan R, Ellis S, Jovanovic L: Improvement in glycemic excursions with a transcutaneous, real-time continuous glucose sensor: a randomized controlled trial. Diabetes Care 2006;29:44–50.

10 Zisser HC, Zisser HC, Bailey TS, Schwartz S, Ratner RE, Wise J: Accuracy of the Seven Continuous Glucose Monitoring System: comparison with frequently sampled venous glucose measurements. J Diabetes Sci Technol 2009;3:1146–1154.

11 Bailey T, Zisser H, Zisser H, Chang A: New features and performance of a next-generation seven-day continuous glucose monitoring system with short lag time. Diabetes Technol Ther 2009;11:749–755.

12 Damiano ER, El-Khatib FH, Zheng H, Nathan DM, Russell SJ: A comparative effectiveness analysis of three continuous glucose monitors. Diabetes Care 2013;36:251–259.

13 Care AD: FDA approves Abbott's FreeStyle Navigator Continuous Glucose Monitoring System: new tool uniquely provides minute-by-minute and trend information that can lead to proactive diabetes management. 2008. https://www.abbottdiabetescare.com/press-room/2008/2008-c.html (accessed January 21, 2013).

14 G4 Platinum Continuous Glucose Monitoring System. San Diego, Dexcom, 2012.

15 Medtronic: Guardian REAL-Time Continous Glucose Monitoring System User Guide. Northridge, Dexcom, 2006.

16 Sartore G, Chilelli NC, Burlina S, Di Stefano P, Piarulli F, Fedele D, Mosca A, Lapolla A: The importance of HbA_{1c} and glucose variability in patients with type 1 and type 2 diabetes: outcome of continuous glucose monitoring (CGM). Acta Diabetol 2012; 49(Suppl 1):S153–S160.

17 Ruedy KJ, Tamborlane WV; Juvenile Diabetes Research Foundation Continuous Glucose Monitoring Study Group: The landmark JDRF continuous glucose monitoring randomized trials: a look back at the accumulated evidence. J Cardiovasc Transl Res 2012; 5:380–387.

18 Klonoff DC, Buckingham B, Christiansen JS, Montori VM, Tamborlane WV, Vigersky RA, Wolpert H; Endocrine Society: Continuous glucose monitoring: an Endocrine Society Clinical Practice Guideline. J Clin Endocrinol Metab 2011;96:2968–2979.

19 Vigersky RA, Fonda SJ, Chellappa M, Walker MS, Ehrhardt NM: Short- and long-term effects of real-time continuous glucose monitoring in patients with type 2 diabetes. Diabetes Care 2012;35:32–38.

20 Dolder CR, Nelson MH: Hypnosedative-induced complex behaviours: incidence, mechanisms and management. CNS Drugs 2008;22:1021–1036.

21 Zisser H, Rivera S, Lane J: Zolpidem-induced sleep eating resulting in significant hyperglycemia in a subject with type 1 diabetes mellitus discovered via continuous glucose monitoring. Clin Diabetes, in press.

22 Schmidt S, Norgaard K: Glucose sensor excludes hypoglycaemia as cause of death. Diabetes Res Clin Pract 2012;96:e30–e32.

23 Dassau E, Jovanovic L, Doyle FJ 3rd, Zisser HC: Enhanced 911/Global Position System Wizard: a telemedicine application for the prevention of severe hypoglycemia – monitor, alert, and locate. J Diabetes Sci Technol 2009;3:1501–1506.

24 Mazze R, Akkerman B, Mettner J: An overview of continuous glucose monitoring and the ambulatory glucose profile. Minn Med 2011;94:40–44.

25 Bergenstal R: Sensor-augmented insulin pumps. The Second Global Diabetes Summit, Columbus, 2012.

26 Medtronic: CareLink Pro Software. 2012. http://www.professional.medtronicdiabetes.com/hcp-products/carelink-pro (accessed January 11, 2013).
27 Poulsen JU, Avogaro A, Chauchard F, Cobelli C, Johansson R, Nita L, Pogose M, Del Re L, Renard E, Sampath S, Saudek F, Skillen M, Soendergaard J: A diabetes management system empowering patients to reach optimised glucose control: from monitor to advisor. Conf Proc IEEE Eng Med Biol Soc 2010; 5270–5271.
28 Beck RW, Tamborlane WV, Bergenstal RM, Miller KM, DuBose SN, Hall CA; T1D Exchange Clinic Network: The T1D Exchange Clinic Registry. J Clin Endocrinol Metab 2012;97:4383–4389.
29 Lucisano J: Application of the implantable continuous glucose monitoring system in a human subject; in Klonoff DC (ed): 11th Annual Diabetes Technology Meeting. Bethesda, Diabetes Technology Society, 2012.
30 Mortellaro M: A wireless, fully implantable continuous glucose sensor. 47th Annual Meeting of the European Association for the Study of Diabetes, Lisbon, 2011.
31 Hasslacher C, Auffarth G, Platten I, Rabsilber T, Smith B, Kulozik F, Knuth M, Nikolaus K, Müller A: Safety and accuracy of a new long-term subconjunctival glucose sensor. J Diabetes 2012;4:291–296.
32 Burnett D, pers. commun. 2012, TheraNova.
33 Judge K, Morrow L, Lastovich AG, Kurisko D, Keith SC, Hartsell J, Roberts B, McVey E, Weidemaier K, Win K, Hompesch M: Continuous glucose monitoring using a novel glucose/galactose binding protein: results of a 12-hour feasibility study with the Becton Dickinson glucose/galactose binding protein sensor. Diabetes Technol Ther 2011;13:309–317.
34 Becton Dickinson: Three-day, in-clinic evaluation of the BD 2nd generation continuous glucose sensor device in type 1 diabetics. 2012. http://clinicaltrials.gov/ct2/show/NCT01645696 (accessed January 11, 2013).
35 Sorensen W: JDRF through the Joint JDRF-Helmsley Charitable Trust Initiative Partners with Medtronic to Advance Continuous Glucose Monitoring towards Artificial Pancreas Systems. New York, JDRF, 2012.
36 Medtronic: Medtronic Inc. Analyst Day Analyst Packet – Morning Session. Minneapolis, Medtronic Inc., 2009.
37 Nielsen JK, Christiansen JS, Kristensen JS, Toft HO, Hansen LL, Aasmul S, Gregorius K: Clinical evaluation of a transcutaneous interrogated fluorescence lifetime-based microsensor for continuous glucose reading. J Diabetes Sci Technol 2009;3:98–109.
38 Müller AJ, Knuth M, Nikolaus KS, Krivánek R, Küster F, Hasslacher C: First clinical evaluation of a new percutaneous optical fiber glucose sensor for continuous glucose monitoring in diabetes. J Diabetes Sci Technol 2013;7:13–23.
39 Smith JL: The pursuit of noninvasive glucose: 'hunting the deceitful turkey'. Mendosa.com, http://www.mendosa.com/noninvasive_glucose.pdf, 2011.
40 Hofmeister R: Prospective noninvasive glucose measurement using a wearable Raman spectrometer; in Klonoff DC (ed): 11th Annual Diabetes Technology Meeting. San Francisco, J Diabetes Sci Technol, 2012, p A65.
41 Chuang H, Trieu MQ, Hurley J, Taylor EJ, England MR, Nasraway SA Jr: Pilot studies of transdermal continuous glucose measurement in outpatient diabetic patients and in patients during and after cardiac surgery. J Diabetes Sci Technol 2008;2:595–602.

Howard Zisser, MD
Director of Clinical Research and Diabetes Technology, Sansum Diabetes Research Institute
Adjunct Professor Department of Chemical Engineering, University of California
15 W. Los Olivos St., Santa Barbara, CA 93105 (USA)
E-Mail hzisser@gmail.com

Bruttomesso D, Grassi G (eds): Technological Advances in the Treatment of Type 1 Diabetes.
Front Diabetes. Basel, Karger, 2015, vol 24, pp 99–109 (DOI: 10.1159/000363481)

Real-Time Continuous Glucose Monitoring in Children and Adolescents

Tadej Battelino[a, b] · Klemen Dovč[a] · Nataša Bratina[a]

[a]Department of Paediatric Endocrinology, Diabetes and Metabolism, UMC – University Children's Hospital, and [b]Faculty of Medicine, University of Ljubljana, Ljubljana, Slovenia

Abstract

Recent large databases of patients with type 1 diabetes in the European Union and the USA have demonstrated that most patients, particularly in the pediatric patient group, do not reach the target values of glycosylated hemoglobin (HbA_{1c}) recommended by professional societies. Diabetes-related technology is associated with improved HbA_{1c} in many but not all randomized controlled trials (RCTs) that included pediatric patients. Recently, a few studies have demonstrated a significant reduction in exposure to hypoglycemia, to which pediatric patients are particularly vulnerable. Scientific evidence supports the use of real-time continuous glucose monitoring (RT-CGM) in all age groups. Data from RCTs for children and adolescents with type 1 diabetes clearly demonstrate a significant reduction in HbA_{1c} as well as a reduction in time spent in and/or frequency of hypoglycemia. However, the effectiveness of RT-CGM depends on its continuous use, and in some pediatric RCTs low compliance with the sensor use precludes significant improvements in metabolic control. RT-CGM with low-glucose threshold insulin suspend seems to effectively prevent and shorten hypoglycemia in all age groups. Several barriers have hindered wider routine use of RT-CGM in children and adolescents, such as poor reimbursement in public insurance systems, insufficient training of diabetes care teams, age-specific behavior peculiarities, and lack of essential motivation for improving diabetes care and outcomes. Evidence-based strategies and quality assurance initiatives can help improve the organization of diabetes care for young patients along with individualized therapy plans that include the use of diabetes-related technology. Finally, RT-CGM integrated into closed-loop insulin delivery systems will enable more patients to reach glycemic targets with less day-to-day hassles.

Immense efforts and finances have been invested in routine diabetes management, clinical research, and development of novel treatment strategies to improve day-to-day metabolic control in millions of patients with diabetes. Despite this, only a minority of patients with type 1 diabetes reach current targets for metabolic control. In the

Type 1 Diabetes Exchange Registry, which has more than 25,000 enrolled patients [1], between 17 and 34% (depending on age, an estimated 25% on average) of the adult patients reached the American Diabetes Association (ADA) target of glycosylated hemoglobin (HbA_{1c}) below 7% [2], and between 23 and 26% of pediatric patients reached the International Society for Pediatric and Adolescent Diabetes (ISPAD) target of HbA_{1c} below 7.5% [3]. Comparable outcomes have been described in large European cohort studies [4, 5], some demonstrating an improvement in metabolic control over time [5] and some no improvement at all [6]. Hypoglycemia likely remains the major limiting factor in reducing HbA_{1c} to the target range for most patients with type 1 diabetes [7], despite the fact that some follow-up studies have reported decreasing incidence [5].

The use of technology in diabetes management has gained considerable ground with continuous subcutaneous insulin infusion (CSII) becoming a major treatment modality [1] often associated with improved metabolic control [1, 8]. More recently, real-time continuous glucose monitoring (RT-CGM) has also entered clinical routine with more than 10% use in the Type 1 Diabetes Exchange adult cohort [1] and around 3% use in pediatric cohorts [1, 9]. This chapter concentrates on results from randomized controlled clinical trials (RCTs) that enrolled children and adolescents alone or combined with adults using RT-CGM as an intervention in type 1 diabetes.

Real-Time Continuous Glucose Monitoring and Glycosylated Hemoglobin A_{1c}

The first RCT using RT-CGM demonstrated a significant decrease in HbA_{1c} with continuous use for 3 months in 156 patients with poor metabolic control (RT-CGM -1.0 ± 1.1 vs. control $-0.4 \pm 1.0\%$, $p = 0.003$) [10] and in the post hoc intention-to-treat analysis of the adolescent subgroup (27 in the RT-CGM group and 27 in the control group; decrease in HbA_{1c} -0.72 ± 1.13 vs. $-0.05 \pm 0.78\%$, adjusted $p = 0.0447$) [11]. Similarly, a separate analysis of 16 adolescent patients in an RT-CGM and 16 adolescent patients in control group (standard pump therapy) demonstrated a statistically significant between-group difference in HbA_{1c} (–0.6%, $p = 0.025$) in an Australian RCT with patient-led use of RT-CGM, which in total included 51 participants for the intention-to-treat analysis (mean end-of-study HbA_{1c} was 0.43% lower in the intervention group compared with the control group, 95% CI: 0.19–0.75%, $p = 0.009$) [12].

The Juvenile Diabetes Research Foundation (JDRF) trial included 56 children and 57 adolescents in an RT-CGM group, and 58 children and 53 adolescents in a control group [13]. Contrary to the results in the adult group (patients older than 24 years) where the mean difference in HbA_{1c} change (–0.53%, 95% CI: –0.71 to –0.35, $p < 0.001$) reached statistical and clinical significance, there was no statistically significant difference in the change in HbA_{1c} between the children and adolescent study groups, save for the number of children reaching HbA_{1c} levels <7% being significantly greater in RT-CGM as compared to the control group (15 vs. 7, respectively; p = 0.01) [13]. However, the post hoc analysis of participants using RT-CGM at least 6 days on average in each age group demonstrated significant improvement in HbA_{1c} over those who used RT-CGM less often (p = 0.02 in the 25-year-old age group, p = 0.002 in the 15- to 24-year-old age group, and p < 0.001 in the 8- to 14-year age group) [14].

A French RTC demonstrated a significant difference only in patients who were fully compliant with the protocol (>70% of RT-CGM use; RT-CGM-CSII 0.96 ± 0.93%, p < 0.001; CSII 0.55 ± 0.93%, p < 0.001; intergroup comparison, p < 0.004), with the pediatric population being too small to reach significance [15]. Another RCT in well-controlled patients (HbA_{1c} <7.5%) that focused on time spent in hypoglycemia and included children and adolescents in an RT-CGM group (n = 27) and a control group (n = 26) demonstrated the between-group difference in HbA_{1c} at 6 months (adjusted for baseline HbA_{1c}, center, and age group) being significantly lower in the RT-CGM group for the whole study population (mean: 6.69 vs. 6.95%, difference in means: –0.27, 95% CI: –0.47 to –0.07, p = 0.008); adjusted mean HbA_{1c} was reduced by 0.23 (6.92 vs. 7.15) in pediatric subjects (10–17 years of age) and by 0.31 (6.51 vs. 6.83) in adults (18–65 years of age) [16].

A large RCT comparing RT-CGM-CSII with the use of multiple daily injections with 443 patients in the primary analysis included 78 children and adolescents in the RT-CGM-CSII group and 78 children and adolescents in the multiple daily injection group [17]. At 12 months, a between-group difference in HbA_{1c} of –0.6% (95% CI: –0.7 to 0.4; p < 0.001) was achieved for the total population, with a pediatric between-group difference in HbA_{1c} of –0.5% (p < 0.001) in favor of the RT-CGM-CSII group, along with significantly more children and adolescents in the RT-CGM-CSII group reaching the age-specific target HbA_{1c} (between-group difference: 25%, p < 0.005). Another French RTC included 178 patients (aged 8–60 years) with poor control (mean starting HbA_{1c} 9%) in the intention-to-treat analysis, 113 in the RT-CGM group (62 patient-led sensor use and 55 physician-led sensor use), and 61 in the control group (multiple daily injections or CSII without RT-CGM). After 12 months, the reduction in HbA_{1c} was significantly greater in the patient-led RT-CGM group (–0.50%, 95% CI: –0.70 to –0.29, p = 0.0006) and physician-led group (–0.45%, 95% CI: –0.66 to –0.24, p = 0.0018) than in the control group (0.02%; 95% CI: –0.18 to 0.23), as well as when the results of both RT-CGM groups were combined (–0.48%, 95% CI: –0.63 to –0.33) versus the control group (p < 0.001) [18]. No separate analysis for the pediatric patients was provided.

A European pediatric RCT focused on the use of RT-CGM from disease onset with 160 participants (age 8.8 ± 4.4 years) randomized 9.6 ± 6 days after the first insulin administration to either sensor-augmented CSII or CSII alone [19]. There was no difference in HbA_{1c} between the groups at 12 months (7.4 ± 1.2% in RT-CGM-CSII vs. 7.6 ± 1.4% in CSII alone). Participants who used RT-CGM at least 3 days per week had significantly lower HbA_{1c} compared to those who used RT-CGM less ($p = 0.032$). Glycemic variability assessed with mean amplitude of glycemic excursions was significantly lower in the RT-CGM-CSII group as compared to CSII alone ($p = 0.037$). There was no incident of severe hypoglycemia in the sensor-augmented CSII group, but 4 incidents in the CSII-alone group ($p = 0.046$).

A recent RCT performed by the Diabetes Research in Children Network (DirecNet) study group focused on the youngest end of the pediatric population. After a 6-week run-in period, 146 children aged 4–9.9 years with a mean HbA_{1c} of 7.9%, and 60% using CSII, were randomized to RT-CGM or standard care for 26 weeks [20]. The primary goal of decreasing HbA_{1c} by ≥0.5% with no severe hypoglycemia was reached by 13 of 69 (19%) children in the RT-CGM group and 19 of 68 (28%) in the control group ($p = 0.17$), with the mean change in HbA_{1c} being -0.1 ± 0.6 in each group ($p = 0.79$). Three events of severe hypoglycemia were recorded in the RT-CGM group versus 6 in the control group (8.6 vs. 17.6 per 100 patient-years, $p = 0.80$). Only 41% of the children wore the sensor ≥6 days during month 6, and the frequency of sensor use was not correlated with the decrease of HbA_{1c}. Results from the quality of life questionnaires did not indicate particular technical difficulties with the sensor; moreover, parental satisfaction with RT-CGM was high. It is therefore difficult to understand why patients either did not use the sensor or did not use the RT-CGM data to improve glycemia on a regular daily basis. The authors suggest that the glycemic targets set by the ADA for this age group were too high and thus prevented a more substantial decrease in HbA_{1c}, along with the 'deep-rooted' unremitting fear of hypoglycemia present in most parents of children with type 1 diabetes.

A smaller feasibility trial focused on toddlers [21]. After 1–2 weeks of run-in to familiarize the families with RT-CGM, 23 families were provided with the necessary knowledge, written instructions on how to use the RT-CGM data for making decisions on management, and sufficient supplies for 6 months. RT-CGM data were downloaded during visits every 4–6 weeks and discussed with the family. Twenty toddlers completed the study with a median use of sensor in the last month of 4.7 days a week with 45% using it ≥6 days weekly. Mean HbA_{1c} did not change ($7.9 \pm 0.8\%$ at baseline vs. $8.0 \pm 0.8\%$ at 26 weeks); however, it decreased by $0.4 \pm 0.7\%$ in the 8 children whose baseline HbA_{1c} was >8.0%, and increased in those with lower initial HbA_{1c}. Only one child experienced severe hypoglycemia, 4 in total (2 on and 2 off RT-CGM). No other severe side effects were reported. The RT-CGM satisfaction scale report at 26 weeks scored an average of 4.1 on a 5-point Likert scale. The authors concluded that RT-CGM was safe and well tolerated by toddlers and liked by their parents [21].

The necessity to successfully integrate RT-CGM data in the day-to-day management of diabetes in children and improve their metabolic control remains the most important imminent task of diabetes teams. It is also likely that the ADA may need to revise their pediatric guidelines and bring them closer to the international ISPAD guidelines [3]. A conclusion that RT-CGM may not work in the pediatric population is not supported by the existing data.

An RTC focused on the impact of RT-CGM on metabolic control in patients using CSII and not achieving target HbA_{1c} [22]. To control for the impact of diabetes education and caregiver-patient contact, a crossover design was used. No written instructions on how to use the RT-CGM data for diabetes management were provided. After a month of run-in, 153 patients (72 children aged 6–18 years) were randomized to either 6 months on RT-CGM followed by a 4-month wash-out and 6 months off RT-CGM, or vice versa. All were included in the intention-to-treat analysis (including 15 that dropped out) for the primary (difference in HbA_{1c} between RT-CGM-on and RT-CGM-off) and secondary outcomes. The mean adjusted difference in HbA_{1c} was –0.43% (95% CI: –0.32 to –0.55, $p < 0.001$; final HbA_{1c} in RT-CGM-on was 8.04%), –0.46% ($p < 0.001$) in pediatric participants and –0.41% ($p < 0.001$) in adult participants. Mean sensor use was 80% (median: 84%) of the required time (mean: 81% over the final 4 weeks), 73% (mean: 74% over the final 4 weeks) in the pediatric group and 86% of the required time (mean: 87% over the final 4 weeks) in the adult group. Interestingly, significantly more boluses were administered on RT-CGM (with no change in the total insulin dose), along with significantly more instances of insulin suspend and temporary basal use, indicating that RT-CGM prompted more active interventions related to diabetes management.

Real-Time Continuous Glucose Monitoring and Hypoglycemia

Not a single RTC that included a pediatric population reported a significant increase in severe hypoglycemia with the use of RT-CGM. Indeed, RTCs that demonstrated a significant decrease in the HbA_{1c} with the use of RT-CGM also showed no significant difference in the rate of severe hypoglycemia [10–18]. The trial comparing RT-CGM-CSII versus CSII alone in a crossover design demonstrated less time spent with a sensor glucose level <3.9 mmol/l during the RT-CGM-on period compared with the RT-CGM-off period (19 vs. 31 min/day, $p < 0.009$) [22]. Similarly, the trial with the primary outcome of time spent <3.5 mmol/l demonstrated significantly shorter duration with RT-CGM as compared to standard management (0.48 ± 0.57 vs. 0.97 ± 1.55 h/day, respectively; ratio of means 0.49, 95% CI: 0.26–0.76; $p = 0.03$). In 53 children and adolescent participants (10–17 years of age) the primary outcome was reduced by 48% with RT-CGM (0.34 vs. 0.65 h/day in control) [16]. When only 44 of 53 pediatric and 53 of 63 adult participants who used RT-CGM for >20 days were analyzed in the post hoc per protocol analysis, the primary outcome of time spent <3.5 mmol/l was reduced by 64% ($p < 0.001$) in pediatric and 50% ($p = 0.02$) in adult participants. This data suggest that RT-CGM may help in reducing exposure to hypoglycemia in all age groups.

Real-Time Continuous Glucose Monitoring with Low-Glucose Threshold Insulin Suspend

RT-CGM may be used as an integrated part of an insulin pump with an option of glucose threshold-triggered temporary insulin suspend. Two recent RCTs investigating the impact of this automatic temporary insulin suspend included pediatric patients. One included participants 16–70 years of age if they had not had more than 1 episode of severe hypoglycemia (resulting in coma or seizures or requiring medical assistance) in the previous 6 months. Participants were required to wear sensors for at least 80% of the time and to have had at least 2 nocturnal hypoglycemic incidents during the 2-week run-in phase to be eligible for randomization to either sensor-augmented CSII with the glucose threshold insulin suspend (threshold-suspend group) or standard sensor-augmented CSII (control group) for 3 months. The low-glucose threshold insulin suspend was initially set to suspend insulin delivery at a sensor glucose value of 70 mg/dl (3.9 mmol/l), and later the setting could range from 70 to 90 mg/dl (5.0 mmol/l). The primary efficacy endpoint was the area under the curve (AUC) for nocturnal hypoglycemia [events of sensor glucose <65 mg/dl (3.6 mmol/l) for consecutive 20 min between 10 p.m. and 8 a.m.]. In 247 randomized patients, the mean (±SD) AUC for nocturnal hypoglycemia was 37.5% less in the threshold-suspend group than in the control group [980 ± 1,200 mg/dl (54.4 ± 66.6 mmol/l) × min vs. 1,568 ± 1,995 mg/dl (87.0 ± 110.7 mmol/l) × min, $p < 0.001$]. There was no change in HbA_{1c} in either group. In the separately analyzed age group of 16–24 years (12 in the threshold-suspend and 14 in the control group), the mean AUC was 1,439 ± 1,711 mg/dl × min versus 1,921 ± 2,625 mg/dl × min for threshold-suspend versus the control group. Interestingly, the rate of nighttime hypoglycemic events was reduced by 31.8% (1.5 ± 1.0 vs. 2.2 ± 1.3 per patient-week, $p < 0.001$), as was the rate of hypoglycemic events during the entire day ($p < 0.001$) [23].

The other RCT included a predominantly pediatric population, with 4 participants in the preschool group (4 to <7 years), 27 in the prepubertal group (7 to <12 years), 34 in the pubertal group (12 to <18 years), and 30 in the adult group (18–50 years), all with a hypoglycemia unawareness score of at least 4 as determined with the modified Clarke questionnaire, randomized to either regular insulin pump therapy or a sensor-augmented insulin pump with low-glucose threshold insulin suspend (set at 60 mg/dl or 3.3 mmol/l) [24]. Prospective data on severe (seizures or coma) and moderate (help from another person with description of symptoms) hypoglycemia were collected 6 months prior to randomization and throughout the 6-month intervention period. Time spent in hypoglycemia was assessed with a 6-day blinded continuous glucose monitor at screening and at 3 and 6 months.

The primary outcome was the combined incidence of severe and moderate hypoglycemia. Out of 100 screened, 49 were assigned to continuation with pump-only therapy and 46 to a sensor-augmented pump with low-glucose insulin suspend function. The baseline rate of severe and moderate hypoglycemia was significantly lower for patients in the pump-only group with an incidence rate per 100 patient-months of 20.7 (95% CI: 13.8–30) as compared with 129.6 (95% CI: 111.1–150.3) in the low-glucose threshold insulin suspend group. After 6 months of intervention, the number of severe and moderate hypoglycemic events decreased from 28 to 16 in the pump-only group and from 175 to 35 in the low-glucose threshold insulin suspend group. The adjusted incidence rate per 100 patient-months was 34.2 (95% CI: 22.0–53.3) for the pump-only group and 9.5 (95% CI: 5.2–17.4) for the low-glucose suspend group, fitted using the 0-inflated Poisson model. The incidence rate ratio was 3.6 (95% CI: 1.7–7.5, $p < 0.001$) in favor of the low-glucose insulin suspend group.

A sensitivity analysis performed in the same way for patients younger than 12 years (15 participants per group) demonstrated an adjusted incidence rate ratio of 5.5 (95% CI: 2.0–15.7, $p < 0.001$), also in favor of the low-glucose insulin suspend group, but the significance was lost when 2 outliers were excluded from the analysis. The time spent in hypoglycemia <70 mg/dl (3.9 mmol/l) and <60 mg/dl (3.3 mmol/l) was significantly shorter in the low-glucose insulin suspend group during the day and at night. HbA_{1c} did not change from baseline in either group: 7.4% (95% CI: 7.2–7.7) in the pump-only ($p = 0.46$) versus 7.5% (95% CI: 7.3–7.7) in the low-glucose insulin suspend group ($p = 0.10$). This study demonstrates that the use of the low-glucose insulin suspend feature on a sensor-augmented insulin pump over 6 months can significantly decrease the incidence of severe and moderate hypoglycemia in a pediatric population with demonstrated hypoglycemia unawareness and therefore at highest risk.

Practical Considerations

Despite the solid scientific evidence for the use of RT-CGM in the pediatric population with type 1 diabetes (table 1), the routine use of sensors remains below 10% even in the most dedicated tertiary institutions. Several factors currently preclude more widespread routine use: insufficient reimbursement in most countries in the European Union (EU) and elsewhere [25], the lack of expertise on the side of diabetes teams, the lack of proper patient-oriented organization of diabetes care, and likely also exaggerated expectations of RT-CGM on the side of patients and their families. With the existing scientific and clinical evidence, the reimbursement in public healthcare systems (such as in the EU countries) should increase in the foreseeable future. Continuous effort from professional associations like ISPAD and others should focus on state-of-the-art education for diabetes healthcare professionals, particularly in the field of diabetes-related technology including RT-CGM. Initiatives like the EU-funded SWEET project [26] will increase the quality of pediatric diabetes centers through unified data collection and benchmarking, thus improving pediatric diabetes care. Finally, dedicated pediatric diabetes teams will have to empower not only young patients and their families, but also caregivers in kindergartens and teachers in schools where these young patients spend a considerable amount of their time [27]. The use of RT-CGM still re-

Table 1. Overview of RCTs on the use of RT-CGM that included a pediatric patient population

Study	Pediatric patients, n	Mean pediatric age, years	Study duration, months	Baseline HbA_{1c}, %	Intervention	Pediatric HbA_{1c} outcome: intervention vs. control, %
Deiss [10], 2006	81 (156)	14.4 (26.8)	3	9.56	RT-CGM vs. SMBG	–0.67, adjusted p = 0.0447 (–0.6, p = 0.003)
O'Connell [12], 2009	55 (32)	16.2 (23.2)	3	7.40	RT-CGM vs. SMBG	–0.6, p = 0.025 (–0.43, p = 0.009)
JDRF [13], 2008	224 under 25 years (317)	14.9 (23.5)	6	7.84	RT-CGM vs. SMBG	NS (–0.53, p < 0.001)
Raccah [15], 2009	51 (115)	NPD (28.5)	6	9.20	RT-CGM vs. SMBG	NPD (–0.41, p < 0.004)
Battelino [16], 2011	53 (120)	NPD (25.8)	6	6.9	RT-CGM vs. SMBG	–0.2% (–0.27, p = 0.008)
Bergenstal [17], 2010	156 (485)	12.2 (32.2)	12	8.3	RT-CGM vs. MDI-SMBG	–0.5, p < 0.001 (–0.6, p < 0.001)
Riveline [18], 2012	24 (178)	NPD (36.4)	12	9.0	RT-CGM vs. SMBG	NPD (–0.50, p < 0.001)
Kordonouri et al. [19], 2010	154 (154)	8.8 (8.8)	12	11.3	RT-CGM vs. SMBG	NS
Mauras [20], 2012	146 (146)	7.5 (7.5)	6	7.9	RT-CGM vs. SMBG	NS
Tsalikian [21], 2012	20 (20)	3.0 (3.0)	6	7.9	RT-CGM vs. SMBG	NS
Battelino [22], 2012	72 (153)	12.0 (28)	6	8.5	RT-CGM vs. SMBG	–0.46, p < 0.001 (–0.43, p < 0.001)
						Pediatric (overall) hypoglycemia outcome: intervention vs. control
Battelino [16], 2011	53 (120)	NPD (25.8)		6.9	RT-CGM vs. SMBG	time in hypoglycemia: 0.48 vs. 0.97 h/day, p = 0.03
Bergenstal [23], 2013	– (247)	NPD (43.2)	3	7.2	threshold RT-CGM vs. no-threshold RT-CGM	NPD (AUC nocturnal hypoglycemic events: –37.5%, p < 0.001)
Ly et al. [24], 2013	65 (95)	18.6 (18.6)	6	7.5	threshold RT-CGM vs. no-threshold RT-CGM	the incidence rate ratio (sum of severe and moderate hypoglycemia): 3.6, p < 0.001

The values in parentheses represent the total study population. NPD = No pediatric data; threshold RT-CGM = sensor-augmented insulin pump with automated low-glucose threshold insulin suspend. NS = Non significant.

quires full compliance from the patient and her/his close environment, and should therefore not be misinterpreted as a form of 'automated' or 'care-free' diabetes care. Age-specific expertise focused on individualized treatment solutions may provide the best outcomes (fig. 1). Continuous technical improvements of subcutaneous sensors and related technologies will also contribute to a higher quality of care.

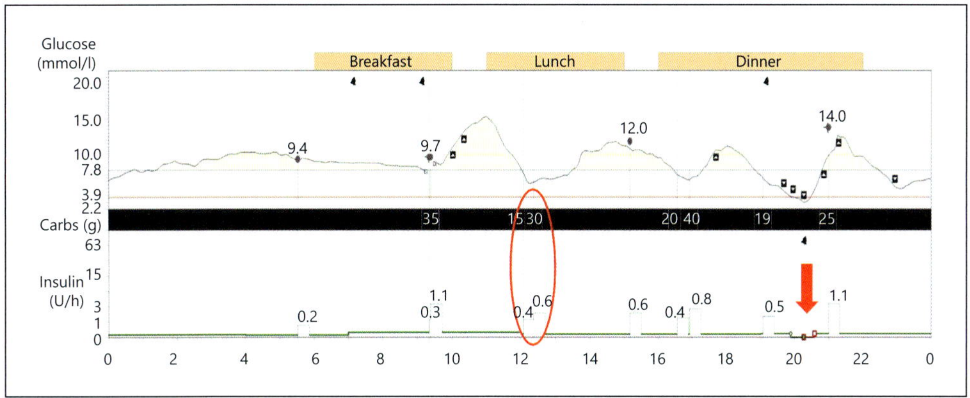

Fig. 1. A part of the daily RT-CGM and CSII download from a 5-year-old girl with type 1 diabetes since the age of 2 years. Her HbA_{1c} at the time of the download was 7.3%. The upper line represents glucose levels from RT-CGM with fingerstick blood glucose measurements indicated with dots close to this line. The wide black strip in the middle contains the number of ingested carbohydrate grams. The lower line represents insulin basal rate infusion with several boluses. Note several composite or 'split' boluses, the one for lunch is encircled. Automated low-glucose threshold insulin suspend occurred just before dinner and is marked with an arrow.

Conclusion

Notwithstanding the data presented in this review, a Cochrane meta-analysis demonstrated limited evidence for the effectiveness of RT-CGM use in children, adults, and patients with poorly controlled diabetes [28]. There are indications that higher compliance with wearing the RT-CGM device improves HbA_{1c} to a larger extent. In selected populations, like the pediatric population, any meta-analysis may introduce several important biases and may not be the best scientific way to judge a particular treatment modality [29]. Careful individual consideration of high-standard RTCs may be needed for a thorough evaluation of RT-CGM in the pediatric population along with designing new additional RTCs focused on this important and highly vulnerable patient group. Furthermore, with wider routine use, sufficient practical experience will eventually accumulate to properly position RT-CGM as a treatment modality. Finally, continuous new development will incorporate RT-CGM into closed-loop insulin delivery systems used at patients' homes [30].

Acknowledgements

The authors were supported in part by the Slovene National Research Agency grants P3-0343 and J3-4116.

References

1 Beck RW, Tamborlane WV, Bergenstal RM, Miller KM, DuBose SN, Hall CA; T1D Exchange Clinic Network: The T1D Exchange Clinic Registry. J Clin Endocrinol Metab 2012;97:4383–4389.

2 American Diabetes Association: Standards of medical care in diabetes – 2013. Diabetes Care 2013; 36(Suppl 1):S11–S66.

3 Rewers M, Pihoker C, Donaghue K, Hanas R, Swift P, Klingensmith GJ: Assessment of glycemic control and adolescents with diabetes. Pediatr Diabetes 2009;10(Suppl 12):71–81.

4 Eeg-Olofsson K, Cederholm J, Nilsson PM, Gudbjornsdottir S, Eliasson B; Steering Committee of the Swedish National Diabetes Register: Glycemic and risk factor control in type 1 diabetes: results from 13,612 patients in a national diabetes register. Diabetes Care 2007;30:496–502.

5 Rosenbauer J, Dost A, Karges B, Hungele A, Stahl A, Bachle C, Gerstl EM, Kastendieck C, Hofer SE, Holl RW; DPV Initiative and the German BMBF Competence Network Diabetes Mellitus: Improved metabolic control in children and adolescents with type 1 diabetes: a trend analysis using prospective multicenter data from Germany and Austria. Diabetes Care 2012;35:80–86.

6 de Beaufort CE, Swift PG, Skinner CT, Aanstoot HJ, Aman J, Cameron F, Martul P, Chiarelli F, Daneman D, Danne T, Dorchy H, Hoey H, Kaprio EA, Kaufman F, Kocova M, Mortensen HB, Njølstad PR, Phillip M, Robertson KJ, Schoenle EJ, Urakami T, Vanelli M; Hvidoere Study Group on Childhood Diabetes 2005: Continuing stability of center differences in pediatric diabetes care: do advances in diabetes treatment improve outcome? The Hvidøre Study Group on Childhood Diabetes. Diabetes Care 2007; 30:2245–2250.

7 Pickup JC: Insulin-pump therapy for type 1 diabetes mellitus. N Engl J Med 2012;366:1616–1624.

8 Dovč K, Telic SS, Lusa L, Bratanic N, Zerjav-Tansek M, Kotnik P, Stefanija MA, Battelino T, Bratina N: Improved metabolic control in pediatric patients with type 1 diabetes: a nationwide prospective 12-year time trends analysis. Diabetes Technol Ther 2014;16:33–40.

9 Ludwig-Seibold CU, Holder M, Rami B, Raile K, Heidtmann B, Holl RW; DPV Science Initiative; German Working Group for Insulin Pump Treatment in Pediatric Patients; German BMBF Competence Network Diabetes: Continuous glucose monitoring in children, adolescents, and adults with type 1 diabetes mellitus: analysis from the prospective DPV diabetes documentation and quality management system from Germany and Austria. Pediatr Diabetes 2012;13:12–14.

10 Deiss D, Bolinder J, Riveline JP, et al: Improved glycemic control in poorly controlled patients with type 1 diabetes using real-time continuous glucose monitoring. Diabetes Care 2006;29:2730–2732.

11 Phillip M, Danne T, Shalitin S, Buckingham B, Laffel L, Tamborlane W, Battelino T; Consensus Forum Participants: Use of continuous glucose monitoring in children and adolescents. Pediatr Diabetes 2012; 13:215–228.

12 O'Connell MA, Donath S, O'Neal DN, Colman PG, Ambler GR, Jones TW, Davis EA, Cameron FJ: Glycaemic impact of patient-led use of sensor-guided pump therapy in type 1 diabetes: a randomised controlled trial. Diabetologia 2009;52: 1250–1257.

13 Juvenile Diabetes Research Foundation Continuous Glucose Monitoring Study Group, Tamborlane WV, Beck RW, Bode BW, Buckingham B, Chase HP, Clemons R, Fiallo-Scharer R, Fox LA, Gilliam LK, Hirsch IB, Huang ES, Kollman C, Kowalski AJ, Laffel L, Lawrence JM, Lee J, Mauras N, O'Grady M, Ruedy KJ, Tansey M, Tsalikian E, Weinzimer S, Wilson DM, Wolpert H, Wysocki T, Xing D: Continuous glucose monitoring and intensive treatment of type 1 diabetes. N Engl J Med 2008;359:1464–1476.

14 Juvenile Diabetes Research Foundation Continuous Glucose Monitoring Study Group, Beck RW, Buckingham B, Miller K, Wolpert H, Xing D, Block JM, Chase HP, Hirsch I, Kollman C, Laffel L, Lawrence JM, Milaszewski K, Ruedy KJ, Tamborlane WV: Factors predictive of use and of benefit from continuous glucose monitoring in type 1 diabetes. Diabetes Care 2009;32:1947–1953.

15 Raccah D, Sulmont V, Reznik Y, Guerci B, Renard E, Hanaire H, Jeandidier N, Nicolino M: Incremental value of continuous glucose monitoring when starting pump therapy in patients with poorly controlled type 1 diabetes: the RealTrend study. Diabetes Care 2009;32:2245–2250.

16 Battelino T, Phillip M, Bratina N, Nimri R, Oskarsson P, Bolinder J: Effect of continuous glucose monitoring on hypoglycemia in type 1 diabetes. Diabetes Care 2011;34:1–6.

17 Bergenstal RM, Tamborlane WV, Ahmann A, Buse JB, Dailey G, Davis SN, Joyce C, Peoples T, Perkins BA, Welsh JB, Willi SM, Wood MA; STAR 3 Study Group: Effectiveness of sensor-augmented insulin pump therapy in type 1 diabetes. N Engl J Med 2010; 363:311–320.

18 Riveline JP, Schaepelynck P, Chaillous L, Renard E, Sola-Gazagnes A, Penfornis A, Tubiana-Rufi N, Sulmont V, Catargi B, Lukas C, Radermecker RP, Thivolet C, Moreau F, Benhamou PY, Guerci B, Leguerrier AM, Millot L, Sachon C, Charpentier G, Hanaire H; EVADIAC Sensor Study Group: Assessment of patient-led or physician-driven continuous glucose monitoring in patients with poorly controlled type 1 diabetes using basal-bolus insulin regimens: a 1-year multicenter study. Diabetes Care 2012;35:965–971.

19 Kordonouri O, Pankowska E, Rami B, Kapellen T, Coutant R, Hartmann R, Lange K, Knip M, Danne T: Sensor-augmented pump therapy from the diagnosis of childhood type 1 diabetes: results of the Paediatric Onset Study (ONSET) after 12 months of treatment. Diabetologia 2010;53:2487–2495.

20 Mauras N, Beck R, Xing D, Ruedy K, Buckingham B, Tansey M, White NH, Weinzimer SA, Tamborlane W, Kollman C: A randomized clinical trial to assess the efficacy and safety of real-time continuous glucose monitoring in the management of type 1 diabetes in young children aged 4 to <10 years. Diabetes Care 2012;35:204–210.

21 Tsalikian E, Fox L, Weinzimer S, Buckingham B, White NH, Beck R, Kollman C, Xing D, Ruedy K; Diabetes Research in Children Network Study Group: Feasibility of prolonged continuous glucose monitoring in toddlers with type 1 diabetes. Pediatr Diabetes 2012;13:301–307.

22 Battelino T, Conget I, Olsen B, Schütz-Fuhrmann I, Hommel E, Hoogma R, Schierloh U, Sulli N, Bolinder J; SWITCH Study Group: The use and efficacy of continuous glucose monitoring in type 1 diabetes treated with insulin pump therapy: a randomised controlled trial. Diabetologia 2012;55: 3155–3162.

23 Bergenstal RM, Klonoff DC, Garg SK, Bode BW, Meredith M, Slover RH, Ahmann AJ, Welsh JB, Lee SW, Kaufman FR; ASPIRE In-Home Study Group: Threshold-based insulin-pump interruption for reduction of hypoglycemia. N Engl J Med 2013;369: 224–232.

24 Ly TT, Nicholas JA, Retterath A, Lim EM, Davis EA, Jones TW: Effect of sensor-augmented insulin pump therapy and automated insulin suspension vs standard insulin pump therapy on hypoglycemia in patients with type 1 diabetes: a randomized clinical trial. JAMA 2013;310:1240–1247.

25 Heinemann L, Franc S, Phillip M, Battelino T, Ampudia-Blasco FJ, Bolinder J, Diem P, Pickup J, Hans Devries J: Reimbursement for continuous glucose monitoring: a European view. J Diabetes Sci Technol 2012;6:1498–1502.

26 Danne T, Lion S, Madaczy L, Veeze H, Raposo F, Rurik I, Aschemeier B, Kordonouri O; SWEET group: Criteria for Centers of Reference for pediatric diabetes – a European perspective. Pediatr Diabetes 2012;13(Suppl 16):62–75.

27 Bratina N, Battelino T: Insulin pumps and continuous glucose monitoring (CGM) in preschool and school-age children: how schools can integrate technology. Pediatr Endocrinol Rev 2010;7(Suppl 3):417–421.

28 Langendam M, Luijf YM, Hooft L, Devries JH, Mudde AH, Scholten RJ: Continuous glucose monitoring systems for type 1 diabetes mellitus. Cochrane Database Syst Rev 2012;1:CD008101.

29 Pickup JC: The evidence base for diabetes technology: appropriate and inappropriate meta-analysis. J Diabetes Sci Technol 2013;7:1567–1574.

30 Nimri R, Muller I, Atlas E, Miller S, Kordonouri O, Bratina N, Tsioli C, Stefanija MA, Danne T, Battelino T, Phillip M: Night glucose control with MD-Logic artificial pancreas in home setting: a single blind, randomized crossover trial-interim analysis. Pediatr Diabetes 2014;15:91–99.

Dr. Tadej Battelino
University Children's Hospital
Bohoričeva 20
SI–1000 Ljubljana (Slovenia)
E-Mail tadej.battelino@mf.uni-lj.si

Bruttomesso D, Grassi G (eds): Technological Advances in the Treatment of Type 1 Diabetes.
Front Diabetes. Basel, Karger, 2015, vol 24, pp 110–127 (DOI: 10.1159/000363482)

Real-Time Continuous Glucose Monitoring in Adult Outpatients

Matteo Bonomo[a] • Giorgio Grassi[b] • Paolo Di Bartolo[c] • Alberto Maran[d]

[a]Diabetes Unit, Niguarda Ca Granda Hospital, Milano, [b]Division of Endocrinology and Metabolism, Department of Internal Medicine, Città della Salute e della Scienza, Torino, [c]Romagna Local Health Unit, Province of Ravenna Diabetes Clinic, Ravenna, and [d]Division of Metabolic Diseases, Department of Medicine, University Hospital of Padova, Padova, Italy

Abstract

With real-time continuous glucose monitoring (RTCGM), the patient has a continuous picture of glucose concentrations – dynamic information with important predictive value. It is in fact a typical 'patient-oriented' tool that permits a more aggressive therapeutic approach and makes it easier to adapt therapy immediately. Currently approved RTCGM devices consist of three main components: a glucose sensor, a transmitter, and a receiver monitor. The system is defined as minimally invasive because it requires insertion into the subcutaneous cellular tissue of a fine needle to measure the glucose in the interstitial fluid directly or via an external sensor. A correct selection of patients is one of the most important factors in determining a successful application of this innovative technology. For this purpose, there are already consensus statements in a number of countries with regard to the indications of these systems. The criteria for identification of candidates are usually divided into three main categories: pediatric/adolescent, adult patients (both in the general population of type 1 diabetes and in specific settings), and pregnant women or women in the preconception period. RTCGM opens up extremely interesting prospects that are destined to radically change the concept of clinical self-management of diabetes. Considering the technical progress towards overcoming the current limitations (essentially: not optimal accuracy, invasiveness, and costs) which currently prevent its widespread use, we can expect wide diffusion of this form of monitoring in the coming years.

Self-Monitoring of Blood Glucose and Continuous Glucose Monitoring

The search for true metabolic optimization, recognized nowadays as essential in order to avoid the chronic complications of diabetes and its progression, must obviously be based on close blood glucose (BG) monitoring. This is the basis for better adaptation of therapeutic interventions, reconciling the goal of glycemic near-normalization with limiting the risk of the hypoglycemia inevitable with any particularly aggressive therapy.

Great progress has been made in recent years with self-monitoring of BG (SMBG), with more sophisticated, accurate, and easy-to-handle tools, and intensified schemes involving frequent measurements before and after meals, at bedtime, and during the night [1]. These strategies, however, all suffer from the limitation of giving 'spot' data. However frequent they may be, these isolated measurements still leave long intervals 'uncovered' during the day – especially at inconvenient times like at work – and even more so at night. They also cannot give a picture of the complex dynamics of the BG profile.

From these considerations it is clear that the possibility of continuous glucose monitoring (CGM) [2] opens up extremely interesting, fresh prospects. CGM has now been introduced in clinical practice, with systems mostly using a subcutaneous needle sensor to measure glucose in the interstitial fluid [3, 4]. Compared to SMBG, CGM (described late on) is a minimally invasive method that provides a large number of measurements: interstitial glucose concentrations are calculated at 5-min intervals (or even more frequently depending on the model used). The information is therefore more complete and, above all, indicates any 'trend' as it arises and the possible relations between phenomena or events that are otherwise hard to interpret. An example is rebound hyperglycemia that may follow asymptomatic hypoglycemic episodes.

If one wants to compare SMBG and CGM, a handy example is the difference between a normal camera and a video camera [3]. The still camera gives a few isolated, but detailed, precise images and needs a person to operate it, while the video camera may give less detail, of inferior quality, but has the advantage of automatically recording, continuously. For the early sensors, this comparison was certainly true, and they had problems of measuring in different environments, i.e. in blood or interstitial fluid [5]. Progress in recent years, however, may soon make this 'alternative' obsolete. Today's video cameras achieve very high definition, and glucose monitoring systems that combine the advantages of dynamic recording with high overall data quality are already on the horizon. Once these are available, CGM will become a fundamental tool for managing patients with complicated diabetes.

'Professional' and 'Real-Time' Continuous Glucose Monitoring

On the topic of CGM, one must make a clear distinction between the retrospective systems: sometimes referred to as 'glycemic Holter monitors' or, more often, as 'professional' (PGM), and real-time glucose monitoring systems (RTCGM). PGM, the first strategy to enter clinical use, has the drawback of not giving an immediate reading; values are recorded and downloaded to the computer later [6]. Interpretation is therefore retrospective and the job of a qualified healthcare provider, the specialist, or another member of the patient's care team. These systems are intended for investigations and back-checks, and are usually not used continuously; the information they provide is extremely useful for 'calibrating' treatment on the basis of recurrent patterns that would be hard to detect with conventional 'one point at a time' monitoring systems.

In other words, PGM provides a series of qualitative and quantitative data such as glucose exposure and variability – often supplied automatically by the software, or calculable if necessary [7, 8] – to add to those already in use for years in the clinical management of the diabetic patient. Besides potential research applications [9], this information can be used in clinical practice to 'reset' the therapeutic regimen periodically by the physician, or in some cases by the patients if they are trained to do so. It also serves to assess the course of glycemic balance, integrating other indicators of medium-term glycemic control, like glycated hemoglobin (HbA_{1c}). In some cases it plays a direct diagnostic role; it can help detect diabetic gastroparesis [10], 'hypoglycemia unawareness' [11, 12], or nondiabetic BG changes, such as the hypoglycemic syndrome [13, 14], glycogenesis [15], or cystic fibrosis [16]. Important information can be obtained for assessing β-cell function after pancreas transplantation (whole organ or islet cells) [17]. It is also a potential tool for education [18]: visual presentation of the effects of different types of food, exercise, therapeutic regimens, or insulin types as graphs certainly helps one understand the variables affecting glycemic balance and, consequently, the possible ways of optimizing behaviors and therapeutic interventions.

Continuous monitoring systems that give the results in real time – RTCGM – have a different role, though with some limits, and only to a certain extent can they help with the issues described for PGM. With these systems, the patient has a continuous picture of the BG and not only the situation at a given moment. The progression can be displayed as little graphs showing recent patterns, with arrows indicating the direction of changes, and their speed. This dynamic information has important predictive value, and a series of alarms – sound or vibration – help the patient take measures to correct excessive swings toward hypo- or hyperglycemia. As we have noted, the information can be interpreted retrospectively in the same way as the 'Holter'-type professional systems, but RTCGM's main advantage is that it enables patients to manage themselves. In fact, it is considered a typical 'patient-oriented' tool. On the one hand, the alarms permit more aggressive therapeutic responses, helping overcome the resistance often shown by patients, as well as by diabetologists, based on their fear of hypoglycemia. The alarms also make it easier to adapt therapy immediately, e.g. by taking extra insulin or (as necessary) more carbohydrates.

Patients have to be properly trained to make full use of these systems for self-management, and the training has to be repeated and periodically updated. If this is overlooked, the risks may be greater than the potential advantages. The patient must have a clear picture of pre- and postprandial glycemic targets and must become familiar with concepts such as correction factors (which may vary at different times of the day), 'residual' insulin, possible differences between the sensor readings and capillary BG resulting from the differences in the glucose concentrations in interstitial tissue and in blood, and the 'lead lag', which may be broad when BG concentrations are changing rapidly. For everyday management it may be useful to give the patient written algorithms. These must be clearly explained and the patient must agree to use them; the clinician should check regularly at outpatient visits that they are being used properly.

Besides these points, we must remember that the sensors still suffer some limits in accuracy. With this in mind, capillary blood tests are therefore mandatory before taking any decisions on therapy based on the monitoring results. However, RTCGM today is an extraordinarily useful tool, especially in situations where particularly tight glycemic control is needed. Constant technological progress in this field will certainly lead to gradual improvement in the performance of these systems, making them increasingly reliable. It will then be possible to extend their indications for even wider use.

Continuous Glucose Monitoring Systems: Technical Aspects

CGM devices that measure interstitial fluid glucose values continuously were first introduced approximately 10 years ago. Early 'professional' CGM systems only provided data for brief periods for retrospective analysis and were quickly followed by RTCGM devices for personal daily use by patients at home.

Currently approved CGM devices consist of three main components: a glucose sensor, a transmitter and a receiver monitor. The glucose sensor is inserted subcutaneously by means of a dedicated device. It detects and measures glucose by means of an enzyme called 'glucose oxidase', which oxidizes the glucose in the interstitial fluid. The hydrogen peroxide produced is separated under the effect of an electric current which generates an electrical signal proportional to the concentration of interstitial glucose. The data is filtered and then a glucose value is provided every 1–5 min on the receiver screen, allowing the user to see current glucose levels and trends [19, 20].

The system is defined as minimally invasive because it requires the inserting a fine needle into the subcutaneous cellular tissue, generally in the abdomen, to measure the glucose in the interstitial fluid directly or via an external sensor.

In 1999, MiniMedM (currently Medtronic) produced the first device to be approved by the FDA – a Holter-style monitor for professional use only that performs measurements every 5 min over a maximum time of 72 h [2]. The sensor is connected via a cable to an external monitor which records the signals from the sensor every 15 min. The results are not visualized in real time, but can be downloaded to a computer for subsequent analysis. The device needs to be calibrated a minimum of 4 times a day using measurements of capillary glycemia. Since 2008, an improved version called 'IProa' has been available that extends the clinical observation up to 6 days [21].

In 2004, the FDA approved the Guardian® monitor, a version of an improved sensor that included a system of alarms not only for hyperglycemia but also for hypoglycemia. One year later, Guardian Real-Time® was available, and it enabled the measurement of glucose to be read in real time, and every 5 min, following a latency period of 2 h. The Paradigm Real-Time® was approved in 2006 as CGMS combined with a continuous subcutaneous insulin infusion device [22]. The MiniMed Paradigm® Veo System includes a continuous subcutaneous insulin infusion with an improved sensor (Enlite®) and is equipped with a low glucose suspend mechanism, which stops insulin delivery automatically whenever glucose levels are too low. All of these systems require a minimum of 2 calibrations a day [23].

The Dexcom SevenD system, approved by the FDA in 2007, enables real-time reading of the measurements of glucose performed every 5 min following a latency period of 2 h over a maximum period of 7 days [24]. The system includes alarms that can be programmed not only for hyperglycemia, but also for hypoglycemia, and needs to be calibrated with values derived from capillary glycemia measurements every 12 h. The new system called the Seven Plus System® has been improved in precision and functions [25].

The Abbott FreeStyle Navigator system was approved by the FDA in 2008. The system is based on Wired Enzyme® technology which uses measurements not dependent on oxygen in place of the peroxide of hydrogen used in the majority of the other devices [26]. It allows real-time reading of glucose determinations after 1 h and up to 5 days. The concentration of glucose is updated every minute and stored for retrospective analyses every 10 min. It requires calibration with at least 4–5 capillary glucose measurements from the start of the monitoring period with the previous version and once daily with the new version. A series of alarms are available for altered levels of glucose, and information is provided on the trends in levels [25].

The GlucoDayS® system (A. Menarini Diagnostics) has been on the market since 2002. Its method of function is based on the technique of microdialysis applied to the interstitial fluid which enables the measurement of the glucose concentration in the subcutaneous tissue [27]. A buffer solution circulates in the subcutaneous interstitial fluid by means of an implanted microfiber which recovers the glucose by dialysis. The glucose is then measured by an enzyme in an extracorporeal device. The level of glucose in the dialyzed liquid is determined each second and a mean value is stored every 3 min. The result is a total of 480 measurements per day. The maximum interval of continuous measurement is 48 h. The data collected by the sensor can be visualized in real time [28].

Calibration

Calibration of the signal with the simultaneous BG level is necessary for the device to estimate the corresponding BG level [29]. This is required to convert the electrical signal registered by the CGM system into a glucose value by using a BG concentration value determined enzymatically. The glucose measured by the CGM in the interstitial tissue must therefore be calibrated by the result of a measurement from a capillary blood sample with a glucose meter. However, if we consider that accuracy of a glucose meter used by a patient in a daily setting can produce deviations up to 20% [30], calibration of the CGM systems could represent a very significant source of error. Depending on the device, this calibration is required 1–3 times per day following the manufacturer's instructions.

Due to the differences caused by dynamic changes in glucose concentration in blood versus interstitial fluid, calibration should be performed ideally during 'steady state' conditions when there are no rapid changes in glycemia. In fact, during rapid variations of glucose values, e.g. after a meal or during physical activity, differences between both compartments occur and this may result in an inaccurate calibration procedure [31, 32].

One limitation of using interstitial fluid glucose is the lag time between serum glucose levels to interstitial glucose levels. While the physiologic lag from serum glucose to interstitial fluid is estimated to be about 5 min [33, 34], the value displayed on the CGM receiver typically lags behind capillary BG by an average of 15 min [35] due to the transit time of interstitial glucose through the sensor membrane (1–2 min) and filtering of the signal by the CGM device (3–12 min) [36]. The lag time is especially relevant during rapid glucose changes (>2 mg/dl/min) and may be different during a rise versus fall in BG [37]. Another component contributing to the lag time is the filter imposed by the sensor software because of 'noisy' sensors. Improving the stability and accuracy of the glucose sensor will reduce filtering and thus lag time [38].

Accuracy

The accuracy of current CGM systems is commonly reported as the mean average relative difference (MARD) relative to a reference glucose measurement (i.e. Yellow Springs Glucose Analyzer), among several other factors [39]. The accepted average for regulatory approval is about <20% over all biologically relevant glucose ranges. A second parameter to evaluate sensor accuracy is the percentage of values according to International Organization for Standardization (ISO) criteria for measuring accuracy: proportion of CGM values within the tolerance of ±15 mg/dl for reference glucose values ≤75 mg/day, and percentage of CGM values within the tolerance of ±20% for reference glucose values ≥75 mg/dl [40].

A correlation analysis, the Clarke error grid analysis (EGA) is another parameter reported in most studies [41]. The chart is divided into therapeutically relevant zones [42]. Points in zones A and B are considered therapeutically acceptable, zone C could lead to unnecessary treatment, and zones D and E could lead to potentially dangerous therapeutic decisions. Because CGM reports continuous BG rather than discreet point values fixed in time, the continuous glucose-EGA, which adds rate EGA, was developed. The rate EGA includes therapeutic error indications for rate and direction of change information that is unique to CGM data [42].

Current sensors are generally less accurate in the first 24 h after insertion, probably due to local tissue changes following tissue trauma at the time of insertion and are generally most accurate during the second to sixth day of wear. The initial sensor instability may be due to the insertion wound causing inflammatory changes with neutrophils and eosinophils consuming oxygen and glucose and generating hydrogen peroxide [43, 44].

The first generation of the Medtronic and Dexcom FDA-approved systems reported an average MARD of 19.7 and 26%, respectively, over the full range, whereas Abbott's first-generation device reported an average MARD of about 12.8% [45]. Since then, significant improvement has been made in sensor accuracy by the companies. Second- and third-generation sensors have shown a similar MARD of 16.2% for Dexcom and 15.9% for the FreeStyle Navigator [46].

Damiano et al. [47] recently reported an average MARD of 11.8 ± 3.8% for the Navigator, and 20.2 ± 6.8 and 16.5 ± 6.7% for the Medtronic Guardian and the Dexcom Seven Plus, respectively.

The Medtronic Enlite and Dexcom G4 have demonstrated significant improvement over the versions reported in the study by Damiano et al. [47] study. Clinical studies with the Enlite sensor by using the Paradigm Veo calibration routine reported an average MARD (over the entire range) of 13.86% [48]. The Dexcom G4 Platinum sensor has been shown to improve accuracy, showing an average MARD of 13.2% as compared to previous versions [49].

The G4 Platinum sensor has been integrated into artificial pancreas systems in different research centers. An advanced CGM called 'G4AP' has been recently developed by Dexcom and the University of Padova to specifically address the heightened performance requirements for future artificial pancreas studies by means of updated denoising and calibration algorithms for improved accuracy and reliability [50].

The results show that the MARD compared with venous plasma glucose was improved from 13.2% with G4 Platinum to 11.7% with G4AP. Accuracy improvements were seen over all days of sensor wear and across the plasma glucose range (40–400 mg/dl). The greatest improvements occurred in the low glucose range (40–80 mg/dl), in euglycemia (80–120 mg/dl), and on the first day of sensor use.

Clinical Use of Continuous Glucose Monitoring: What Evidence?

Real-Time Continuous Glucose Monitoring in the General Type 1 Diabetes Mellitus Population

The impact of RTCGM on metabolic control, measured in terms of improvement in HbA_{1c}, is amply documented in adults with type 1 diabetes [51–53]. In recent years, several reports have been published on the validity of real-time systems to be used directly by the patient. The first randomized controlled trial by Deiss et al. [51] was published in 2006; at the end of a 3-month observation period in a mixed population of adults and children with type 1 diabetes, not well controlled (HbA_{1c} >9%); HbA_{1c} decreased significantly more in the CGM group than in the patients using conventional SMBG. In a third group where the monitor was employed intermittently for 3 days every 2 weeks, the results were midway between the other two.

Two further randomized controlled trials, of particular interest on account of the sample size and the trial duration, were sponsored by the Juvenile Diabetes Research

Foundation (JDRF). In the first, published in the *New England Journal of Medicine* in 2008 [52], a mixed population of adults, adolescents, and children with different initial levels of metabolic compensation were managed for 26 weeks with either CGM or conventional SMBG. Patients in the control group measured their BG more than 6 times a day. Changes in the main endpoint, HbA_{1c}, differed widely with age: among adults there was a significant difference in favor of the CGM group (>25 years), but not in younger patients. Metabolic control in adolescents in particular was almost the same with both strategies, and in children the situation fell midway between these two groups, though with no significant differences. The secondary endpoints were the percentage of patients with HbA_{1c} <7% and the number of episodes of major hypoglycemia among these cases. The difference was significant not only in adults but also in children, whose parents were responsible for managing the information. The authors suggested the differences in the three age groups were related to compliance with the treatment; the sensors were used at least 6 days a week by 80% of the adults and 50% of the children, but this rate was only 30% for the adolescents.

The second JDRF trial [53] also enrolled a mixed population of adults and children, but at the beginning of the trial they all had good metabolic control (HbA_{1c} <7.0%). This time the primary endpoints were not only HbA_{1c}, but also the time spent with BG ≤70 mg/dl and the frequency of major hypoglycemic episodes. The results with CGM were significantly better for HbA_{1c} and for a combined outcome of HbA_{1c} changes and hypoglycemia measurements. In these patients, who were already well managed, there is evidence that CGM can give additional benefit.

There is some experimental evidence that, with time, RTCGM can help type 1 diabetes patients reach and maintain optimal levels of HbA_{1c} more effectively and safely than with traditional BG management. Any assessment of the 'efficacy' of RTCGM in terms of glycemic control, hypoglycemia, and quality of life must, however, be based on careful analysis in systematic reviews and/or meta-analysis which take into consideration all available evidence as a whole. 'Official' reviews like those published by Cochrane [54] and the Agency for Healthcare Quality Research (AHQR) [55] have special weight, especially for 'payers'. In the AHQR systematic review, analysis of the studies showed a drop in HbA_{1c} from baseline to the end of the trial of 0.26% in favor of RTCGM compared to SMBG in the whole population. In adult patients the drop was bigger with 0.38%, while in children it was only 0.13%. Here again, the improvement in glycemic control was more marked in patients who complied best with the use of the continuous BG sensor; 60% compliance was considered adequate in adults and children, giving a difference between HbA_{1c} RTCGM and SMBG of –0.36% [55].

The success of this strategy is thus clearly related to certain factors, such as how well the patient's glycemia is controlled, with more marked improvement in patients with higher baseline HbA_{1c} [6]; the other factor is constant use of the device [54, 56]. It is therefore essential to identify the features that can predict a patient's ability to comply with treatment.

Some of the studies mentioned documented a significant direct relation between the patient's pretrial home BG testing rates and compliance with RTCGM [57, 58]. Patients who are already used to checking their BG at least 4 times a day seem significantly more likely to use RTCGM as instructed. It has been reported, however, that patients who do not normally check their BG properly themselves are more likely to drop out of the studies [57].

Another important point is that in the trials mentioned, patients were invited to wear the device for a week before enrolment. This 'test period' is extremely useful to exclude patients who are unlikely to succeed, i.e. those who feel the device is too intrusive in their daily life and cannot appreciate the benefits of having continuous information on BG oscillations [58].

Real-Time Continuous Glucose Monitoring in Specific Settings

RTCGM in Pregnancy

The great potential of CGM systems in pregnant women with diabetes mellitus was evident from the moment they started to be used in clinical practice, at the beginning of the last decade, in view of the importance of tight glycometabolic control throughout pregnancy in order to minimize the risks of maternal and fetal complications [59]. Most studies and reports, however, refer to the use of these systems in a 'retrospective' approach to gain further knowledge of the physiology of glycemic homeostasis in pregnancy, i.e. normal values at different times of day, timing of postprandial peaks [60, 61], and their changes in diabetic women [62], with their patterns during pregnancy [63].

Isolated reports have suggested that CGM could help predict fetal malformations [64] or macrosomia at birth [65]. CGM findings are also useful as a basis for therapeutic decisions. An Australian study in 2007 [66], for instance, in a series of women with gestational and pregestational type 1 and 2 diabetes, found that treatment changes were much more frequent when the physicians based their decisions on CGM rather than SMBG. Kestila et al. [67] recorded more aggressive therapy, with more use of insulin, in gestational diabetes mellitus checked periodically by continuous monitoring. Pilot studies on small series [68] have also indicated better maternal metabolic control and better pregnancy outcomes in women who used 'professional-type' intermittent monitoring systems.

There is only one report of a randomized controlled trial, by Murphy et al. [69] in Cambridge, in which retrospective CGM was used as an educational tool for women with types 1 and 2 pregestational diabetes mellitus. The system was used at intervals of 4–6 weeks, and the data served as a basis for discussing the therapeutic approach with the women; in comparison with a group managed using a standard approach, metabolic control, birth weight, and macrosomia were all better.

So far we have only referred to 'professional' use of CGM in pregnancy for documentation and to gain knowledge to inform the medical team and guide therapeutic decisions. However, like in other fields, real-time use – i.e. patient-oriented – seems to offer the most interesting prospects. As these systems offer several extremely useful features, i.e. they show the patterns and dynamics of BG levels and action can be taken to forecast and correct abnormal excursions at an early stage, they also have alarms to signal risky BG levels in both absolute terms and as short-term tendencies. This information can enable a physician to take whatever aggressive action is needed to achieve optimal metabolic control within the narrow limits desirable in pregnancy; with conventional therapies – even intensified – this can be problematic because of the fear of hypoglycemia.

Despite these considerations, experience to date with RTCGM in pregnancy is extremely limited, permitting no firm conclusions. In 2010, a case report was published by Secher et al. [70]. Although obviously only anecdotal, it is nevertheless interesting as the group compared three successive pregnancies of a woman with type 1 diabetes; in the first she used multiple daily injections, in the second a micropump, and in the third a sensor-augmented pump. The first and second pregnancies were both complicated by preeclampsia and there were important neonatal complications in the first. In the third, however, with real-time monitoring the outcome was totally positive.

An Italian group had a similar experience in 2008 [71] with a young woman with type 1 diabetes mellitus whose first pregnancy had been managed with a micropump, and in which the infant suffered immediate postpartum hypoglycemia, requiring neonatal ICU admission. Early in her second pregnancy she asked for a sensor-augmented pump. At week 22, when RTCGM was started, her BG levels improved substantially (fasting and postprandial) and HbA_{1c} fell gradually, reaching 4.8% at the last measurement in pregnancy; at week 38 she had an induced vaginal delivery, with no perinatal complications.

In 2013 a Danish group reported the first randomized controlled trial in pregnancies complicated by types 1 and 2 diabetes mellitus [72]. They compared the metabolic control and obstetric-neonatal outcomes with two therapeutic approaches: the first was defined as 'routine', though it was closely followed with SMBG, and the second involved intermittent CGM as well as SMBG. The results were no different for the two groups, but intermittent use of the sensor meant that management could not be 'patient-oriented', although this should be the main aim of real-time monitoring. In this case, it would perhaps be more appropriate to speak of an 'unblinded' professional use: in the experimental group patients did not use a self-management algorithm and the monitor was simply applied for 6 days 5 times during the pregnancy (weeks 8, 12, 21, 27, and 33). The results were then interpreted by a member of the team, and discussed with the patient. The main aim of the intervention was not so much metabolic optimization as safety in avoiding hypoglycemia, as the alarm was set to go off at low BG levels, not for hyperglycemia.

To conclude, RTCGM systems offer a series of potential advantages in pregnancy which should greatly help achieve optimal glycometabolic control, which is essential for an optimal maternal-fetal outcome in these cases. The current lack of evidence to back their use probably reflects more the planning and methodological limitations of the studies to date than any real doubt about their validity. This should be clearly confirmed in the next few years by an international multicenter trial promoted by the JDRF – the CONCEPTT Trial [73]. This is now in its early phase, but it should enroll more than 300 women with type 1 diabetes mellitus: both women who are planning a pregnancy and some who are already pregnant. They will be randomly allocated to an experimental arm in which their current intensive insulin therapy (multiple daily injections or continuous subcutaneous insulin infusion) will be flanked by uninterrupted RTCGM. The control group will continue capillary self-monitoring.

RTCGM and Sport

Many of the potential advantages of CGM in pregnancy hold for sport, too. This is an area where this approach could open up new horizons; however, one must distinguish between retrospective utilization, as a research tool for professionals, and 'patient-oriented' use, intended to help diabetic athletes manage their disorder themselves. In the former case, CGM should provide useful further knowledge of glycemic homeostasis during different sports, in physiological conditions, and in diabetes mellitus, providing indications for optimal therapeutic management. In contrast, real-time use could help patients enormously by enabling them to practice sports with maximum safety. This would also help break down the barriers that have always existed to sports considered 'risky'.

Interesting information has been obtained, for instance, on the frequency, intensity, and timing of glycemic excursions – mostly in the direction of hypoglycemia – during and after intense aerobic activity, e.g. spinning [74], long-distance races [75], cycling, swimming [76], cross-country skiing [77], and scuba diving [78, 79]. The use of CGM in residential sports camps has made it possible to investigate mixed sports, like football or hockey [77], and in some experimental protocols the athletes alternated medium-intensity exercise with short bouts of intense effort [80].

The findings as a whole indicate more fully than traditional study methods that glucose concentrations fall gradually during prolonged aerobic activity, with a high frequency of hyper- and hypoglycemic swings, often asymptomatic. Several interesting reports have described frequent hypoglycemic episodes after exercise – sometimes many hours later, especially in the middle of the night. According to Iscoe et al. [76], this tendency is less marked when the exercise includes short high-intensity bouts; however, other studies have not shown this [81].

Clearly, the information from these retrospective analyses of CGM findings is extremely useful for planning the management of sports, so as to prevent BG swings during and after the effort, making even demanding situations safer for the diabetic athlete. But the most promising application of this technology is clearly in real time. Various reports, mostly of isolated cases or only small numbers, have been published in the last few years on the use of RTCGM in different sports. A team of cyclists with type 1 diabetes took part in the latest editions of the 'Race across America' [82], and in other less-demanding cycling races, always with excellent results. Other diabetic sportsmen and women have benefited from continuous monitoring during high-altitude trekking [83, 84]. Monitoring on the basis of a specific algorithm to manage insulin therapy and carbohydrate intake has been valuable in team sports like football, basketball, and volleyball [85].

There is still ample room for exploration and development of the use of RTCGM for diabetic athletes performing at various levels. Like all other fields where this technology is applied, however, the reliability of the findings is an essential point. The accuracy of the main sensors tested is the same, in general, as in situations not involving sport. A good correlation has been shown during effort between the data provided by the monitor and the capillary BG values, both in absolute terms [86], and as the size of the drop in BG [87]. Nevertheless, in a camp for type 1 diabetic adolescents practicing different sports, Adolfsson et al. [77] found that measurements were less accurate in the hypoglycemic range (MARD: 43%) than for hyperglycemia (MARD: 18%). That study also reported a loss of accuracy during more strenuous effort. The time lag widely reported for the sensor's readings on interstitial fluid, and already evident in resting conditions, has been confirmed for diabetic athletes. The drop in BG during medium-intensity prolonged exercise [87] and its rapid rise during intense anaerobic activity [88] may be detected with some delay, and may seem smaller in the real-time recording.

On the topic of using sensors during sports in 'extreme' environmental conditions, such as high-altitude mountaineering or scuba diving, an important study by Adolfsson et al. [89] appeared in 2012, reproducing high- or low-pressure situations in a hyperbaric chamber. The accuracy of the Enlite sensor was satisfactory in hypobaric conditions (MARD: 14.9% at 51 kPa/383 mm Hg, 0.5 atm, corresponding to 5,500 m altitude) and hyperbaric conditions (MARD: 6.7% at 404 kPa/3,030 mm Hg, 4.0 atm, corresponding to 30 m depth).

We can therefore conclude that at present, a real-time sensor is reliable enough to be useful in various sports, bearing in mind the limits outlined here, especially the time lag. It is, however, always advisable to check capillary blood before deciding on any corrections to therapy.

Progress is fast in this field and we can expect measurements to become more accurate, so that in the short term these tools should become extremely valuable for diabetic athletes both for recreational and competitive sports.

Characteristics of Patients Eligible for Real-Time Continuous Glucose Monitoring

The identification of the characteristics of eligible patients for RTCGM systems is intended to contribute to the production of effective recommendations for their clinical use. As is known, a correct selection of patients is one of the most important factors in determining a successful application of innovative technological devices as real-time glucose monitors.

Based on the limited evidence presented in the previous paragraphs, there are already consensus statements in a number of countries with regard to the indications of these systems. Taking into account that clinical guidelines and consensus documents from scientific societies impact not only on clinical practice, but also on health policy decisions, their implementation would ensure homogeneous care pathways and high quality standards, supporting reimbursement decisions through informed processes.

Actually, the indications given by some European authorities for RTCGM use vary little from country to country [40, 90–93]. In almost all documents they are differentiated between adults and children and pregnancy and pregnancy planning is considered separately; there is always a threshold of HbA_{1c}, although not uniform, and hypoglycemia is usually cited as a main indication if present in severe form or in case of unawareness [94]. The most complete and documented recommendations in this field have been published in recent years in France jointly by the Société Francophone du Diabète (SFD), the EVADIAC Group, and the Société Française d'Endocrinologie (SFE) [90], and in Germany by the German Diabetes Association [40].

In Italy an expert panel has recently defined the 'Consensus document on the selection of patients eligible for real-time continuous glucose monitoring' [95], whose conclusions, reported below, resume in substance many points already present in the other European papers. According to this document, considering the different metabolic patterns, patterns of treatment, lifestyle, and clinical evidence available, the criteria for identification of candidates can be divided into three categories: pediatric/adolescent, adults, and pregnant women or women in preconception.

Indications for Real-Time Continuous Glucose Monitoring

Patients <18 years old with type 1 diabetes mellitus:

- Treatment with insulin pump therapy
- Hypoglycemia:
  Severe → RTCGM strongly recommended
  Frequent, recurrent, undetected → RTCGM recommended
- Need to perform more than 10 SMBG per day
- High glycemic variability, regardless of HbA_{1c}
- HbA_{1c} <7% (<53 mmol/mol) in which it is necessary to minimize the risk of hypoglycemia

Adults with type 1 diabetes mellitus:

- Treatment with insulin pump therapy and HbA_{1c} >8% (>64 mmol/mol), notwithstanding intensive management, appropriate therapeutic education and intensive SMBG
- Hypoglycemia:
  Severe → RTCGM strongly recommended
  Frequent, recurrent, undetected → RTCGM recommended
- Unstable diabetes for which frequent emergency room visits and hospitalizations are needed
- In the presence of a discrepancy between the BG levels observed with SMBG and HbA_{1c}

Pregnancy (clinical evidence is in development, more crucial is the expert opinion):

- Preconception: HbA_{1c} >7.0% (>53 mmol/mol), notwithstanding intensive treatment and management with multiple daily injections or a pump, appropriate therapeutic education and intensive SMBG
- Pregnancy in course: HbA_{1c} >6.0% (>42 mmol/mol), notwithstanding intensive treatment and management with multiple daily injections or a pump, appropriate therapeutic education and intensive SMBG

Prospects

We have already summarized the conclusions at the end of each section of this chapter. Apart from its specific indications and applications, RTCGM definitely offers enormous potential, and is destined to radically change the concept of clinical self-management of diabetes, opening up new horizons on the way to true metabolic optimization. The current limitations that prevent its widespread use are essentially (1) the accuracy of the sensor measurement, which since it is still not optimal, confirmation on capillary blood is always needed before taking any therapeutic action; (2) the invasiveness of the system, requiring painful subcutaneous needle access and continuous wearing of a sensor-transmitter unit; (3) the persistent need for calibration with finger-sticking, and (4) the presence of alarms. All these factors interfere with a patient's daily life, sometimes limiting acceptance of the system and hence compliance. Additionally, patients and medical personnel must be taught to use the technique properly. Finally, there are the costs. However, many of these critical points are gradually getting smoothed out, and we are convinced that progress will be rapid in the next few years, helping overcome restrictions on reimbursement by healthcare authorities and insurance companies. As Jay Skyler wrote in 2009 in an editorial in *Diabetes Technology and Therapeutics* [96], the prospects for CGM today are probably similar to that of SMBG in the late 1970s or early 1980s: 'at a junction where adoption is about to explode'. As happened with SMBG, therefore, we can expect wide diffusion of this form of continuous monitoring in the coming years, and the technique will be routinely used by growing numbers of type 1 (and maybe not only type 1) diabetic patients.

References

1 Olansky L, Kennedy L: Finger-stick glucose monitoring: issues of accuracy and specificity. Diabetes Care 2010;33:948–949.

2 Mastrototaro J: The MiniMed Continuous Glucose Monitoring System (CGMS). J Pediatr Endocrinol Metab 1999;12(Suppl 3):751–758.

3 Klonoff DC: Continuous glucose monitoring: roadmap for 21st century diabetes therapy. Diabetes Care 2005;28:1231–1239.

4 Vaddiraju S, Burgess DJ, Tomazos I, Jain FC, Papadimitrakopoulos F: Technologies for continuous glucose monitoring: current problems and future promises. J Diabetes Sci Technol 2010;4:1540–1562.

5 Aussedat B, Dupire-Angel M, Gifford R, Klein JC, Wilson GS, Reach G: Interstitial glucose concentration and glycemia: implications for continuous subcutaneous glucose monitoring. Am J Physiol Endocrinol Metab 2000;278:E716–E728.
6 Blevins TC: Professional continuous glucose monitoring in clinical practice 2010. J Diabetes Sci Technol 2010;4:440–456.
7 Clarke W, Kovatchev B: Statistical tools to analyze continuous glucose monitor data. Diabetes Technol Ther 2009;11(Suppl 1):S45–S54.
8 Rodbard D: Interpretation of continuous glucose monitoring data: glycemic variability and quality of glycemic control. Diabetes Technol Ther 2009; 11(Suppl 1):S55–S67.
9 Muchmore D, Sharp M, Vaughn D: Benefits of blinded continuous glucose monitoring during a randomized clinical trial. J Diabetes Sci Technol 2011;5:676–680.
10 Tanenberg RJ, Pfeifer MA: Continuous glucose monitoring system: a new approach to the diagnosis of diabetic gastroparesis. Diabetes Technol Ther 2000;2(Suppl 1):S73–S80.
11 Kaufman FR, Austin J, Neinstein A, Jeng L, Halvorson M, Devoe DJ, Pitukcheewanont P: Nocturnal hypoglycemia detected with the continuous glucose monitoring system in pediatric patients with type 1 diabetes. J Pediatr 2002;141:625–630.
12 Kubiak T, Hermanns N, Schreckling HJ, Kulzer B, Haak T: Assessment of hypoglycaemia awareness using continuous glucose monitoring. Diabet Med 2004;21:487–490.
13 Wang X: Application of the Continuous Glucose Monitoring System (CGMS) in the 72-hour fast test in two patients with hypoglycemia. Diabetes Technol Ther 2004;6:883–886.
14 Conrad SC, Mastrototaro JJ, Gitelman SE: The use of a continuous glucose monitoring system in hypoglycemic disorders. J Pediatr Endocrinol Metab 2004; 17:281–288.
15 Hershkovitz E, Rachmel A, Ben-Zaken H, Phillip M: Continuous glucose monitoring in children with glycogen storage disease type I. J Inherit Metab Dis 2001;24:863–869.
16 O'Riordan SM, Hindmarsh P, Hill NR, Matthews DR, George S, Greally P, Canny G, Slattery D, Murphy N, Roche E: Validation of continuous glucose monitoring in children and adolescents with cystic fibrosis: a prospective cohort study. Diabetes Care 2009;32:1020–1022.
17 Faradji RN, Monroy K, Riefkohl A, Lozano L, Gorn L, Froud T, Cure P, Baidal D, Ponte G, Messinger S: Continuous glucose monitoring system for early detection of graft dysfunction in allogenic islet transplant recipients. Transplant Proc 2006;38:3274–3276.
18 Nardacci EA, Bode BW, Hirsch IB: Individualizing care for the many: the evolving role of professional continuous glucose monitoring systems in clinical practice. Diabetes Educ 2010;36:4S–19S.
19 Mastrototaro JJ: The MiniMed continuous glucose monitoring system. Diabetes Technol Ther 2000; 2(Suppl 1):S13–S18.
20 Garg S, Zisser H, Schwartz S, Bailey T, Kaplan R, Ellis S, Jovanovic L: Improvement in glycemic excursions with a transcutaneous, real-time continuous glucose sensor: a randomized controlled trial. Diabetes Care 2006;29:44–50.
21 Ryan MT, Savarese VW, Hipszer B, Dizdarevic I, Joseph M, Shively N, Joseph JI: Continuous glucose monitor shows potential for early hypoglycemia detection in hospitalized patients. Diabetes Technol Ther 2009;11:745–747.
22 Mastrototaro J, Lee S: The integrated MiniMed Paradigm real-time insulin pump and glucose monitoring system: implications for improved patient outcomes. Diabetes Technol Ther 2009;11(Suppl 1): S37–S43.
23 Skyler JS: Continuous glucose monitoring: an overview of its development. Diabetes Technol Ther 2009;11(Suppl 1):S5–S10.
24 Bailey T, Zisser H, Chang A: New features and performance of a next-generation seven-day continuous glucose monitoring system with short lag time. Diabetes Technol Ther 2009;11:749–755.
25 McGarraugh G: The chemistry of commercial continuous glucose monitors. Diabetes Technol Ther 2009;11(Suppl 1):S17–S24.
26 Danne T, de Valk HW, Kracht T, Walte K, Geldmacher R, Solter L, von dem Berge W, Welsh ZK, Bugler JR, Lange K: Reducing glycaemic variability in type 1 diabetes self-management with a continuous glucose monitoring system based on wired enzyme technology. Diabetologia 2009;52:1496–1503.
27 Varalli M, Marelli G, Maran A, Bistoni S, Luzzana M, Cremonesi P, Caramenti G, Valgimigli F, Poscia A: A microdialysis technique for continuous subcutaneous glucose monitoring in diabetic patients (part 2). Biosens Bioelectron 2003;18:899–905.
28 Maran A, Crepaldi C, Tiengo A, Grassi G, Vitali E, Pagano G, Bistoni S, Calabrese G, Santeusanio F, Leonetti F: Continuous subcutaneous glucose monitoring in diabetic patients: a multicenter analysis. Diabetes Care 2002;25:347–352.
29 Bequette BW: Continuous glucose monitoring: real-time algorithms for calibration, filtering, alarms. J Diabetes Sci Technol 2010;4:404–418.
30 Freckmann G, Schmid C, Baumstark A, Pleus S, Link M, Haug C: System accuracy evaluation of 43 blood glucose monitoring systems for self-monitoring of blood glucose according to DIN EN ISO 15197. J Diabetes Sci Technol 2012;6:1060–1075.

31 Kulcu E, Tamada JA, Reach G, Potts RO, Lesho MJ: Physiological differences between interstitial glucose and blood glucose measured in human subjects. Diabetes Care 2003;26:2405–2409.

32 Clarke WL, Kovatchev B: Continuous glucose sensors: continuing questions about clinical accuracy. J Diabetes Sci Technol 2007;1:669–675.

33 Steil GM, Rebrin K, Mastrototaro J, Bernaba B, Saad MF: Determination of plasma glucose during rapid glucose excursions with a subcutaneous glucose sensor. Diabetes Technol Ther 2003;5:27–31.

34 Basu A, Dube S, Slama M, Errazuriz I, Amezcua JC, Kudva YC, Peyser T, Carter RE, Cobelli C, Basu R: Time lag of glucose from intravascular to interstitial compartment in humans. Diabetes 2013;62:4083–4087.

35 Cengiz E, Sherr JL, Weinzimer SA, Tamborlane WV: New-generation diabetes management: glucose sensor-augmented insulin pump therapy. Expert Rev Med Devices 2011;8:449–458.

36 Rebrin K, Sheppard NF Jr, Steil GM: Use of subcutaneous interstitial fluid glucose to estimate blood glucose: revisiting delay and sensor offset. J Diabetes Sci Technol 2010;4:1087–1098.

37 Voskanyan G, Barry Keenan D, Mastrototaro JJ, Steil GM: Putative delays in interstitial fluid (ISF) glucose kinetics can be attributed to the glucose sensing systems used to measure them rather than the delay in ISF glucose itself. J Diabetes Sci Technol 2007;1:639–644.

38 Keenan DB, Mastrototaro JJ, Voskanyan G, Steil GM: Delays in minimally invasive continuous glucose monitoring devices: a review of current technology. J Diabetes Sci Technol 2009;3:1207–1214.

39 Zueger T, Diem P, Mougiakakou S, Stettler C: Influence of time point of calibration on accuracy of continuous glucose monitoring in individuals with type 1 diabetes. Diabetes Technol Ther 2012;14:583–588.

40 Liebl AL, Henrichs HR, Heinemann L, Freckmann G, Biermann E, Thomas A; CGM Working Group Diabetes Technology of the German Diabetes Association: Continuous glucose monitoring: evidence and consensus statement for clinical use. J Diabetes Sci Technol 2013;7:500–519.

41 Clarke WL, Anderson S, Farhy L, Breton M, Gonder-Frederick L, Cox D, Kovatchev B: Evaluating the clinical accuracy of two continuous glucose sensors using continuous glucose-error grid analysis. Diabetes Care 2005;28:2412–2417.

42 Clarke WL, Anderson S, Kovatchev B: Evaluating clinical accuracy of continuous glucose monitoring systems: continuous glucose-error grid analysis (CG-EGA). Curr Diabetes Rev 2008;4:193–199.

43 Gifford R, Batchelor MM, Lee Y, Gokulrangan G, Meyerhoff ME, Wilson GS: Mediation of in vivo glucose sensor inflammatory response via nitric oxide release. J Biomed Mater Res 2005;A75:755–766.

44 Klueh U, Liu Z, Feldman B, Henning TP, Cho B, Ouyang T, Kreutzer D: Metabolic biofouling of glucose sensors in vivo: role of tissue microhemorrhages. J Diabetes Sci Technol 2011;5:583–595.

45 Weinstein RL, Schwartz SL, Brazg RL, Bugler JR, Peyser TA, McGarraugh GV: Accuracy of the 5-day FreeStyle Navigator Continuous Glucose Monitoring System: comparison with frequent laboratory reference measurements. Diabetes Care 2007;30:1125–1130.

46 Kovatchev B, Anderson S, Heinemann L, Clarke W: Comparison of the numerical and clinical accuracy of four continuous glucose monitors. Diabetes Care 2008;31:1160–1164.

47 Damiano ER, El-Khatib FH, Zheng H, Nathan DM, Russell SJ: A comparative effectiveness analysis of three continuous glucose monitors. Diabetes Care 2013;36:251–259.

48 Keenan DB, Mastrototaro JJ, Zisser H, Cooper KA, Raghavendhar G, Lee SW, Yusi J, Bailey TS, Brazg RL, Shah RV: Accuracy of the Enlite 6-day glucose sensor with Guardian and Veo calibration algorithms. Diabetes Technol Ther 2012;14:225–231.

49 Christiansen M, Bailey T, Watkins E, Liljenquist D, Price D, Nakamura K, Boock R, Peyser T: A new-generation continuous glucose monitoring system: improved accuracy and reliability compared with a previous-generation system. Diabetes Technol Ther 2013;15:881–888.

50 Garcia A, Rack-Gomer AL, Bhavaraju NC, Hampapuram H, Kamath A, Peyser T, Facchinetti A, Zecchin C, Sparacino G, Cobelli C: Dexcom G4AP: an advanced continuous glucose monitor for the artificial pancreas. J Diabetes Sci Technol 2013;7:1436–1445.

51 Deiss D, Bolinder J, Riveline JP, Battelino T, Bosi E, Tubiana-Rufi N, Kerr D, Phillip M: Improved glycemic control in poorly controlled patients with type 1 diabetes using real-time continuous glucose monitoring. Diabetes Care 2006;29:2730–2732.

52 Juvenile Diabetes Research Foundation Continuous Glucose Monitoring Study, Tamborlane WV, Beck RW, Bode BW, Buckingham B, Chase HP, Clemons R, Fiallo-Scharer R, Fox LA, Gilliam LK: Continuous glucose monitoring and intensive treatment of type 1 diabetes. N Engl J Med 2008;359:1464–1476.

53 Juvenile Diabetes Research Foundation Continuous Glucose Monitoring Study Group, Beck RW, Hirsch IB, Laffel L, Tamborlane WV, Bode BW, Buckingham B, Chase P, Clemons R, Fiallo-Scharer R, Fox LA, Gilliam LK, Huang ES, Kollman C, Kowalski AJ, Lawrence JM, Lee J, Mauras N, O'Grady M, Ruedy KJ, Tansey M, Tsalikian E, Weinzimer SA, Wilson DM, Wolpert H, Wysocki T, Xing D: The effect of continuous glucose monitoring in well-controlled type 1 diabetes. Diabetes Care 2009;32:1378–1383.

54 Langendam M, Luijf YM, Hooft L, DeVries JH, Mudde AH, Scholten RJ: Continuous glucose monitoring systems for type 1 diabetes mellitus. Cochrane Database Syst Rev 2012;1:CD008101.
55 Yeh HC, Brown TT, Maruthur N, Ranasinghe P, Berger Z, Suh YD, Wilson LM, Haberl EB, Brick J, Bass EB: Comparative effectiveness and safety of methods of insulin delivery and glucose monitoring for diabetes mellitus: a systematic review and meta-analysis. Ann Intern Med 2012;157:336–347.
56 Pickup JC, Freeman SC, Sutton AJ: Glycaemic control in type 1 diabetes during real time continuous glucose monitoring compared with self monitoring of blood glucose: meta-analysis of randomised controlled trials using individual patient data. BMJ 2011; 343:d3805.
57 Juvenile Diabetes Research Foundation Continuous Glucose Monitoring Study Group, Beck RW, Buckingham B, Miller K, Wolpert H, Xing D, Block JM, Chase HP, Hirsch I, Kollman C, Laffel L, Lawrence JM, Milaszewski K, Ruedy KJ, Tamborlane WV: Factors predictive of use and of benefit from continuous glucose monitoring in type 1 diabetes. Diabetes Care 2009;32:1947–1953.
58 Juvenile Diabetes Research Foundation Continuous Glucose Monitoring Study Group: Effectiveness of continuous glucose monitoring in a clinical care environment: evidence from the Juvenile Diabetes Research Foundation Continuous Glucose Monitoring (JDRF-CGM) trial. Diabetes Care 2010;33:17–22.
59 Jovanovic L: Continuous glucose monitoring during pregnancy complicated by gestational diabetes mellitus. Curr Diab Rep 2001;1:82–85.
60 Yogev Y, Ben-Haroush A, Chen R, Rosenn B, Hod M, Langer O: Diurnal glycemic profile in obese and normal weight nondiabetic pregnant women. Am J Obstet Gynecol 2004;191:949–953.
61 Siegmund T, Rad NT, Ritterath C, Siebert G, Henrich W, Buhling KJ: Longitudinal changes in the continuous glucose profile measured by the CGMS in healthy pregnant women and determination of cut-off values. Eur J Obstet Gynecol Reprod Biol 2008; 139:46–52.
62 Ben-Haroush A, Yogev Y, Chen R, Rosenn B, Hod M, Langer O: The postprandial glucose profile in the diabetic pregnancy. Am J Obstet Gynecol 2004;191: 576–581.
63 Murphy HR, Rayman G, Duffield K, Lewis KS, Kelly S, Johal B, Fowler D, Temple RC: Changes in the glycemic profiles of women with type 1 and type 2 diabetes during pregnancy. Diabetes Care 2007;30: 2785–2791.
64 Kerssen A, de Valk HW, Visser GH: Forty-eight-hour first-trimester glucose profiles in women with type 1 diabetes mellitus: a report of three cases of congenital malformation. Prenat Diagn 2006;26: 123–127.
65 Kerssen A, de Valk HW, Visser GH: Increased second trimester maternal glucose levels are related to extremely large-for-gestational-age infants in women with type 1 diabetes. Diabetes Care 2007;30:1069–1074.
66 McLachlan K, Jenkins A, O'Neal D: The role of continuous glucose monitoring in clinical decision-making in diabetes in pregnancy. Aust NZ J Obstet Gynaecol 2007;47:186–190.
67 Kestila KK, Ekblad UU, Ronnemaa T: Continuous glucose monitoring versus self-monitoring of blood glucose in the treatment of gestational diabetes mellitus. Diabetes Res Clin Pract 2007;77:174–179.
68 Yogev Y, Ben-Haroush A, Chen R, Kaplan B, Phillip M, Hod M: Continuous glucose monitoring for treatment adjustment in diabetic pregnancies – a pilot study. Diabet Med 2003;20:558–562.
69 Murphy HR, Rayman G, Lewis K, Kelly S, Johal B, Duffield K, Fowler D, Campbell PJ, Temple RC: Effectiveness of continuous glucose monitoring in pregnant women with diabetes: randomised clinical trial. BMJ 2008;337:a1680.
70 Secher AL, Schmidt S, Nørgaard K, Mathiesen ER: Continuous glucose monitoring-enabled insulin-pump therapy in diabetic pregnancy. Acta Obstet Gynecol Scand 2010;89:1233–1237.
71 Mion E, Brambilla MC, Pisoni MP, Corica D, Bonomo M: Monitoraggio del glucosio real-time in gravidanza: l'esperienza di due gravidanze a confronto. G Ital Diabetol 2008;28:184–186.
72 Secher AL, Ringholm L, Andersen HU, Damm P, Mathiesen ER: The effect of real-time continuous glucose monitoring in pregnant women with diabetes: a randomized controlled trial. Diabetes Care 2013;36:1877–1883.
73 Feig D: Continuous glucose monitoring in women with type 1 diabetes in pregnancy trial (CONCEPTT). http://cctn.jdrf.ca/research-clinical-trials/jdrf-cctn-clinical-trials1/.
74 Iscoe KE, Campbell JE, Jamnik V, Perkins BA, Riddell MC: Efficacy of continuous real-time blood glucose monitoring during and after prolonged high-intensity cycling exercise: spinning with a continuous glucose monitoring system. Diabetes Technol Ther 2006;8:627–635.
75 Cauza E, Hanusch-Enserer U, Strasser B, Ludvik B, Kostner K, Dunky A, Haber P: Continuous glucose monitoring in diabetic long distance runners. Int J Sports Med 2005;26:774–780.
76 Iscoe KE, Corcoran M, Riddell MC: High rates of nocturnal hypoglycemia in a unique sports camp for athletes with type 1 diabetes: lessons learned from continuous glucose monitoring systems. Can J Diabetes 2008;32:182–189.

77 Adolfsson P, Nilsson S, Lindblad B: Continuous glucose monitoring system during physical exercise in adolescents with type 1 diabetes. Acta Paediatr 2011; 100:1603–1609.
78 Adolfsson P, Ornhagen H, Jendle J: Accuracy and reliability of continuous glucose monitoring in individuals with type 1 diabetes during recreational diving. Diabetes Technol Ther 2009;11:493–497.
79 Bonomo M, Cairoli R, Verde G, Morelli L, Moreo A, Delle Grottaglie M, Brambilla MC, Meneghini E, Aghemo P, Corigliano G, Marroni A: Safety of recreational scuba diving in type 1 diabetic patients: the Deep Monitoring Programme. Diabetes Metab 2009; 35:101–107.
80 Iscoe KE, Riddell MC: Continuous moderate-intensity exercise with or without intermittent high-intensity work: effects on acute and late glycaemia in athletes with type 1 diabetes mellitus. Diabet Med 2011;28:824–832.
81 Maran A, Pavan P, Bonsembiante B, Brugin E, Ermolao A, Avogaro A, Zaccaria M: Continuous glucose monitoring reveals delayed nocturnal hypoglycemia after intermittent high-intensity exercise in nontrained patients with type 1 diabetes. Diabetes Technol Ther 2010;12:763–768.
82 Demma LH, Bode B: The utility of a continuous glucose monitoring system for elite cyclist during the Race across America. Infusystem 2007;4:8.
83 de Mol P, de Vries ST, de Koning EJ, Gans RO, Tack CJ, Bilo HJ: Increased insulin requirements during exercise at very high altitude in type 1 diabetes. Diabetes Care 2011;34:591–595.
84 Valletta JJ, Chipperfield AJ, Clough GF, Byrne CD: Metabolic regulation during constant moderate physical exertion in extreme conditions in type 1 diabetes. Diabet Med 2012;29:822–826.
85 Riddell MC, Milliken J: Preventing exercise-induced hypoglycemia in type 1 diabetes using real-time continuous glucose monitoring and a new carbohydrate intake algorithm: an observational field study. Diabetes Technol Ther 2011;13:819–825.
86 Iscoe KE, Campbell JE, Jamnik V, Perkins BA, Riddell MC: Efficacy of continuous real-time blood glucose monitoring during and after prolonged high-intensity cycling exercise: spinning with a continuous glucose monitoring system. Diabetes Technol Ther 2006;8:627–635.
87 Wilson DM, Beck RW, Tamborlane WV, Dontchev MJ, Kollman C, Chase P, Fox LA, Ruedy KJ, Tsalikian E, Weinzimer SA: The accuracy of the FreeStyle Navigator Continuous Glucose Monitoring System in children with type 1 diabetes. Diabetes Care 2007; 30:59–64.
88 Davey RJ, Ferreira LD, Jones TW, Fournie PA: Effect of exercise-mediated acidosis on determination of glycemia using CGMS. Diabetes Technol Ther 2006; 8:516–518.
89 Adolfsson P, Ornhagen H, Eriksson BM, Cooper K, Jendle J: Continuous glucose monitoring – a study of the Enlite sensor during hypo- and hyperbaric conditions. Diabetes Technol Ther 2012;14:527–532.
90 Benhamou PY, Catargi B, Delenne B, Guerci B, Hanaire H, Jeandidier N, Leroy R, Meyer L, Penfornis A, Radermecker RP: Real-time continuous glucose monitoring (CGM) integrated into the treatment of type 1 diabetes: consensus of experts from SFD, EVADIAC and SFE. Diabetes Metab 2012;38(Suppl 4):S67–S83.
91 Hammon PJ, Amiel SA, Dayan CM, Kerr D, Pickup J, Shaw J: ABCD Position Status on continuous glucose monitoring: use of glucose sensing in outpatient clinical diabetes care. Pract Diabetes Int 2010;27:2.
92 Andersson M, Eliasson B, Gustafsson J, Hanas R: Guidelines for the clinical use of CGM in Sweden. 2009. Letter to Tandvårds-Och Läkemedelsförmånsverket.
93 Positionspapier des Insulinpumpenausschusses der OEDG zur kontinuierlichen Glukosemessung (CGMS – Continuous Glucose Monitoring). http://www.oedg.org/1102_positionspapier.html.
94 Heinemann L, Franc S, Phillip M, Battelino T, Ampudia-Blasco FJ, Bolinder J, Diem P, Pickup J, Hans Devries J: Reimbursement for continuous glucose monitoring: a European view. J Diabetes Sci Technol 2012;6:1498–1502.
95 Grassi G, Aragona M, Bonomo M, Bruttomesso D, Cherubini V, De Feo E, Di Bartolo P, Lepore G, Pitocco D, Schiaffini R: Consensus document of an expert panel on the selection of patients eligible for real-time continuous glucose monitoring. G Ital Diabetol Metab 2014;34:5–13.
96 Skyler JS: CGM – a technology in evolution. Diabetes Technol Ther 2009;11:63–64.

Dr. Matteo Bonomo
Diabetes Unit, Ospedale Niguarda Cà Granda
Piazza Dell'Ospedale Maggiore 3
IT–20162 Milano (Italy)
E-Mail matteo.bonomo@ospedaleniguarda.it

Bruttomesso D, Grassi G (eds): Technological Advances in the Treatment of Type 1 Diabetes.
Front Diabetes. Basel, Karger, 2015, vol 24, pp 128–142 (DOI: 10.1159/000363486)

Subcutaneous Insulin Pump

Giuseppe Lepore[a] · Letizia Tommaselli[b]

[a]USC Malattie Endocrine e Diabetologia, A.O. Papa Giovanni XXIII Bergamo, Bergamo, and [b]Dipartimento di Biomedicina Clinica e Molecolare, Unità Operativa di Endocrinologia, Università degli studi di Catania, Catania, Italy

Abstract

Over the last 20 years, continuous subcutaneous insulin infusion (CSII) has become a viable alternative to multiple daily insulin injections (MDI) in type 1 diabetic patients. Both randomized controlled trials and observational studies have found lower glycated hemoglobin (HbA_{1c}) levels, less severe hypoglycemic episodes, smaller blood glucose fluctuations, and a better quality of life in CSII-treated adult patients with type 1 diabetes in comparison to MDI treatment. CSII requires care by skilled professionals, careful selection of patients, meticulous patient monitoring, and thorough patient education. Although obviously more expensive than MDI, CSII may be cost-effective when elevated HbA_{1c} levels or continued disabling hypoglycemia persist despite optimized MDI therapy. More recently, sensor-augmented pumps (SAPs) have become available. These combine the technology of an insulin pump with a continuous glucose sensor. The best results with SAPs can be expected in patients who use the glucose sensor frequently, draw adequate conclusions from the data, and make immediate therapeutic decisions. Randomized controlled studies have provided evidence that SAPs can improve HbA_{1c} without increasing severe hypoglycemic episodes in patients with type 1 diabetes with elevated baseline HbA_{1c}, and that the frequency and duration of hypoglycemic events can be reduced in patients with satisfactory baseline HbA_{1c}, increasing treatment satisfaction.

The first insulin pump prototype, devised by Arnold Kadish in 1963, was a very large device worn as a backpack that delivered glucagon and insulin. A handier version was developed by Dean Kamen in the late 1970s. Early portable pumps were large and quite complicated to use. They offered a single basal rate, plus a stepped-up rate of infusion to cover meals. Insulin was delivered through a nylon cannula implanted in the abdominal wall. Some pumps even required the use of a screwdriver in order to adjust the flow rate of insulin. Technological advancements during the 1990s transformed continuous subcutaneous insulin infusion (CSII) into a viable alternative to multiple daily injections (MDI).

Current Insulin Pump Technology

At present a typical insulin pump consists of the main device (including controls, processing module, and batteries), a disposable insulin reservoir, and a disposable infusion set made by a cannula for subcutaneous insertion and a tubing system connecting the pump to a Teflon cannula or a stainless steel needle. Insulin pumps deliver rapid-acting insulin both as slow continuous and adjustable infusion rates over 24 h (basal rate) and as bolus doses that can be given at meals or to correct hyperglycemia.

Smart pumps deliver up to 48 basal rates/day according to selected time schedules, adjust insulin dose with a precision of 0.025 U/h, and can deliver standard insulin boluses, extended boluses, or a combination of the two. Most pumps can interface with personal computers for programming or data recording. The connection to a computer simplifies record keeping and can be used as an interface to diabetes management software. Moreover, some pumps are connected to a blood glucose meter. Most recent pump models have an automated bolus calculator which helps calculate the insulin dose on the basis of current blood glucose, intake of carbohydrate, carbohydrate-to-insulin ratio, insulin sensitivity factor, and duration of insulin action [1]. Even if automated bolus calculators have the same basic functions, there are differences in setup protocols and algorithms used to calculate correction boluses. Recently, a new type of pump, called the 'patch pump', has been developed. Patch pumps are 'tubing less' pumps, in which the insulin reservoir and infusion set are housed in the same unit. They are made of a disposable infusion pump attached at the infusion site and a remote device that controls the pump wirelessly. Patch pumps are smaller and more discrete compared to conventional insulin pumps. A comparison between current insulin pumps is shown in table 1.

Basal Rate and Bolus Calculation

Before starting therapy, the initial basal rate and bolus doses must be determined. The approximate total daily dose of insulin if a patient is switching from MDI to an insulin pump may be derived from MDI doses, but should be reduced by 20% owing to pharmacokinetic differences between the two modalities. The basal rate is calculated at 50% of that value. It is preferable that initially only one rate is used for the entire 24-hour period and that variations of rates are introduced later. An appropri-

Table 1. Comparison of current insulin pumps

Pump	Animas Vibe	Accu-Chek Spirit Combo Roche	Dana Diabecare R	Medtronic Veo (554,754)	Insulet OmniPod	Tandem Diabetes t: slim
Size, mm	51×77×18	88×56×21	75×45×19	76.2×5.1×20.3 91.4×50.8×20.3	Pod: 61×41×18 Pad: 66×110×26	79.5×50.8×15.2
Weight, g	110	110	63	100 (554) 108 (754)	OP: 34 PDM: 113	112
Reservoir size, U	200	315	300	176 (554) 300 (754)	200	300
Basal increment, U	0.025	0.1	0.01	0.025	0.05	0.001
Total basal	12/day	24/day	24/day	48/day	48/day	16/day
Temporary basal	–90 to +200% in 10% increments for 0.5–24 h	in 10% increments from 0 to 250% for 15 min to 24 h	±0–200% for 1–12 h	±0.1 U increment as single basal rate for 0.5–24 h or as % of current basal	% or U/h (1–12 h, in 30-min increments)	0–250% of current basal (in increments of 1%), 6 temporary basal rates; duration: 15 min to 72 h
Bolus increments, U	0.05, 0.1, 1, 5	0.1, 0.2, 0.5, 1, 2	0.05, 0.1, 0.5, 1	0.025, 0.1, 0.5, 1	0.05, 0.1, 0.5, 1	0.05–25
Bolus type	standard, extended, combination	standard, extended, multiwave	standard, extended, combination	standard, extended, combination	normal, extended, combination	normal, quick, extended
Bolus calculator	yes	yes	yes	yes	yes	yes
Software download	ezManager Max, Diasend software	Accu-Chek 360 Diabetes Management System or Accu-Chek Smart Pix device reader	DANA Manager software	Medtronic CareLink® Therapy Management System	OmniPod extension for the CoPilot Health Management System	t: connect Diabetes Management Application
CSII-CGM integrated system	yes	no	yes	no	no	no

ate basal rate keeps blood glucose levels stable overnight and when the patient has not eaten or bolused recently. Once the initial flat basal rate has been established, the remainder of the insulin total daily dose may be divided into bolus doses. The bolus dose before a meal is based on the carbohydrate content of the meal, carbohydrate-to-insulin ratio, current blood glucose, and insulin sensitivity factor (which is blood glucose decrease per unit of insulin and is calculated as 1,800: total daily insulin dose). The insulin sensitivity factor is also used to correct hyperglycemia between meals. Actually, many patients use an automated bolus calculator to estimate bolus doses.

Clinical Efficacy and Safety

The potential advantages of CSII with respect to MDI include lower glycated hemoglobin (HbA_{1c}) and hence less long-term complications of diabetes, smaller blood glucose fluctuations, fewer episodes of severe hypoglycemia, and improved quality of life (QoL).

Glucose Control

Several observational studies have compared HbA_{1c} levels before and after CSII therapy. The National Institute for Health and Clinical Excellence (NICE) in the 'Review of technology appraisal guidance concerning CSII' reported 46 studies that compared levels of HbA_{1c} before and after CSII therapy: all of the studies in the adult age group showed a statistically significant decrease in levels of HbA_{1c} (range: 0.2–1.4%) after initiation of CSII therapy. Moreover, NICE found 4 randomized controlled trials (RCTs) in type 1 diabetes mellitus that compared CSII with analogue MDI therapy (3 NPH-based and 1 glargine-based); in the studies of adult patients with type 1 diabetes mellitus, there was little evidence of a statistically significant difference between CSII and MDI therapy in terms of HbA_{1c} reduction [2].

In a more recent meta-analysis, Yeh et al. [3] evaluated 19 RCTs in children or adults that compared CSII with MDI. In adults with type 1 diabetes mellitus, HbA_{1c} levels decreased more with CSII than with MDI (mean difference: –0.30%; 95% CI: –0.58 to –0.02). The pooled estimate was influenced by 1 study in which participants had a higher HbA_{1c} level at enrolment (9.3%) compared with that of the other studies (7.7–8.2%). Most studies point out the fact that CSII superiority depends on patients' pre-CSII glycemic profile.

In a retrospective analysis of data from 17 diabetes outpatient clinics, Fahlén et al. [4] showed that switching from MDI without long-acting analogues to CSII improved metabolic control, particularly in patients with higher levels HbA_{1c} and BMI at baseline. Another possible advantage of CSII therapy in type 1 diabetes is the decrease of glucose excursions. The variability of blood glucose concentration throughout the day and night not only affects QoL, but also may represent an independent risk factor for diabetic complications [5]. A randomized cross-over study demonstrated that CSII reduces glucose variability compared to MDI therapy using glargine as basal insulin, in spite of similar HbA_{1c} levels [6].

Hypoglycemia

Pickup and Sutton [7] in a meta-analysis of 22 studies compared severe hypoglycemia and glycemic control during CSII and MDI. Severe hypoglycemia was reduced during CSII compared with MDI, with a rate ratio of 2.89 (95% CI: 1.45–5.76) for RCTs and 4.34 (95% CI: 2.87–6.56) for before/after studies (rate ratio: 4.19, 95% CI: 2.86–6.13, for all studies). The reduction was greatest in those with the highest initial severe hypoglycemia rates on MDI ($p < 0.001$). The mean difference in HbA_{1c} between treatments was less for RCTs [0.21% (0.13–0.30)] than in before/after studies [0.72% (0.55–

0.90)], but strongly related to the initial HbA_{1c} on MDI ($p < 0.001$). Differently from Pickup and Sutton, another meta-analysis, which evaluated 15 randomized trials of CSII versus MDI, did not show significant a difference in severe (pooled odds ratio: 0.48, 95% CI: 0.23–1.00) or nocturnal hypoglycemia (pooled odds ratio: 0.82, 95% CI: 0.33–2.03). Patients with type 1 diabetes using CSII had slightly lower HbA_{1c} (random-effects weighted mean difference: –0.2%, 95% CI: –0.3 to –0.1, compared with MDI). Adolescents and adults with type 1 diabetes enrolled in crossover trials had fewer minor hypoglycemic episodes with CSII than MDI (–0.08 episodes/patient/week, 95% CI: –0.21 to 0.06), but the difference was not significant [8]. Twenty-six observational studies comparing the rate of severe hypoglycemic episodes in people on CSII or MDI therapy were evaluated in the NICE review. Of the 10 studies in the adult/mixed age groups, 8 reported statistically significant decreases in the rate of severe hypoglycemic episodes during CSII. The rate ratios were in the range 0.07–0.40. The remaining 2 studies could not be analyzed since there were no hypoglycemic episodes [2].

Ketoacidosis

Patients on CSII have a smaller subcutaneous insulin depot with respect to patients treated with MDI; therefore, ketosis can develop rapidly if insulin infusion is interrupted. Early studies indicated a high rate of ketoacidosis with CSII at some centers, but more recent observations failed to find more ketoacidosis in patients on CSII [2].

Long-Term Complications

Few studies have reported on the long-term microvascular or macrovascular outcomes with CSII. In a 3-year multicenter retrospective observational study, 110 type 1 diabetic patients treated with CSII were compared with 110 patients treated with MDI matched at baseline for age, sex, diabetes duration, and HbA_{1c}. At entry, 90 patients in each group had a normal albumin excretion rate and 20 had persistent microalbuminuria. The albumin excretion rate [median (95% CI)] was similar at baseline [6.0 μg/min (9–21) in the CSII group vs. 4.4 (8–16) in the MDI group, NS] and significantly lower in the patients treated with CSII, both at year 2 and at year 3 of follow-up [4.7 μg/min (6–12) vs. 6.4 (13–29), $p < 0.002$]. Nine patients progressed to microalbuminuria in the MDI group while only 1 did in the CSII group. Nine patients regressed to normoalbuminuria in the CSII group, whereas only 2 regressed to normoalbuminuria in the MDI group [9].

Quality of Life

The effect of CSII therapy on QoL was considered by few RCTs. Generally, these studies showed improved diabetes mellitus-specific QoL favoring CSII [10]. In fact, the use of insulin pumps yielded QoL benefits, such as flexibility, autonomy, more freedom to engage in athletic activities, and improved sleep and socialization. Most likely, the decrease of severe hypoglycemic episodes improves QoL in patients experiencing frequent and disabling episodes.

Pregnancy in Women with Type 1 Diabetes

Pregnant women with type 1 diabetes mellitus have an increased risk of congenital malformations, obstetrical complications, and perinatal morbidity and mortality. It has been demonstrated that maintenance of near-normoglycemia during the preconception period and pregnancy can reduce the risk of these complications. Despite the use of intensive self-monitoring of blood glucose (SMBG) and the introduction of insulin analogues, the frequency of fetal complications remains higher than in the normal population. At present it remains controversial whether during pregnancy CSII has advantages over MDI. A systematic review comparing the efficacy of the two insulin regimens in pregnant women with preexisting diabetes identified only 2 studies. There was a significant increase in mean birthweight associated with CSII as opposed to MDI. However, taking into consideration the lack of significant difference in rate of macrosomia, this is not viewed by the authors as clinically significant. No significant differences were found in perinatal mortality (RR: 2.00, 95% CI: 0.20–19.91), fetal anomaly (RR: 1.07, 95% CI: 0.07–15.54), maternal hypoglycemia (RR: 3.00, 95% CI: 0.35–25.87), or maternal hyperglycemia (RR: 7.00, 95% CI: 0.39–125.44) [11]. Recently, 2 retrospective studies, involving 144 and 99 type 1 diabetic pregnant women, respectively, showed that CSII and MDI are equivalent in terms of metabolic control and fetal-maternal outcomes [12, 13].

Sensor-Augmented Insulin Pump Therapy

Despite the widespread use of insulin pumps and multiple injection regimens and the availability of insulin analogues, intensive treatment of type 1 diabetes often does not achieve optimum glucose control. Administration of insulin, with no reference to glucose data, is a common cause of poor diabetes control. SMBG has an established role in achieving target glucose values, but standard SMBG gives limited information on glucose variability. Furthermore, postprandial hyperglycemia and asymptomatic nocturnal hypoglycemia often go unrecognized even in type 1 diabetes mellitus patients who measure blood glucose levels several times daily. Continuous glucose monitoring (CGM) is bound to redefine current concepts of glycemic control and optimal diabetes management. New CGM technology provides real-time information on glucose levels and the rate and direction of glucose changes, and, furthermore, sends message alerts in the presence of a trend towards hypo- or hyperglycemia.

The combination of an insulin pump and CGM, also referred to as sensor-augmented pump (SAP) therapy, constitutes a new dimension of diabetes therapy. In some pump models, CGM data are wirelessly transferred from the glucose sensor to the pump, which displays glucose values and trends (fig. 1).

An SAP is usually offered to patients after consideration of several factors such as patient willingness and ability to use this technology appropriately, age of patients, and glycemic control at baseline. The benefits of CGM stem from how sensor data are utilized.

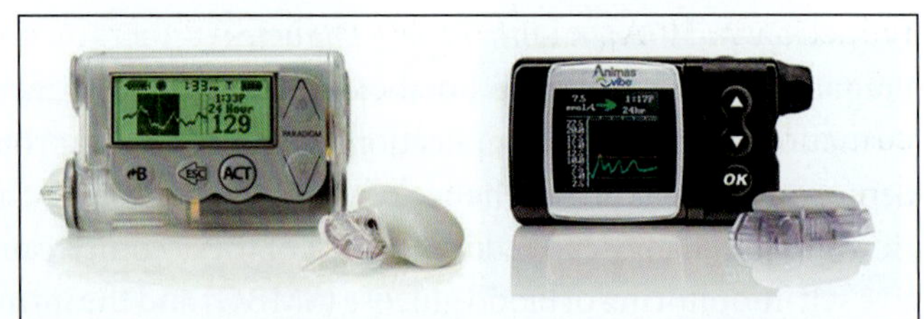

Fig. 1. SAPs currently marketed.

Education

Thorough and frequent analysis of sensor data enhance the assessment of glucose patterns and trends, and is expected to improve glucose control. Patients, personally or together with the caring team, can review sensor data from graphs visualized directly on the CGM receiver or downloaded to a computer. Warnings in case of acute glycemic deteriorations should prevent hypoglycemic events and inappropriate postprandial hyperglycemia, improve meal insulin dosing, and help insulin administration during and after exercise.

In 2008, referring to patient selection for CSII, Hirsch et al. [14] suggested that a multifaceted Web-based program be established for physicians, diabetes educators, registered dieticians, and patients. Depending on the target audience, topics extended from calibration and alarm setting to interpreting data and adjusting therapy. Printed materials and other media platforms were also recommended.

The availability of algorithms for patients and families can be very important. The Diabetes Research in Children Network (DirecNet) Study Group published guidelines that included algorithms that help make decisions on the basis of glucose values read in real time or downloaded from the sensor [15].

Other investigators have used a different approach [16]. No treatment protocols or fixed algorithms were provided to the patients, and therapy adjustments were made in partnership with subjects at clinic visits. It remained the medical responsibility of the treating physician to guide the subject in reaction to real-time CGM values and hyper- and hypoglycemic alerts. Subjects were encouraged to make self-adjustments to their treatment, and examples of therapy changes were provided in the patient diary.

Influence of Age

The JDRF study [17] found that SAPs did not improve HbA_{1c} in the age groups 8–14 and 15–24 years. Further analysis, however, found that the lack of effect was due to a shorter period of CGM use in children and adolescents compared with the adult group. In 1 year, the STAR 3 study [18] found HbA_{1c} levels in SAP-treated subjects were lower than in the injection therapy group. Among children there was an absolute reduction in HbA_{1c} of 0.4 ± 0.9% in the SAP therapy group and an increase of 0.2 ± 1.0% in the MDI group. Several other RCTs have confirmed that SAPs improve glucose control at no increased risk of hypoglycemia in pediatric patients [19–21]. Therefore, age does not seem to be a factor for the success of SAP therapy.

Frequency of Use

Frequent use of sensor data is very important. In the STAR 3 study, sensor use for 41–60% of the time was associated with a reduction of 0.64% in HbA_{1c} levels, and sensor use over 80% doubled the benefit [18]. In the STAR 1 study, lower HbA_{1c} levels were observed only in patients who used the sensor 60% or more of the time [22].

A recent meta-analysis on the use of real-time CGM compared with SMBG in type 1 diabetes included 6 trials with 449 patients randomized to CGM and 443 to SMBG. HbA_{1c} was 0.3% lower among CGM users (95% CI: –0.43 to –0.17%). By means of a best-fit regression model, investigators showed that for every 1-day increase of sensor use per week, the decrease in HbA_{1c} was 0.15% [23]. The report of the Agency for Healthcare Research and Quality (AHRQ) in 2012 also confirmed that real-time CGM is most effective in patients wearing the sensor at least 60% of the time. Thus, sensor compliance may be a marker for overall treatment adherence and explain HbA_{1c} reduction [24].

Glycemic Control at Baseline

Meta-analysis of RCTs of real-time CGM versus SMBG indicated that the best effect on HbA_{1c} occurs in patients who use the sensor most frequently and/or who have the highest baseline HbA_{1c} level [23]. The most appropriate and cost-effective use of real-time CGM in pump users should therefore be in those who have not achieved target HbA_{1c} levels despite a period of intensive CSII therapy. This conclusion, however, has not been shared by others [25]. The Endocrine Society clinical practice guideline recommends the use of real-time CGM also in subjects with good glycemic control (HbA_{1c} <7%) because real-time CGM use can reduce the frequency of biochemical hypoglycemia and help to maintain HbA_{1c} levels at <7.0% compared with standard blood glucose measurement.

In 2009, JDRF conducted a separate, concurrent randomized trial to evaluate the efficacy and safety of CGM in adults with type 1 diabetes who already had successfully achieved HbA_{1c} levels <7.0% with intensive insulin therapy (mostly in CSII therapy). The CGM group was able to maintain HbA_{1c} levels at baseline values. Time per day with glucose levels in the range of 70–180 mg/dl increased significantly. This beneficial effect was maintained in the 6-month extension study [26]. Moreover, all of the other HbA_{1c} outcomes favored the CGM group over the control group.

Hypoglycemia

SAP therapy does not seem to lower the risk of severe hypoglycemia, but several studies have reported decreasing HbA_{1c} levels without increasing the rate of severe hypoglycemia or the time spent in nonsevere hypoglycemia [18, 26, 27].

The threshold-suspend feature of SAPs can minimize the risk of hypoglycemia, interrupting insulin delivery at a preset glucose value. A multicenter open-label RCT on 247 hypoglycemia-prone patients demonstrated that a SAP with a low-glucose suspend function (Medtronic Paradigm Veo System; Medtronic Minimed, Northridge, Calif., USA) reduced nocturnal hypoglycemia without increasing HbA_{1c} or the risk of ketoacidosis [28].

An RCT evaluated the incidence of severe and moderate hypoglycemia with a SAP with the low-glucose suspend function compared with standard insulin pump therapy in 95 patients with type 1 diabetes. After 6 months of treatment, the rates of severe and moderate hypoglycemic episodes decreased from 28 to 16 in the pump-only group versus 175 to 35 in the low-glucose suspension group. The adjusted incidence rate per 100 patient-months was 34.2 (95% CI: 22.0–53.3) for the pump-only group versus 9.5 (95% CI: 5.2–17.4) for the low-glucose suspension group. There was no change in HbA_{1c} in either group [29].

Quality of Life

SAP therapy has the potential to improve diabetes treatment satisfaction and to reduce the perceived magnitude of diabetes-related problems, hypoglycemia fear, and hypoglycemia-avoidant behavior, which are all critical to treatment adherence. Several randomized controlled studies examining QoL in real-time CGM versus conventional treatment found no differences in generic and diabetes-specific QoL scores [30, 31]. Otherwise, separate multiple regression analyses on 334 adult patients and 147 pediatric patients participating in the STAR 3 study demonstrated that most patient perceptions, including overall treatment satisfaction/preference, improved significantly in the SAP therapy arm, especially among adult patients and the caregivers of pediatric patients [32]. Perceived clinical efficacy was a primary determinant of overall treatment satisfaction/preference only for adults, reflecting an emphasis on long-term outcomes in addition to immediate concerns. A recent follow-up study that investigated the metabolic and psychosocial effects of SAP therapy in adults with type 1 diabetes 36 months after the start of therapy substantially confirmed these findings [33]. Healthcare providers could enhance the benefits of therapy by considering patients' perceptions and preferences regarding therapy and by emphasizing the benefits that are most meaningful to each subject.

Pregnancy

Real-time CGM use in pregnancy in women with type 1 diabetes seems promising, but large well-controlled randomized trials are needed to better assess the true impact of this technology on pregnancy. A recent consensus panel of the American Association of Clinical Endocrinologists recommended real-time CGM for all women with type 1 diabetes during pregnancy [34]. However, there have been no trials to evaluate whether real-time CGM actually improves pregnancy outcomes. Murphy et al. [35] recently studied a small group of patients with type 1 diabetes during a 24-hour hospital admission at 12–16 weeks of gestation and again at 28–32 weeks. Insulin infusion rates were calculated using individualized algorithms adjusted manually at 15-min intervals by a research nurse in response to CGM values. They reported excellent overnight euglycemia, but more problematic postprandial control. Clearly, more work is needed before the results can be generalized to a broader group of patients in real-life settings.

Disadvantages of Continuous Subcutaneous Insulin Infusion and Sensor-Augmented Pumps

Some disadvantages have been recognized with CSII therapy. Major concerns when using CSII are pump malfunctioning, needle dislodgement, and catheter occlusion without the patient realizing there is a problem. This can lead to serious consequences, such as severe hyperglycemia. According to Guilhem et al. [36], 232 out of 640 insulin pumps malfunctioned within a median time of 15.1 months. Therefore, this study found a 36% rate of insulin pump failure not due to user errors. According to these authors, complete pump breakdown is the most common event, but failures due to tubing obstruction or leakage at the infusion site are very frequent. Another concern is the risk of epidermal complications, and the most common problem when using the insulin pump is skin infection at the catheter site. Erythema, subcutaneous nodules, or abscesses requiring antibiotic treatment and/or surgical drainage can also develop at the site of injection. Lenhard and Reeves [37] followed 78 children and adolescents and found that 20–21% reported allergic skin reactions, while 29–36% reported skin infections. In order to prevent skin infections, care should be taken to use topical disinfectants before the insertion of the catheter needle and to rotate the catheter every 2–3 days.

Wearing a noticeable mechanical device could affect one's feelings about his or her body image and sense of social acceptance. The public image of being noticed with an insulin pump could cause feelings of being different and less acceptable. Ritholz et al. [38] evaluated psychosocial issues related to diabetes, approaches to self-care, self-perceptions, and social interactions among insulin pump users with type 1 diabetes: women were more concerned than men about body image and social acceptance with pump use. Most of the problems that patients can encounter (e.g. negative body image due to a device attached) with SAPs are the same already experienced with CSII pumps.

While RT-CGM alarms have obvious potential utility in preventing and minimizing hypoglycemia, clinical experience indicates that with some patients, this benefit is counterbalanced by an increased frequency of hypoglycemia due to excessive postprandial bolusing. A major focus of education and follow-up care of the patient using real-time CGM will need to be addressed to reduce this risk.

Cost-Effectiveness

CSII therapy incurs costs for the pump, consumables such as batteries, reservoirs, and infusion sets, and requires specially trained personnel. There are additional costs for education of patients starting pump therapy. Although obviously more expensive than MDI, CSII may be cost-effective in specific situations.

NICE conducted a systematic review of papers on the cost-effectiveness of CSII use and found 11 publications [39]. Except for 2 studies, all publications used the Centre for Outcomes Research (CORE) Diabetes Model, an Internet-based, interactive computer model for determining the long-term health outcomes and economic consequences of implementing different treatment policies or interventions in type 1 and type 2 diabetes mellitus.

Three studies were performed in the UK and showed a gain in quality-adjusted life-years (QALYs) for people receiving CSII compared with MDI therapy at an increased cost. The incremental cost-effectiveness ratios for CSII compared with MDI therapy were GBP 34,330 per QALY gained for the lower value of decrease in HbA_{1c} levels, GBP 16,842 per QALY gained for the upper value of decrease in HbA_{1c} levels (–1.29%), and GBP 22,897 per QALY gained for the intermediate decrease in HbA_{1c} levels. NICE noted that only pronounced decreases in HbA_{1c} levels, contingent on a baseline level well above 7.5% on optimized MDI treatment, brought the incremental cost-effectiveness ratios down to a level considered acceptable.

Recently the cost-effectiveness of SAP therapy was evaluated combining estimates from the STAR 3 trial and the literature to populate the CORE Diabetes Model [40]. For a 65% use of 3-day and 6-day sensors, the incremental cost-effectiveness ratios were USD 229,675 per QALY (95% CI: 139,071–720,865) and USD 168,104 per QALY (95% CI: 102,819–523,161), respectively. The ratios ranged from USD 69,837 to 211,113 per QALY with different strategies for incorporating utility benefits resulting from less fear of hypoglycemia with SAP therapy. The authors concluded that despite superior clinical benefits of SAPs compared with MDI, SAP therapy does not appear to be economically attractive in the USA for adults with type 1 diabetes in its current state of development. However, further clinical developments that reduce disposable costs of the system could significantly improve its economic attractiveness.

Indications

The literature reports many reasons for starting CSII such as unsatisfactory metabolic control, a marked dawn phenomenon, recurrent ketoacidosis, severe hypoglycemia, high HbA_{1c}, frequent or unpredictable hypoglycemia during optimized MDI, hypoglycemia unawareness, low insulin requirement, unpredictable swings in blood glucose levels, personal preference, desire for fewer injections, desire for a better QoL, and pregnancy. However, CSII has elevated costs. The cost-effectiveness analysis suggests reserving the use of pump therapy for indications for which there is robust evidence of benefit. NICE recommends CSII therapy as a treatment option for adults with type 1 diabetes mellitus provided that attempts to achieve target HbA_{1c} levels with MDI result in the person experiencing disabling hypoglycemia, or HbA_{1c} levels have remained high (i.e. ≥8.5%) on MDI therapy (including, if appropriate, the use of long-acting insulin analogues) despite a high level of care [39].

With regard to SAP therapy, reimbursement exists for certain clinical indications in some European countries. A recent commentary described the different reimbursement situations across Europe for this innovative but costly technology as a prelude to establishing more uniform use. According to many healthcare professionals and potential CGM users, national health services and health insurance organizations are reluctant to reimburse CGM. In summary, the main indications for reimbursement are bad metabolic control generally defined as HbA_{1c} ≥8%, severe hypoglycemia, frequent hypoglycemic events, unawareness hypoglycemia, and before and during pregnancy [41].

Conclusions

Both RCTs and observational studies have found lower HbA_{1c} levels, less severe hypoglycemic episodes, and a better QoL in CSII-treated adults with type 1 diabetes with respect to MDI treatment. In RCTs, the differences in favor of CSII were smaller than in observational studies. CSII requires care by skilled professionals, careful selection of patients, meticulous patient monitoring, and thorough patient education. Moreover, candidates for CSII must be strongly motivated to improve glucose control and be willing to work with their healthcare provider in assuming substantial responsibility for their day-to-day care. Therefore, in this context, RCTs do not represent the best methodology for evaluating the efficacy of CSII treatment in routine clinical practice. Although obviously more expensive than MDI, CSII may be cost-effective in specific situations such as elevated HbA_{1c} levels or continued disabling hypoglycemia despite optimized MDI therapy.

CGM can improve CSII. Although CGM is not a treatment in itself, it is a technology that increases information. The best results with SAPs can be expected in patients who use the sensor frequently, draw adequate conclusions from the data, and make immediate therapeutic decisions. It is essential that both patients and clinicians receive adequate training in interpreting and responding to CGM data. Randomized controlled studies have provided evidence that SAPs can improve HbA_{1c} results without increasing severe hypoglycemic episodes in patients with type 1 diabetes with elevated baseline HbA_{1c}, and that the frequency and duration of hypoglycemic events can be reduced in patients with satisfactory baseline HbA_{1c}, increasing treatment satisfaction.

References

1 Gross TM, Kayne D, King A, Rother C, Juth S: A bolus calculator is an effective means of controlling postprandial glycemia in patients on insulin pump therapy. Diabetes Technol Ther 2004;5:365–369.

2 NHS National Institute for Health and Clinical Excellence: Continuous Subcutaneous Insulin Infusion for the Treatment of Diabetes Mellitus. NICE Technol Appraisal Guidance. London, NICE, 2011, vol 151, pp 1–30.

3 Yeh HC, Brown TT, Maruthur N, Ranasinghe P, Berger Z, Suh YD, Wilson LM, Haberl EB, Brick J, Bass EB, Golden SH: Comparative effectiveness and safety of methods of insulin delivery and glucose monitoring for diabetes mellitus: a systematic review and meta-analysis. Ann Intern Med 2012;157:336–347.

4 Fahlén M, Eliasson B, Oden A: Optimization of basal insulin delivery in type 1 diabetes: a retrospective study on the use of continuous subcutaneous insulin infusion and insulin glargine. Diabet Med 2005;22: 382–386.

5 Ceriello A: The emerging role of post-prandial hyperglycaemic spikes in the pathogenesis of diabetic complications. Diabet Med 1998;15:188–193.

6 Bruttomesso D, Crazzolara D, Maran A, Costa S, Dal Pos M, Girelli A, Lepore G, Aragona M, Iori E, Valentini U, Del Prato S, Tiengo A, Buhr A, Trevisan R, Baritussio A: In type 1 diabetic patients with good glycaemic control, blood glucose variability is lower during continuous subcutaneous insulin infusion than during multiple daily injections with insulin glargine. Diabet Med 2008;25:326–332.

7 Pickup JC, Sutton AJ: Severe hypoglycaemia and glycaemic control in type 1 diabetes: meta-analysis of multiple daily insulin injections compared with continuous subcutaneous insulin infusion. Diabet Med 2008;25:765–774.

8 Fatourechi MM, Kudva YC, Murad MH, Elamin MB, Tabini CC, Montori VM: Clinical review: hypoglycemia with intensive insulin therapy: a systematic review and meta-analyses of randomized trials of continuous subcutaneous insulin infusion versus multiple daily injections. J Clin Endocrinol Metab 2009;94:729–740.

9 Lepore G, Bruttomesso D, Bonomo M, Dodesini AR, Costa S, Meneghini E, Corsi A, Nosari I, Trevisan: Continuous subcutaneous insulin infusion is more effective than multiple daily insulin injections in preventing albumin excretion rate increase in type 1 diabetic patients. Diabet Med 2009;26:602–608.

10 Hoogma RP, Hammond PJ, Gomis R, Kerr D, Bruttomesso D, Bouter KP, Wiefels KJ, de la Calle H, Schweitzer DH, Pfohl M, Torlone E, Krinelke LG, Bolli GB; 5-Nations Study Group: Comparison of the effects of continuous subcutaneous insulin infusion (CSII) and NPH-based multiple daily insulin injections (MDI) on glycaemic control and quality of life: results of the 5-Nations trial. Diabet Med 2006;23: 141–147.

11 Farrar D, Tuffnell DJ, West J: Continuous subcutaneous insulin infusion versus multiple daily injections of insulin for pregnant women with diabetes. Cochrane Database Syst Rev 2007;3:CD005542.

12 Bruttomesso D, Bonomo M, Costa S, Dal Pos M, Di Cianni G, Pellicano F, Vitacolonna E, Dodesini AR, Tonutti L, Lapolla A, Di Benedetto A, Torlone E: Type 1 diabetes control and pregnancy outcomes in women treated with continuous subcutaneous insulin infusion (CSII) or with insulin glargine and multiple daily injections of rapid-acting insulin analogues (glargine-MDI). Diabetes Metab 2011;37: 426–431.

13 Gonzàlez-Romero S, Gonzàlez-Molero I, Fernàndez-Abellàn M, Dominguez-Lòpez ME, Ruiz-de-Adana S, Olveira G, Soriguer F: Continuous subcutaneous insulin infusion versus multiple daily injections in pregnant women with type 1 diabetes. Diabetes Technol Ther 2010;12:263–269.

14 Hirsch IB, Armstrong D, Bergenstal R, Buckingham B, Childs B, Clarke WL, Peters A, Wolpert H: Clinical application of emerging sensor technologies in diabetes management: consensus guidelines for continuous glucose monitoring (CGM). Diabetes Technol Ther 2008;10:232–245.

15 Diabetes Research in Children Network (DirecNet) Study Group: Use of the DirecNet Applied Treatment Algorithm (DATA) for diabetes management with a real-time continuous glucose monitor (the FreeStyle Navigator). Pediatr Diabetes 2008;9:142–147.

16 Battelino T, Conget I, Olsen B, Schütz-Fuhrmann I, Hommel E, Hoogma R, Schierloh U, Sulli N, Bolinder J; Switch Study Group: The use and efficacy of continuous glucose monitoring in type 1 diabetes treated with insulin pump therapy: a randomised controlled trial. Diabetologia 2012;55:3155–3162.

17 Beck RW, Buckingham B, Miller K, Wolpert H, Xing D, Block JM, Chase HP, Hirsch I, Kollman C, Laffel L, Lawrence JM, Milszewski K, Ruedy KJ, Tamborlane WV: Factors predictive of use and of benefit from continuous glucose monitoring in type 1 diabetes. Diabetes Care 2009;32:1947–1953.

18 Bergenstal RM, Tamborlane WV, Ahmann A, Buse JB, Dailey G, Davis SN, Joyce C, Peoples T, Perkins BA, Welsh JB, Willi SM, Wood MA; STAR 3 Study Group: Effectiveness of sensor-augmented insulin-pump therapy in type 1 diabetes. N Engl J Med 2010; 363:311–320.
19 Scaramuzza AE, Iafusco D, Rabbone I, Bonfanti R, Lombardo F, Schiaffini R, Buono P, Toni S, Cherubini V, Zuccotti GV; Diabetes Study Group of the Italian Society of Paediatric Endocrinology and Diabetology: Use of integrated real-time continuous glucose monitoring/insulin pump system in children and adolescents with type 1 diabetes: a 3-year follow-up study. Diabetes Technol Ther 2011;13: 99–103.
20 Battelino T, Phillip M, Bratina N, Nimri R, Oskarsson P, Bolinder J: Effect of continuous glucose monitoring on hypoglycemia in type 1 diabetes. Diabetes Care 2011;34:795–800.
21 Larson NS, Pinsker JE: The role of continuous glucose monitoring in the care of children with type 1 diabetes. Int J Pediatr Endocrinol 2013;2013:8.
22 Hirsch IB, Abelseth J, Bode BW, Fischer JS, Kaufman FR, Mastrototaro J, Parkin CG, Wolpert HA, Buckingham BA: Sensor-augmented insulin pump therapy: results of the first randomized treat-to-target study. Diabetes Technol Ther 2008; 10:377–383.
23 Pickup JC, Sutton AJ: Severe hypoglycemia and glycemic control in type 1 diabetes: meta-analysis of multiple daily insulin injections compared with continuous subcutaneous insulin infusion. Diabet Med 2008;25:765–774.
24 Golden SH, Sapir TJ: Methods for insulin delivery and glucose monitoring: comparative effectiveness. Manag Care Pharm 2012;18(Suppl 6):S1–S17.
25 Klonoff DC, Buckingham B, Christiansen JS, Montori VM, Tamborlane WV, Vigersky RA, Wolpert H; Endocrine Society: Continuous glucose monitoring: an Endocrine Society Clinical Practice Guideline. J Clin Endocrinol Metab 2011;96: 2968–2979.
26 The Juvenile Diabetes Research Foundation Continuous Glucose Monitoring Study Group: Sustained benefit of continuous glucose monitoring on A_{1C}, glucose profiles, and hypoglycemia in adults with type 1 diabetes. Diabetes Care 2009;32:2047–2049.
27 Hermanides J, Nørgaard K, Bruttomesso D, Mathieu C, Frid A, Dayan CM, Diem P, Fermon C, Wentholt IM, Hoekstra JB, DeVries JH: Sensor-augmented pump therapy lowers HbA(1c) in suboptimally controlled type 1 diabetes; a randomized controlled trial. Diabet Med 2011;28:1158–1167.
28 Bergenstal RM, Klonoff DC, Garg SK, Bode BW, Meredith M, Slover RH, Ahmann AJ, Welsh JB, Lee SW, Kaufman FR; ASPIRE In-Home Study Group: Threshold-based insulin-pump interruption for reduction of hypoglycemia. N Engl J Med 2013;369: 224–232.
29 Ly TT, Nicholas JA, Retterath A, Lim EM, Davis EA, Jones TW: Effect of sensor-augmented insulin pump therapy and automated insulin suspension vs standard insulin pump therapy on hypoglycemia in patients with type 1 diabetes: a randomized clinical trial. JAMA 2013;310:1240–1247.
30 Juvenile Diabetes Research Foundation Continuous Glucose Monitoring Study Group, Beck RW, Lawrence JM, Laffel L, Wysocki T, Xing D, Huang ES, Ives B, Kollman C, Lee J, Ruedy KJ, Tamborlane WV: Quality-of-life measures in children and adults with type 1 diabetes: Juvenile Diabetes Research Foundation Continuous Glucose Monitoring Randomized Trial. Diabetes Care 2010;33:2175–2177.
31 Mauras N, Beck R, Xing D, Ruedy K, Buckingham B, Tansey M, White NH, Weinzimer SA, Tamborlane W, Kollman C; Diabetes Research in Children Network (DirecNet) Study Group: A randomized clinical trial to assess the efficacy and safety of real-time continuous glucose monitoring in the management of type 1 diabetes in young children aged 4 to <10 years. Diabetes Care 2012;35:204–210.
32 Peyrot M, Rubin RR; STAR 3 Study Group: Treatment satisfaction in the Sensor-Augmented Pump Therapy for A_{1C} Reduction 3 (STAR 3) trial. Diabet Med 2013;30:464–467.
33 Schmidt S, Nørgaard K: Sensor-augmented pump therapy at 36 months. Diabetes Technol Ther 2012; 14:377–383.
34 Blevins TC, Bode BW, Garg SK, Grunberger G, Hirsch IB, Jovanovic L, Nardacci E, Orzeck EA, Roberts VL, Tamborlane WV; AACE Continuous Glucose Monitoring Task Force, Rothermel C: Statement by the American Association of Clinical Endocrinologists Consensus Panel on continuous glucose monitoring. Endocr Pract 2010;16:730–745.
35 Murphy HR, Elleri D, Allen JM, Harris J, Simmons D, Rayman G, Temple R, Dunger DB, Haidar A, Nodale M, Wilinska ME, Hovorka R: Closed-loop insulin delivery during pregnancy complicated by type 1 diabetes. Diabetes Care 2011;34:406–411.
36 Guilhem I, Balkau B, Lecordier F, Malécot JM, Elbadii S, Leguerrier AM, Poirier JY, Derrien C, Bonnet F: Insulin pump failures are still frequent: a prospective study over 6 years from 2001 to 2007. Diabetologia 2009;52:2662–2664.
37 Lenhard MJ, Reeves GD: Continuous subcutaneous insulin infusion: a comprehensive review of insulin pump therapy. Arch Intern Med 2001;161:2293–2300.

38 Ritholz MD, Smaldone A, Lee J, Castillo A, Wolpert H, Veinger K: Perceptions of psychosocial factors and the insulin pump. Diabetes Care 2007;30:549–554.

39 National Institute for Clinical Excellence (NICE): Guidance on the Use of Continuous Subcutaneous Insulin Infusion for the Treatment of Diabetes Mellitus (review of Technology Appraisal Guidance No. 57). NICE Technology Appraisal Guidance 151. London, NICE, 2008.

40 Kamble S, Schulman KA, Reed SD: Cost-effectiveness of sensor-augmented pump therapy in adults with type 1 diabetes in the United States. Value Health 2012;15:632–638.

41 Heinemann L, Franc S, Phillip M, Battelino T, Ampudia-Blasco FJ, Bolinder J, Diem P, Pickup J, De Vries H: Reimbursement for continuous glucose monitoring: a European view. J Diabetes Sci Technol 2012;6:1498–1502.

Dr. Giuseppe Lepore
USC Malattie Endocrine e Diabetologia
Piazza OMS 1
IT–24126 Bergamo (Italy)
E-Mail glepore@hpg23.it

Bruttomesso D, Grassi G (eds): Technological Advances in the Treatment of Type 1 Diabetes.
Front Diabetes. Basel, Karger, 2015, vol 24, pp 143–150 (DOI: 10.1159/000363488)

Continuous Subcutaneous Insulin Infusion and Sensor-Augmented Pump Therapy in Children and Adolescents

Ivana Rabbone[a] · Giulio Frontino[b] · Riccardo Bonfanti[b]

[a]Department of Pediatrics, Universiy of Turin, Turin, and [b]Pediatric Diabetologic Unit, Scientific Institute San Raffaele, Milan, Italy

Abstract

Continuous subcutaneous insulin infusion (CSII) therapy is safe and effective in all age groups of type 1 diabetic patients. It may be elective therapy in neonatal diabetes and in preschool patients. Randomized trials in children and adolescents in CSII therapy have shown a significant improvement in treatment satisfaction without a substantial change in glycosylated hemoglobin A_{1c} (HbA_{1c}). Elevated levels of HbA_{1c} not only at the start of CSII, but also during the follow-up, may be an important indicator of pump discontinuation. Sensor-augmented pump therapy (SAP) has a more beneficial effect in reducing HbA_{1c} values, hyperglycemic excursions, and glycemic variability in children and adolescents with type 1 diabetes. Data on the safety and feasibility of SAP in preschool children have also been published. The low glucose suspend (LGS) function and its evolution, the predictive LGS, represent semiautomated processes able to prevent severe hypoglycemic events and extreme glucose fluctuations also in type 1 diabetes children and adolescents.

Over the last 5 years, technology has made a significant impact on insulin therapy in children and adolescents. This is represented first and foremost by the use of continuous subcutaneous insulin infusion (CSII) in all age groups, and secondly by the recent introduction of continuous glucose monitoring systems (CGMS). CSII is an effective, well-tolerated, and safe therapy, and its use in groups of younger patients is increasing, although it requires a high level of commitment.

Neonatal Diabetes

Neonatal diabetes is a rare pediatric disease. There is very limited data regarding the optimal insulin treatment in these patients [1]. However, pump therapy in newborns could be considered the gold standard of insulin therapy by providing more flexibility in the administration of very small insulin doses, especially in the context of unpredictable feeding patterns and frequent changes in nutrient intake. In this rare form of diabetes mellitus, CSII is safe and effective in obtaining adequate metabolic control with no described episodes of diabetic ketoacidosis or severe hypoglycemia. Furthermore, in cases of identified Kir 6.2 mutations which result in a diagnosis of permanent neonatal diabetes mellitus, CSII may represent a useful tool when switching from insulin to glibenclamide treatment. The possibility to administer minute insulin doses in case of hyperglycemia may reduce the risk of diabetic ketoacidosis while shifting from one treatment to the other [2].

Evidence-Based Medicine

Studies assessing CSII use in toddlers, preschool children, and adolescents are helpful in underlining some of the benefits and complications associated with CSII use [3, 4]. A recent meta-analysis comparing CSII and multiple daily injections (MDI) demonstrated a statistically significant reduction (–0.3%) in glycosylated hemoglobin A_{1c} (HbA_{1c}) in those using CSII compared to that of the MDI population [5]. A randomized trial in children and adolescents (7–17 years of age) showed a significant improvement in treatment satisfaction without a substantial change in HbA_{1c} [6]. Insulin pump therapy is an option for many patients who aim to increase their treatment satisfaction. A recent Italian multicenter study (VIPKIDS) showed that CSII in adolescents with type 1 diabetes was associated with a higher health-related quality of life than those using MDI [7].

Pump Initiation and Patient Selection

Discussing the best therapeutic options with the patients and their families and the improvement of diabetes educational resources have been important for limiting the economic burdens derived from the management of one of the most common chronic diseases in the world. Over time, starting pump therapy at an early disease stage appears to have no added benefit for glycemic control than starting later. The timing of CSII initiation should be tailored to the individual patient by the diabetes care team [8]. Children and adolescents have a circadian distribution of insulin needs according to different ages. Therefore, prediction of an optimal pattern a priori can improve initiation and clinical follow-up of CSII in these

Table 1. Indications for pump use in children of different ages

Preschool and school-age children
Recurrent hypoglycemia
Wide fluctuations in blood glucose levels
Very low insulin needs and difficulty in splitting the dose
Needle phobia
Puberty and adolescence
Dawn phenomenon
Insulin resistance
Recurrent hypoglycemia
Impaired metabolic control
Improvement of quality of life

Table 2. Characteristics of Italian hospitals qualified and licensed to prescribe CSII

Pediatric diabetes team specialized in using and teaching CSII therapy
Medical availability 24 h/day and 7 days/week
Collaboration among all the medical figures involved in the care of a child with a pump (i.e. general practitioner, family pediatrician, ER doctors, etc.)

patients [9]. It is therefore important to carefully select patient candidates (and caregivers when considering preschool- and school-aged children) for CSII therapy.

International and Italian Guidelines

According to international recommendations [10], the indications to start CSII therapy are represented by the following: recurrent severe hypoglycemia, wide fluctuations in blood glucose levels regardless of HbA_{1c}, suboptimal diabetes control, microvascular complications and/or risk factors for macrovascular complications, and adequate metabolic control but with an insulin regimen that compromises lifestyle. In the Italian recommendations for insulin pump use in children [11], specific indications according to patient age were taken into consideration (table 1). The criteria that qualify a patient as a candidate for pump therapy may in fact differ as every age may have different metabolic characteristics. In very young children the main risk is hypoglycemia, while in adolescents the dawn phenomenon and/or insulin resistance are more characteristic [9, 12]. Beyond patient indications, both the diabetes team (table 2) and patient/family prerequisites (table 3) have to be assessed. The main contraindication to CSII therapy is the lack of one of the characteristics specified in tables 2 and 3, regardless of the indications.

Table 3. Patient/family characteristics of the patients who qualified as candidates for pump therapy

Consent to wear the pump
Motivation of patient and family
Education about therapy and glycemic control
Willingness to check blood sugar levels often

Dropouts

When taking costs into consideration, especially in a period of crisis for the healthcare economy, it is essential to avoid dropouts. Female gender, females older than 10 years, and poor metabolic control at pump initiation are associated with a higher risk for pump discontinuation [13]. HbA_{1c} not only at the start of CSII, but also during follow-up, may be an important indicator which may aid in identifying patients at greater risk of discontinuing CSII therapy [14]. Nevertheless, discontinuation of CSII should be considered if contraindications should arise during follow-up.

Sensor-Augmented Pump Therapy

Sensor-augmented pump therapy (SAP) is represented by the contemporary use of CSII and CGMS in order to further improve glucose control by employing both technologies. While self-monitoring of blood glucose can only assess single instantaneous glucose values, SAP allows the patient to also evaluate glucose trends and adjust insulin administration accordingly.

Evidence-Based Medicine

Although SAP therapy has been introduced only recently, several controlled trials and meta-analyses have been published on this topic, such as a recent report regarding a 3-year survey in Italian patients [15]. In particular, most recent reports from the Agency for Healthcare Research and Quality (AHRQ) report that SAP use in children and adolescents improves HbA_{1c} by 0.6% with a reduction of the time spent in a hypoglycemic state [16]. This is a significant achievement in insulin therapy: if the patient is able to adequately use an SAP, near normalization of glucose values (HbA_{1c} 6–6.5%) may be achieved with a significant reduction in hypoglycemic events (compared to the DCCT/EDIC report) [17]. Moreover, the STAR3 group has published a report involving children and adolescents confirming the beneficial effect of SAP therapy in reducing HbA_{1c} values, hyperglycemic excursions, and glucose variability in a rapid and safe manner [18].

SAP therapy has been used in children and adolescents from diabetes onset in the ONSET Study. This study involved 154 patients: 62 patients belonged to the group employing a SAP system and 69 patients to the group performing conventional insulin pump therapy with self-monitoring of blood glucose. At 24 months of treatment, 52.4% continued to use the SAP system with no difference in terms of metabolic control. Children in the SAP group showed a significant but small difference in the rate of fall of C-peptide secretion [19].

International Guidelines

International and national guidelines have been published for the use of SAP therapy in children and adolescents [20, 21]. SAP therapy has an indication in the following patients:

- Children and adolescents with HbA_{1c} above target with a correctly applied intensive insulin therapy
- Children and adolescents with HbA_{1c} <7% in order to maintain metabolic control to reduce hypoglycemic risk
- Children and adolescents with frequent severe hypoglycemic events and/or hypoglycemia unawareness

SAP therapy has been used in very young children with diabetes (<6 years of age). Frontino et al. [22] have published data on the safety and feasibility of SAPs in preschool children, confirming that SAP therapy is a feasible therapeutic option in these children. In this study, preschool children were able to use a SAP continuously for 6 months. Furthermore, unpublished follow-up data from the same group has shown continuous SAP compliance for up to 12 months (40% of children) with adequate metabolic control and very few episodes of hypoglycemia, confirming data obtained from older patients.

Limiting Factors

The implementation of this technology is currently constrained due to several significantly limiting factors:

- Compliance: a limited percentage of patients is able to use SAP therapy in the medium/long-term. No more than 40% of patients are able to use SAP for more than 6 months, and this percentage decreases especially in adolescent patients. Compliance is essential as it is widely demonstrated that CGMS are to be used at least 6 days a week in order to significantly improve metabolic control.
- Lag time: current glucose sensors show a delay in glucose determination of at least 5–15 min. The lag time combined with a response in insulin absorption of at least 1 h determine a significant delay in any response of the SAP system to rapid glucose oscillations.

- Dimension: the size and weight of the components of SAP therapy (CSII and CGMS) are still significant for young children and adolescents. As suggested by an ISPAD report, it is necessary to 'rethink' the system for pediatric use [21].
- Burnout: an adequately used SAP requires a truly motivated patients and parents. The need to process plenty of information, the frequent patient-device interaction, potentially disturbing alarms, and several advanced functions may be overwhelming and lead the patient to suspend SAP therapy. At present, the medium-term benefits of SAP are likely not sufficient to overcome the devices' demands on the patient.
- Cost: SAP therapy bears important costs for healthcare systems. The yearly expenses for SAP therapy are 50 times greater than MDI therapy. This represents a significant problem in times of economic crisis.
- A recent German publication showed that <4% of patients use SAP therapy continuously [23]. However, other reports have shown that 30% of patients are compliant at 1 year of therapy [24]. Considering the potential benefits of this technology, all these limiting factors should be addressed in order to achieve more widespread use of SAP therapy.

Hypoglycemia Prevention

The next step in the development of SAP technology is related to improving synergy between CSII and CGMS by means of partial or continuous control algorithms.

The low glucose suspend (LGS) function represents the first semiautomated process to be implemented in SAP therapy for the prevention of severe hypoglycemic events. It is well-known that hypoglycemia may determine seizures, coma, or death in bed secondary to cardiac arrhythmia caused by hypoglycemia itself. Due to these potentially critical consequences, a fear of hypoglycemia may develop, representing a major limiting factor in achieving metabolic control.

Danne et al. [25] have reported that the use of LGS for 6 weeks in a cohort of 21 patients with type 1 diabetes (mean age: 10.8 years) was able to significantly reduce hypoglycemic excursions: the time spent in a hypoglycemic state was reduced from 101 to 58 min/day, without a significant modification in mean glucose.

The evolution of this system is represented by predictive LGS, with a suspension of insulin delivery for 30 min in case of a predicted hypoglycemia in the subsequent 30 min. Differently from LGS, the purpose of this function is to prevent the hypoglycemic event per se [26].

The control-to-range algorithm, defined as sensor-guided insulin treatment optimizing glycemia within a predefined target range by preventing extreme glucose fluctuations, represents a further technological step forward. Clinical trials to assess the feasibility of this algorithm in a 'at-home' setting are promising and under way. The creation of newer efficient predictive algorithms and accurate glucose sensors represent a closer move towards the development of an artificial pancreas, one of the most relevant achievements of diabetes technology research and indeed the future of insulin therapy.

Conclusions

Intensive basal-bolus insulin therapy is the best treatment for type 1 diabetes patients in all age groups. SAP more than CSII therapy represents the gold standard for achieving the best glycemic control and the lowest glycemic variability. Therefore, SAP or CSII represent the first therapeutic choice in newborns and preschool diabetic children, and are worthy alternatives for older children and adolescents.

References

1 Bharucha T, Brown J, McDonnell C, Gebert R, McDougall P, Cameron F, Werther G, Zacharin M: Neonatal diabetes mellitus: Insulin pump as an alternative management strategy. J Paediatr Child Health 2005;41:522–526.

2 Olinder AL, Kernell A, Smide B: Treatment with CSII in two infants with neonatal diabetes mellitus. Pediatr Diabetes 2006;7:284–288.

3 Berghaeuser MA, Kapellen T, Heidtmann B, Haberland H, Klinkert C, Holl RW: Continuous subcutaneous insulin infusion in toddlers starting at diagnosis of type 1 diabetes mellitus. A multicenter analysis of 104 patients from 63 centres in Germany and Austria. Pediatric Diabetes 2008;9:590–595.

4 Maniatisa K, Klingensmith GJ, Sloverr H, Mowry CJ, Chase HP: Continuous subcutaneous insulin infusion therapy for children and adolescents: an option for routine diabetes care. Pediatrics 2001;107:351–356.

5 Misso ML, Egberts KJ, Page M, O'Connor D, Shaw J: Continuous subcutaneous insulin infusion (CSII) versus multiple insulin injections for type 1 diabetes mellitus. Cochrane Database Syst Rev 2010;1: CD005103.

6 Doyle EA, Weinzimer SA, Steffen AT, Ahern JAH, Vincent M, Tamborlane WV: A randomized, prospective trial comparing the efficacy of continuous subcutaneous insulin infusion with multiple daily injections using insulin glargine. Diabetes Care 2004;27:1554–1558.

7 Cherubini V, Gesuita R, Bonfanti R, Franzese A, Frongia AP, Iafusco D, Iannilli A, Lombardo F, Rabbone I, Salvatoni A, Scaramuzza A, Schiaffini R, Sulli N, Toni S, Tumini S, Mosca A, Carle F; VIPKIDS Study Group: Health-related quality of life and treatment preferences in adolescents with type 1 diabetes. The VIPKIDS study. Acta Diabetol 2014;51:43–51.

8 Shalitin S, Lahav-Ritte T, Lebenthal Y, Devries L, Phillip M: Does the timing of insulin pump therapy initiation after type 1 diabetes onset have an impact on glycemic control? Diabetes Technol Ther 2012; 14:389–397.

9 Holterhus PM, Bokelmann J, Riepe F, Heidtmann B, Wagner V, Rami-Merhar B, Kapellen T, Raile K, Quester W, Holl RW; German/Austrian DPV-Initiative and the German Pediatric CSII Working Group: Predicting the optimal basal insulin infusion pattern in children and adolescents on insulin pumps. Diabetes Care 2013;36:1507–1511.

10 Phillip M, Battelino T, Rodriguez H, Danne T, Kaufman F: Use of insulin pump therapy in the pediatric age-group. Diabetes Care 2007;30:1653–1662.

11 Pinelli L, Rabbone I, Salardi S, Toni S, Scaramuzza A, Bonfanti R, Cherubini V, Franzese A, Frongia AP, Lafusco D, Sulli N, Tumini S, Curto O, Miassimelli M; Diabetes Study Group of the Italian Society of Paediatric Endocrinology and Diabetology: Insulin pump therapy in children and adolescents with type 1 diabetes: the Italian viewpoint. Acta Biomed 2008; 79:57–64.

12 Rabbone I, Bobbio A, Berger K, Trada M, Sacchetti C, Cerutti F: Age-related differences in metabolic response to continuous subcutaneous insulin infusion in pre-pubertal and pubertal children with type 1 diabetes mellitus. J Endocrinol Invest 2007;30:477–483.

13 De Vries L, Grushka Y, Lebenthal Y, Shalitin S, Phillip M: Factors associated with increased risk of insulin pump discontinuation in pediatric patients with type 1 diabetes. Pediatr Diabetes 2011;12:506–512.

14 Lombardo F, Scaramuzza A, Iafusco D: Failure of glycated hemoglobin drop after continuous subcutaneous insulin infusion initiation may indicate patients who discontinue: a 4-year follow-up study in children and adolescents with type 1 diabetes. Acta Diabetol 2012;49:S99–S105.

15 Scaramuzza A, Iafusco D, Rabbone I, Bonfanti R, Lombardo F, Schiaffini R, Buono P, Toni S, Cherubini V, Zuccotti GV: Use of integrated real time continuous glucose monitoring/insulin pump system in children and adolescents with type 1 diabetes: a 3-year follow-up study. Diabetes Technol Ther 2011; 13:99–103.

16 Yeh HC, Brown TT, Maruthur R, Ranasinghe P, Berger Z, Suh YD, Wilson NM, Haberl EB, Bass EB, Brick J, Golstein SH: Comparative effectiveness and safety of methods of insulin delivery and glucose monitoring for diabetes mellitus: a systematic review and meta-analysis. Ann Intern Med 2012;157:336–347.

17 White NH, Cleary PA, Dabms W, Golstein D, Malone J, Tamborlane WV: Beneficial effect of intensive therapy of diabetes during adolescence: outcomes after the conclusion of Diabetes Control and Complication Trial (DCCT). J Pediatr 2001;139: 804–812.

18 Slover RH, Welsh JB, Criego A, Weinzimer SA, Willi SM, Wood A, Tamborlane WV: Effectiveness of sensor-augmented pump therapy in children and adolescents with type 1 diabetes in STAR3 study. Pediatr Diabetes 2012;13:6–11.

19 Kordonouri O, Hartmann E, Pankowska E, Rami B, Kapellen T, Coutant R, Lange K, Danne T: Sensor augmented pump from the onset of type 1 diabetes: late follow-up results of the Pediatric Onset Study. Pediatr Diabetes 2012;13:515–518.

20 Bonfanti R, Buono P, Cardella F, Cherubini V, D'Annunzio G, Frezza A, Frongia P, Iafusco D, Lombardo F, Marinaro A, Moniciotti C, Rabbone V, Scaramuzza A, Schiaffini R, Toni S, Tumini S, Zucchini S: Consensus guidelines: raccomandazioni per l'autominitoraggio e l'autocontrollo in bambini ed adolescenti con diabete di tipo 1. Acta Biomedica 2011;82:5–46.

21 Phillip M, Danne T, Shatlin S, Buckingham B, Laffel l, Tamborlane W, Battelino T: Use of continuous glucose monitoring in children and adolescents. Pediatr Diabetes 2012;13:215–228.

22 Frontino G, Bonfanti R, Scaramuzza A, Rabbone I, Meschi F, Rigamonti A, Battaglino R, Favalli V, Bonura C, Scicignano S, Gioia E, Zuccotti GV, Cerutti F, Chiumello G: Sensor-augmented pump therapy in very young children with type 1 diabetes: an efficacy and feasibility observational study. Diabetes Technol Ther 2012;14:762–764.

23 Ludwing-Seibold PH, Holder M, Rami B, Raile K, Heidtmann D, Holl RW; DPV Science Initiative; German Working Group for insulin pump treatment in pediatric patients; German BMBF Competence Network Diabetes: Continuous glucose monitoring in children, adolescents, and adults with type 1 diabetes mellitus: analysis from the prospective DPV diabetes documentation and quality management system from Germany and Austria. Pediatr Diabetes 2012;13:12–14.

24 Norggard K, Scaramuzza A, Bratina N, Lalic NM, Jaroz-Chobot P, Kokcis P, Jasinskiene E, de Block C, Carrette O, Castenada J, Cohen O: Routine sensor-augmented pump therapy in type 1 diabetes: the INTERPRET study. Diabetes Technol Ther 2013;15: 273–280.

25 Danne T, Kordonouri O, Holder M, Haberland H, Golemborsky S, Remus K, Blasig S, Wadien T, Zierov S, Hartman R, Thomas A: Prevention of hypoglycaemia by using low glucose suspend function in sensor-augmented pump therapy. Diabetes Technol Ther 2011;13:1129–1134.

26 Buckingham BA, Cameron F, Calhoun P, Maahs M, Wilson DM, Chase HP, Baquette BW, Lum J, Sibayan J, Beck RW, Kollman C: Outpatient safety assessment of in-home predictive low glucose suspend system with type 1 diabetes subjects at risk of nocturnal hypoglycemia. Diabetes Tech Therap 2013;15:622–627.

Ivana Rabbone, MD
Department of Pediatrics, University of Turin
Piazza Polonia 94
IT–10126 Turin (Italy)
E-Mail ivana.rabbone@unito.it

Bruttomesso D, Grassi G (eds): Technological Advances in the Treatment of Type 1 Diabetes.
Front Diabetes. Basel, Karger, 2015, vol 24, pp 151–165 (DOI: 10.1159/000363511)

Predictive Low Glucose Suspend: An Option for Routine Outpatient Care

Thomas Danne[a] · Olga Kordonouri[a] · Andreas Thomas[b]

[a]Children's Hospital auf der Bult, Hannover, and [b]Medtronic GmbH, Meerbusch, Germany

Abstract

In type 1 diabetes, severe hypoglycemia is a barrier to optimal metabolic control. The combination of a continuous glucose sensor and an insulin pump with a mechanism of automatic shut-off in the presence of low glucose values [low glucose suspend (LGS)] can be used to reduce the risk of hypoglycemia. In a prospective study, we investigated the effect of the LGS algorithm on the frequency of hypoglycemic episodes in children and adolescents with type 1 diabetes under real-life conditions. We found that 2-hour insulin shut-off increased glucose levels by approximately 35 mg/dl/h and significantly decreased the number of hypoglycemic episodes. Reactive ketoacidosis was not detected, even in the presence of serious patient errors (e.g. calibration-associated errors). The ASPIRE (Automation to Simulate Pancreatic Insulin Response) study showed that these conclusions can be extended to adult patients. As children are at greatest risk for hypoglycemia, it is important to study the safety and efficacy of predictive LGS in this population.

Hypoglycemia, besides being frightening, is a major obstacle in the achievement of euglycemia and the prevention of long-term complications. The Diabetes Control and Complications Trial (DCCT) convincingly established a link between tight glucose control and avoidance of long-term complications, but also underscored the between link aggressive management of diabetes and an increase in the number of hypoglycemic episodes. Indeed, the DCCT reported a threefold increase in severe hypoglycemia in intensively treated patients. Hypoglycemia is also reported to be the cause of death in 2–4% of type 1 diabetic patients. In addition to type 1 diabetes, hypoglycemia is also relatively common in type 2 diabetes, with prevalence rates of 70–80% in patients using insulin to achieve good metabolic control [1].

The use of real-time or personal continuous glucose monitoring (CGM) provides data on hypoglycemia that may otherwise go unnoticed to the patient. Hypoglycemia is particularly challenging because it may occur when the patient is distracted, unaware, or asleep [2, 3]. Hypoglycemia can lead to hyperglycemia and contribute to glucose variability due to the release of counterregulatory hormones and to overtreatment with glucose. In rare cases, severe prolonged hypoglycemia remains a considerable risk to the patient and can result in cardiac arrhythmias, neurological sequelae, and even death [4–8].

Rationale for Suspension of Insulin to Prevent Severe Hypoglycemia

Hypoglycemia is frightening to patients and their families. It has been estimated that about 55% of severe hypoglycemic episodes occur during sleep. Acutely, diminished brain function during a hypoglycemic episode is a danger to the patient. In addition, recurrent hypoglycemia may cause long-lasting damage to the brain, resulting in impairment of memory or other cognitive functions.

In addition to the effects on cognition, recurrent hypoglycemia also impairs natural defense mechanisms against hypoglycemia, creating a vicious cycle. Normally, hypoglycemia triggers a series of hormonal and neural responses designed to bring glucose concentration towards normal and maintain brain metabolism. A component of this counterregulatory response is the secretion of epinephrine, which generates 'neurogenic' symptoms (e.g. palpitations, sweating, and anxiety) that warn the patient of the impending threat; however, after severe hypoglycemia the body's natural responses are depressed, impairing the exit from hypoglycemia. Prolonged hypoglycemia is a precursor of seizure activity. In children, CGM tracings have shown that nocturnal seizures are preceded by 2.25–4 h of glucose levels <60 mg/dl [9]. The JDRF study [10] reported an average time spent on hypoglycemia as follows: 62 min at a glucose level <70 mg/dl, 30 min <60 mg/dl, and even 7 min <50 mg/dl.

The integration of an insulin pump with a CGM system [so-called 'sensor-augmented pump therapy' (SAP)] can improve the management of diabetes, as indicated by several randomized controlled trials which found a significant reduction in glycated hemoglobin (HbA_{1c}) levels during SAP with respect to intensive insulin therapy by multiple daily injections or pump alone [10–13].

Real-time CGM offers the possibility of proactively avoiding hypoglycemic episodes through adjustable alert limits [14–16]; however, patients do not always react to the alerts. This is the rationale for developing automated insulin delivery systems where withdrawal of insulin infusion with impending hypoglycemia would be a first clinically relevant step.

General Considerations for Automatic Insulin Delivery

Several physiological considerations need to be taken into account when comparing continuous subcutaneous insulin infusion (CSII) in patients with type 1 diabetes to the nondiabetic situation. Insulin should ideally be released first in high concentrations into the portal circulation (where approx. 50% is extracted for glycogen production and inhibition of gluconeogenesis) before it reaches the peripheral circulation. Also, to mimic the secretion pattern of pancreatic β-cells, at mealtime a short insulin peak (hunger-induced in the cephalic phase) should be followed by a sustained (glucose concentration-dependent) secretion, while between meals glucose levels should be regulated by small amounts of insulin released in a pulsatile fashion. Thus, CSII should deliver human insulin into the portal system on the basis of local glucose concentrations to avoid excessive insulin concentrations and hypoglycemia. In addition, rapid changes in insulin sensitivity, as following physical exercise, should be taken into consideration. With current technologies, such an ideal closed loop can only be created under artificial laboratory conditions, while several compromises are made for real-life outpatient conditions.

A physiological insulin infusion into the portal vein is theoretically possible through an umbilical access which is usually not available after the neonatal period. However even the intraperitoneal route from an implanted pump or via an abdominal port is a compromise. This access remains reserved for rare indications such as subcutaneous insulin resistance and presently leaves the subcutaneous route (CSII) as the only option for routine outpatient care.

This results in several consequences for designing algorithms for hypoglycemia prevention and closing the loop. To mimic more closely the β-cell and to compensate for the delay due to subcutaneous absorption, human regular insulin usually has been replaced by rapid-acting insulin analogues, but even these new insulins do not have the quick onset of action and the short period of activity that would be needed for near-physiological regulation and the requirements of closed-loop technologies. In addition, the nonphysiologic subcutaneous route delays the suppression of hepatic glucose output. Thus, the automated response to low or falling glucose levels would require intravenous glucose or a bihormonal pump with simultaneous insulin and glucagon infusion [17]. The latter approach has been tried but needs a complex system with two reservoirs and delivery sites, and faces stability issues regarding glucagon. It also appears that glucagon may not always be effective (e.g. after alcohol consumption).

A minimum requirement for the continuous adjustment of insulin delivery is the presence of a continuous glucose sensor. Ideally, this sensor should measure blood glucose which would necessitate an implanted access. Currently available sensors analyze the glucose concentration in the subcutaneous tissue, which may result in a significant delay in case of rapid changes in the glucose concentration. In general the fine-tuning of glucose via the interstitial glucose values appears feasible due to the close relationship between cerebral and interstitial glucose values.

Architecture of a Closed Loop System

The hardware design for an outpatient system for continuous glucose regulation has to make use of currently available insulin pumps and glucose sensors (fig. 1). While these components are readily available on the market, the crucial link between them

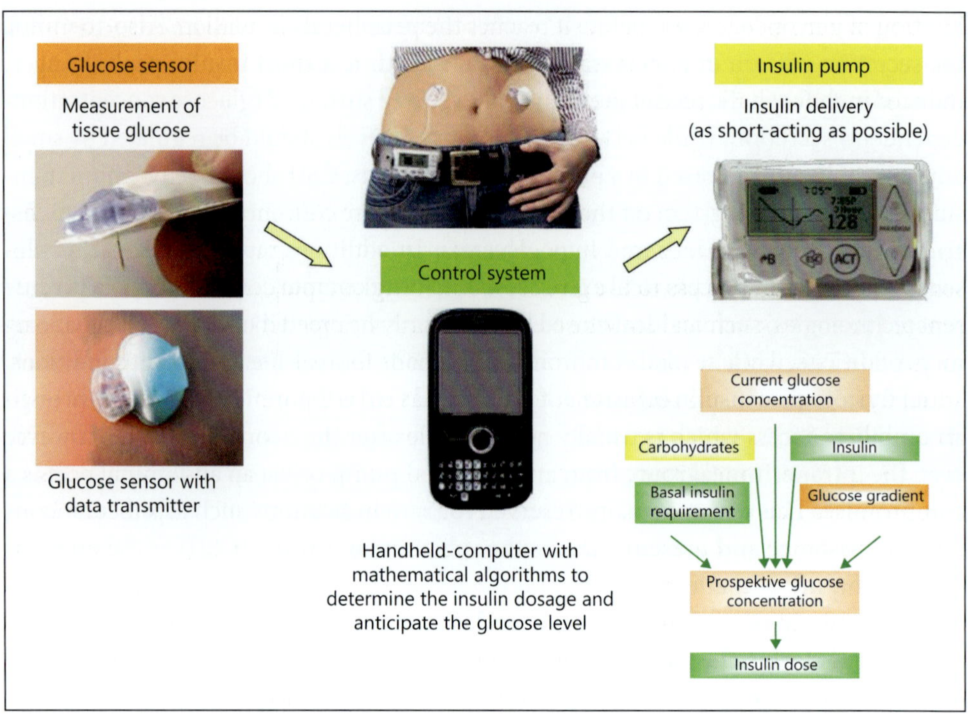

Fig. 1. Components and design of a closed-loop system with an external insulin pump, external glucose sensor, and handheld computer that contains the algorithm for regulation of insulin delivery. The diagram at bottom right shows factors to consider in the calculation of the insulin dose.

is the software that can be preinstalled on one of the devices or an additional handheld computer or smartphone. These software algorithms, which change subcutaneous insulin delivery on the basis of measured glucose, need to consider the compromises and limitations mentioned above. Under inpatient conditions, those algorithms have already been tested in a system called 'Biostator', which infuses glucose or insulin intravenously. In addition to the problems related to the subcutaneous site, the lack of regulating glucagon needs to be figured in as well.

Methodology of Continuous Glucose Monitoring

Current methods of CGM include the use of subcutaneous glucose sensors which convert glucose from the subject's interstitial fluid into an electronic signal, the strength of which is proportional to the amount of glucose concentration. In the electrochemical method, glucose is chemically converted into gluconic acid and hydrogen peroxide with the help of biocatalytical enzymes (e.g. glucose oxidase):

$$\text{Glucose} + O_2 + H_2O \rightarrow \text{Gluconic acid} + H_2O_2 \qquad (1)$$

Hydrogen peroxide is then oxidized over a platinum electrode with a voltage between 600 and 900 mV, and the released electrons generate a current that is proportional to the amount of converted glucose:

$$H_2O_2 \rightarrow 2\,H^+ + O_2 + 2\,e^- \quad (2)$$

At the physiological glucose concentration (40–400 mg/dl, 2.2–22.2 mmol/l) such a current is in the nanoampere range. The prerequisite for the electrochemical measurement is a direct access to the glucose-containing compartment. Thus, the glucose sensor (an electrochemical enzyme electrode that is wrapped in an oxygen-containing membrane) needs to be placed in the subcutaneous tissue to have access to the interstitial fluid. A second prerequisite is that there has to be equilibrium between interstitial and blood glucose, as rapid blood glucose changes may otherwise lead to a time lag of 5–25 min. In addition, individual factors such as glucose absorption rates or insulin action need to be taken into consideration when algorithms for predictive glucose management are developed. Due to variable rates of sensor 'drift', the sensor needs to be calibrated and recalibrated in certain intervals with conventional blood glucose measurements. The sensor is attached to a transmitter which sends the interstitial glucose information via radio or blue tooth signals to a screen that provides continuous real-time glucose values, as well as high/low glucose alerts.

Algorithms for Calculating Insulin Delivery in Closed-Loop Systems

While there is agreement that most of the modern pump models fulfil the mechanical and technical prerequisites regarding precision and reliability of insulin delivery, the current generation of glucose sensors still needs improvements both in accuracy and reliability. Meanwhile, a great effort has been made to develop algorithms dictating insulin dosing not only on the basis of the current glucose estimates, but also on the basis of values predicted 2–3 h ahead. This requires the regulation of both glucose concentration (C_{Gluc}) and insulin concentration (C_{Ins}). Basically, glucose homeostasis is regulated by a system of interconnected regulatory circuits. In the nondiabetic human, the pancreatic β- and α-cells are the regulatory units for secreting either insulin or glucagon, targeting glucose levels of 70–140 mg/dl (3.9–7.8 mmol/l). However, these regulatory circuits have a certain time lag. Thus, in addition to glucose concentration, additional factors like the time-dependent absorption of nutrients and variation of insulin action after subcutaneous infusion (as well as type of rapid insulin), amount of physical exercise, or other stress have to be considered when predicting the necessary insulin dose. Moreover, the insulin concentration that still is active in the organism needs to be figured in. Further complexity arises from glucose sensor-related issues such as the physiological difference between measurement in interstitial fluid compared to blood as well as potential bias related to sensor calibration (fig. 2). Therefore, it is necessary to develop a mathematical formula like in the example shown below. This formula de-

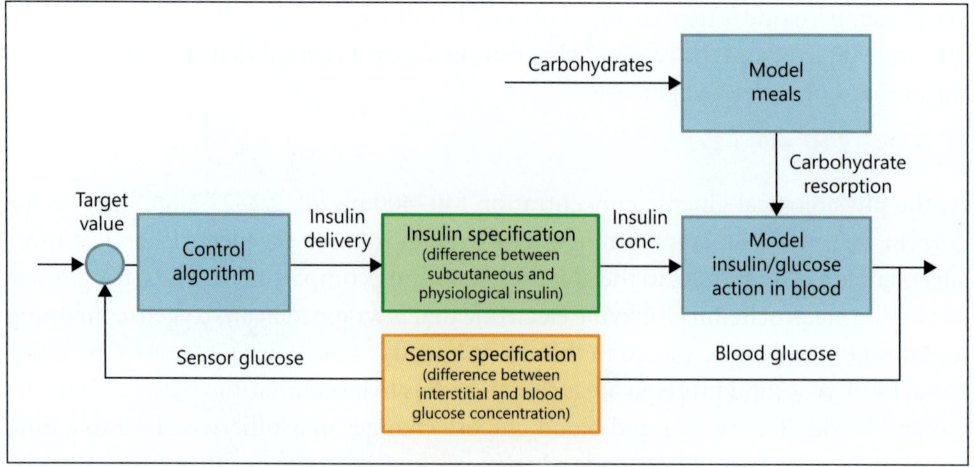

Fig. 2. Control cycle for a closed-loop system, with subcutaneous glucose measurement and insulin delivery in subcutaneous tissue. conc. = Concentration.

scribes the control cycle for a closed-loop system and the physiological glucose regulation (fig. 2–4).

For those readers interested in the mathematical details, one algorithm is explained in detail as an example. One approach for predictive glucose management is the so-called 'PID control' imitating the physiological insulin secretion pattern where 'P' represents the proportional regulation, 'I' the integral regulation, and 'D' derivative regulation [18]. These three phases correspond to the feedback behavior of the β-cell [fig. 3, compare the picture of physiological secretion pattern (top left) with the mathematical reproduction (top right)]. It can be calculated as follows:

- The proportional phase (P) considers the difference between the current glucose value and the target glucose ($C_{sensor} - C_{target}$); the resulting insulin delivery is proportional to the glucose level:

$$P = K_p \times [C_{sensor} - C_{target}] \quad (3)$$

where C_{Sensor} = glucose concentration sensor, C_{target} = target glucose concentration, and K_p = proportionality factor.

- Increment phase I (slow second-phase rise of insulin secreation) is proportional to the difference between the current sensor glucose level and target glucose ($C_{sensor} - C_{target}$):

$$dI/dt = K_p \times [C_{sensor} - C_{target}] \,/\, T_I \quad (4)$$

where T_I = time parameter for increment phase.

- Response phase (derivative, rapid first-phase rise of insulin secreation); the resulting insulin delivery is proportional to the rate of glucose change over the time (D):

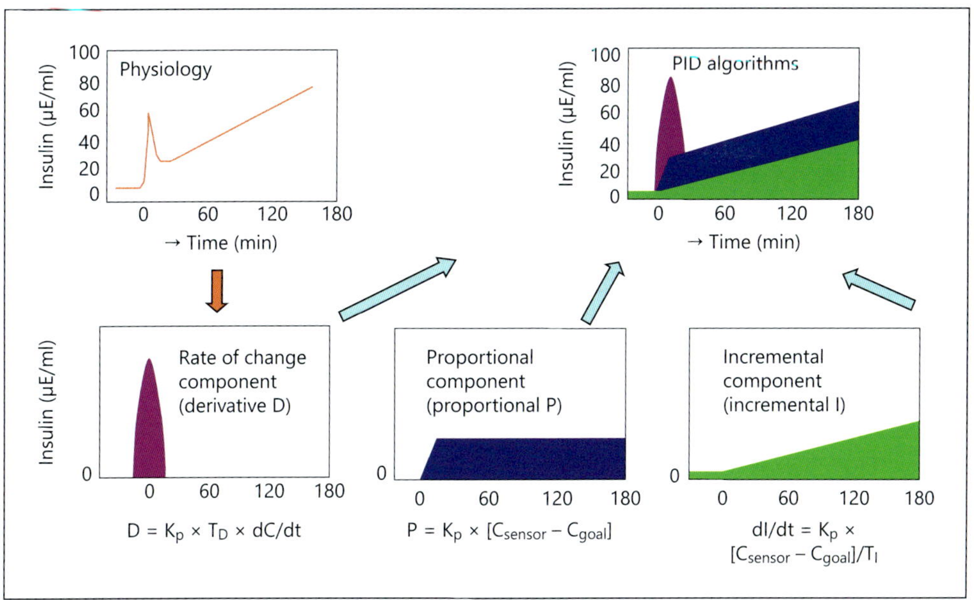

Fig. 3. Model of insulin secretion from the β-cell according to the PID model [18].

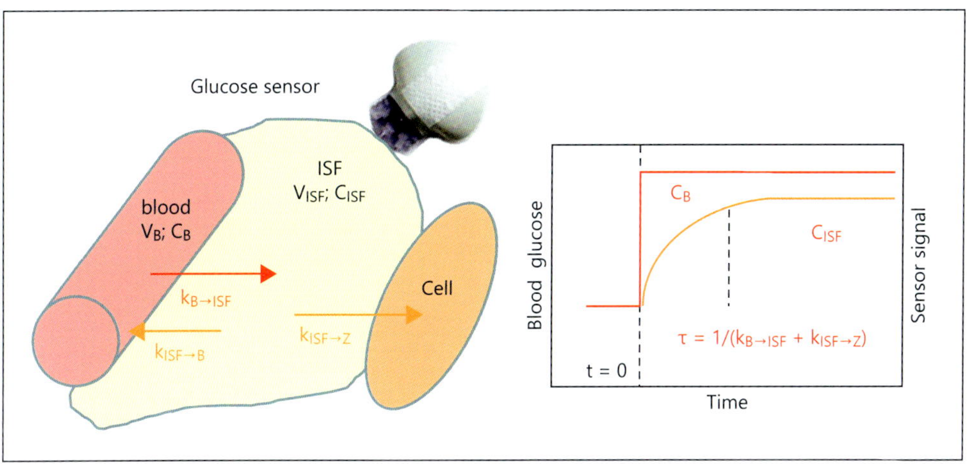

Fig. 4. Continuity model for the exchange of glucose between blood and interstitial fluid.

$$D = K_p \times T_D \times dC / dt \quad (5)$$

where dC/dt = change of glucose concentration/time, and T_D = time parameter for the derivative phase.

The relative amount of insulin delivered in each component is balanced by the three parameters K_p, T_I, and T_D. All three parameters have to be adjusted individually: K_p (in mIU/min/mg/dl, IU = international insulin unit) determines the insulin secretion rate as a reaction of the basal glucose level, T_I (in min) determines the proportion of the increment phase, and T_D determines the proportion of the derivative phase.

The complete algorithm for delivery is the sum of the three parts (fig. 3):

$$PID = P + I + D \quad (6)$$

Thus, the necessary insulin dose is calculated from the current glucose concentration, the glucose target and the parameters K_p, T_I, and T_D. As mentioned above, the use of glucose sensors placed in the subcutaneous tissue requires an adjustment for the glucose concentration C_{ISF} (ISF = interstitial fluid) being different from the blood glucose concentration C_B (B = blood), when the blood glucose is changing. This can be expressed in a simple model of continuity (fig. 4). The figure shows the physiological flow between blood and interstitial tissue with flow rates k between both compartments. This flow results in a change of the glucose concentration C in the blood or interstitial volume V. Following the time-dependent rate of change in the glucose concentration in the subcutaneous tissue depends on the glucose exchange between blood and interstitial fluid represented by the glucose flow rate $k_{B \to ISF}$, $k_{ISF \to B}$, and the drainage of glucose in the body cells (Z) $k_{ISF \to Z}$ (glucose consumption). An increase of the insulin concentration results in an increase of glucose consumption in the peripheral cells. The ensuing equation is:

$$dC_{ISF} / dt = -(k_{ISF \to Z} + k_{B \to ISF}) \times C_{ISF} + k_{ISF \to B} \times V_B / V_{ISF} \times C_B \quad (7)$$

where C_B = glucose concentration in blood, C_{ISF} = glucose concentration in the interstitial fluid, V_B = blood volume, V_{ISF} = interstitial volume, $k_{B \to ISF}$ = flow rate blood → interstitial space, $k_{ISF \to B}$ = flow rate interstitial space → blood, and $k_{ISF \to Z}$ = glucose consumption in the peripheral cells.

The relationship of glucose concentration in the interstitial fluid to concentration in the blood is the concentration (C_{ISF}/C_B). After reaching glucose homeostasis, the glucose concentration in the interstitial fluid can be calculated as follows:

$$C_{ISF} = C_B \times [k_{ISF \to B} \times V_B / V_{ISF}] / (k_{ISF \to Z} + k_{B \to ISF}) \quad (8)$$

The time lag between blood and interstitial fluid depends on the two flow rates $k_{B \to ISF}$ and $k_{ISF \to Z}$, and can be expressed as:

$$\tau_{Sensor} = 1 / (k_{B \to ISF} + k_{ISF \to Z}) \quad (9)$$

This time constant is calculated to be the time necessary to reach 63% of the equilibrium. When using an enzymatic electrochemical glucose sensor, the sensor current I_{sig} is proportional to the glucose concentration in the interstitial space:

$$I_{sig} = \alpha \times C_{ISF} \quad (10)$$

Here α is a parameter expressing the sensitivity of the sensor (in nA/mg/dl) which changes over time. As the glucose sensor is calibrated, the measured glucose concentration is calculated, accounting for the calibration factors F_{cal} as follows:

$$C_{sensor\ glucose} = F_{cal} \times I_{sig} \quad (11)$$

Using the PID model, the necessary insulin delivery per time period is calculated as:

$$I_{dose}(t) = K_p \times F_{Err} + 1 / T_I \int F_{Err} \times dt + T_D{}^s \quad (12)$$

F_{Err} is the resulting error due to the deviation from the blood glucose, i.e. the difference between the current glucose level and target glucose level, and K_p, T_I, T_D are the individual adjustable parameters in the PID model. In addition, equation 12 does not account for the subcutaneous insulin delivery, thus the relationship between sensor glucose $C_{sensor\ glucose}$ and blood glucose C_B needs to be adjusted as follows:

$$C_{sensor\ glucose} / C_B = F_{kal} \times K_{sensor} / (\tau_{Sensor}\ s + 1) \quad (13)$$

This results in the following relationship between insulin level in blood (I_{blood}) to insulin dose (I_{dose}):

$$I_{blood} / I_{dose} = K_{Ins} / [(\tau_{blood}\ s + 1) \times (\tau_{ISF}\ s + 1)] \quad (14)$$

This formula allows the prediction of the glucose concentration during closed-loop control as a result of a given insulin dose. Different complex models of glucose metabolism have been developed by various groups on the basis of these equations like the MPC-algorithm (model predictive control [19], or the hypoglycemic predictive algorithms [20]). These different models and algorithms essentially all calculate the same parameters: how to change the insulin infusion rate depending on time and given glucose concentration. Differences in the algorithms result in the degree that parameters such as insulin sensitivity, insulin action, carbohydrate intake, physical exercise, stress, etc., are taken into account and to what degree a prediction horizon is calculated. Mathematical approaches that are used in the algorithms include fuzzy logic [21] and neuronal networks [22].

Trials with Automatic Suspension of Insulin Delivery

Despite the development of real-time glucose sensors with hypoglycemic alarms, many patients sleep through these alarms. Therefore, pilot studies investigated the feasibility of using real-time CGM to discontinue insulin pump therapy when hypoglycemia was predicted [23]. The efficacy of automatic suspension of insulin delivery in induced hypoglycemia among subjects with type 1 diabetes was evaluated in the ASPIRE (Automation to Simulate Pancreatic Insulin Response) study, which tested the experimental design of an exercise provocation by ergometer in adults [24, 25]. In this randomized crossover study, subjects used a sensor-augmented insulin pump system with a low glucose suspend (LGS) feature that automatically stops insulin delivery for 2 h following a sensor glucose value ≤70 mg/dl. Subjects fasted overnight and exercised until their plasma glucose value reached ≤85 mg/dl on different occasions separated by washout periods lasting 3–10 days. Exercise sessions were done with the LGS feature turned on (LGS-on) or with continued insulin delivery regardless of sensor glucose value (LGS-off). The order of LGS-on and LGS-off sessions was randomly assigned. YSI glucose data were used to compare the duration and severity of hypoglycemia from successful LGS-on and LGS-off sessions, and to estimate the risk of rebound hyperglycemia after pump suspension. Fifty subjects attempted 134 sessions, 98 of which were successful. The length of hypoglycemia was less during LGS-on than during LGS-off (mean ± SD = 138.5 ± 76.68 vs. 170.7 ± 75.91 min, $p = 0.006$). Compared with LGS-off sessions, mean nadir YSI glucose was higher (59.5 ± 5.72 vs. 57.6 ± 5.69 mg/dl, $p = 0.015$) during LGS-on, as was mean end-observation YSI glucose (91.4 ± 41.84 vs. 66.2 ± 13.48 mg/dl, $p < 0.001$). Most (53.2%) end-observation YSI glucose values in the LGS-on sessions were in the 70–180 mg/dl range, and none was >250 mg/dl. This study in adults demonstrated that automatic suspension of insulin delivery significantly reduced duration and severity of induced hypoglycemia without causing rebound hyperglycemia.

The Low Glucose Suspend Approach

The first insulin pump equipped with a number of features to actively manage glucose levels was the Paradigm® Veo™ System (Medtronic Inc.). It is equipped with a LGS feature that leads to an interruption in the supply of insulin for a period of up to 120 min. This occurs when the glucose value falls below an adjustable hypoglycemia threshold (set by the patient and healthcare provider) and the patient does not respond to the alert (e.g. during sleep or in an environment with very loud background noise), and turns off insulin suspension to resume insulin delivery. After LGS is triggered, if the patient fails to respond by resuming insulin delivery, insulin suspension will last for 120 min, after which insulin delivery will be automatically resumed for 4 h, even if the sensor glucose value falls below the set LGS threshold again. However, if at the 4-hour period of time the glucose value reaches the LGS threshold, another cycle of 120-min suspension followed by 4 h of insulin delivery will be resumed. The goal of this algorithm, with insulin delivery cycling on and off, is to prevent the occurrence of diabetic ketoacidosis after LGS events [26].

The Pediatric Low Glucose Suspend Feasibility Study

The aim of our investigation was to determine whether number, duration, and degree of hypoglycemic episodes could be reduced through the use of the LGS feature under real-life conditions, using a hypoglycemia alert level of 75 mg/dl (4.2 mmol/l) and a LGS threshold of 70 mg/dl (3.9 mmol/l), and what effects the use of LGS had on metabolic control in pediatric patients. Twenty-one children and youth with type 1 diabetes (1–18 years of age, duration of diabetes ≥12 months, and CSII ≥3 months) from three diabetes centers in Germany with experience in CSII, CGM, and SAP were included in the study [27].

Before starting, patients and parents were trained on the use of the Veo system. Two phases were compared with each other in this prospective study. The first phase (2 weeks) consisted of SAP without the use of LGS, as previous research has shown that such CGM time is sufficient to determine the hypoglycemia rate in terms of statistical safety [28, 29]. The second phase lasted 6 weeks, as no previous experience on the behavior of patients using the LGS algorithm was available. The hypoglycemia alert was set at 75 mg/dl (4.2 mmol/l) and thus slightly higher than commonly defined for hypoglycemia. The rationale was the inherent 'time lag' between blood glucose and sensor glucose (measured in interstitial tissue), and the possibility that during a phase of rapidly decreasing blood glucose concentration, a sensor glucose reading of 75 mg/dl (4.2 mmol/l) may correspond to blood glucose values <70 mg/dl (3.9 mmol/l).

All patients used the glucose sensor >90% of the time over 8 weeks. The baseline HbA_{1c} level was 7.8 ± 1.1% (DCA 2000). A total of 445 LGS activations occurred in which the insulin supply was interrupted or 0.89 ± 0.67 LGS activations per patient per day (LGS/patient/day). When subdivided into day- and nighttime, the results were 0.38 ± 0.32 LGS/patient/day for the time between 10.00 p.m. and 6.00 a.m., and 0.49 ± 0.43 LGS/patient/day for the time between 6.00 a.m. and 10.00 p.m. If all LGS alerts are counted, including those confirmed by patients, and those during which no interruption in insulin delivery occurred, there were 853 events ≤70 mg/dl (3.9 mmol/l). When these alerts are included in the total, the average comes to 2.56 ± 1.86 LGS/patient/day. In contrast to the total number of LGS alerts and the total number of LGS activations, the complete cycle occurred primarily during sleep time (84.4% of the 120-min interruptions).

Comparing the glycemic parameters during the two phases of the investigation, a significant improvement in all parameters of hypoglycemia was observed with LGS, while average glucose or occurrence of hyperglycemia remained unchanged. Using the Device Satisfaction Survey, the majority of patients and their parents evaluated the management of hypoglycemia and the Veo system very positively, although patients with a high number of alerts tended to be a little less content. This study showed that with LGS the risk for hypoglycemia can be reduced without compromising the safety of CSII in children with type 1 diabetes.

The occurrence of severe hypoglycemia has been labeled as the rate limiting step in achieving optimal metabolic control [30]. The LGS algorithm was effective using 70 mg/dl (4.2 mmol/l) as the threshold for the onset of LGS. This value allowed for a reduction in time spent and number of episodes of <70 mg/dl without a concomitant rise in hyperglycemia. Even though not all hypoglycemic episodes were avoided with this LGS threshold, it is possible that setting a higher LGS threshold of 80 mg/dl (4.4

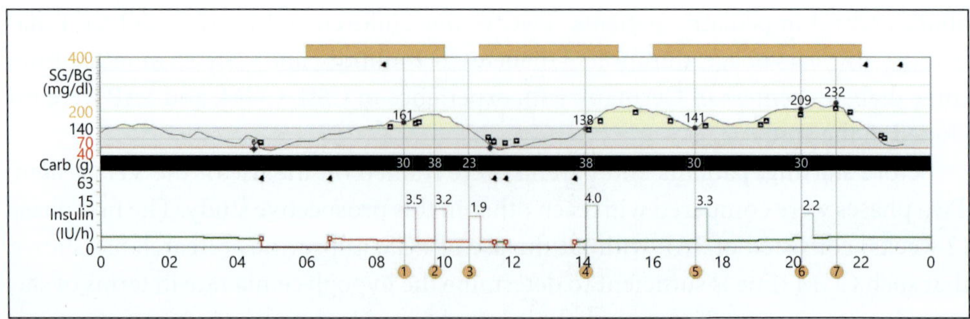

Fig. 5. Example for prevention of a severe hypoglycemic episode by switching off the insulin supply after an LGS alert not noticed by patient. For both cases, an interruption of 2 h occurred at 4:40 a.m. and 11:45 a.m. [27].

mmol/l) or 90 mg/dl (5.0 mmol/l) may be successful in reducing low glycemic excursions even further. This may be desirable for example in patients prone to hypoglycemia or young children at greater risk for neurocognitive consequences. However, potential hypoglycemia reduction by setting the threshold higher has to be balanced with the occurrence of more LGS alerts.

Increasing the overall number of alerts may affect a patient's sensitivity to the alerts and the overall patient acceptance of the device. In a 6-hour cycle, the 2-hour suspended insulin delivery is followed by 4 h of basal insulin delivery. In the absence of intervention, this 6-hour cycle continues indefinitely. For the period of the study, 5 patients cycled twice and 1 patient cycled 3 times. During the LGS time, there was an elevation in glucose concentration of 68.4 ± 13.1 mg/dl (3.8 ± 0.73 mmol/l) after the 2-hour interruption or a rate of approximately 35 mg/dl/h. Reactive ketoacidosis is not to be expected, even in the presence of serious patient errors (e.g. calibration-associated errors). We observed a case of sensor failure due to an extension of the sensor implantation time way beyond the recommended duration. The erroneous low glucose readings due to sensor failure prompted subsequent interruptions in the insulin supply during the night, but did not result in DKA. The elevated morning glucose could be readily corrected in the morning as would have been the case without LGS. The study provided evidence that by using the LGS function in children, severe hypoglycemia may be prevented in many cases (fig. 5). Our data are in line with three other major studies with the LGS that have been published to date: the UK User Evaluation [31], the CareLink Data Mining [32], and the Australian Hypoglycemia Prevention Study [33]. Common findings across studies show that when the LGS is set between 50 and 70 mg/dl, most individuals have an LGS event every day or every other day, but in more than 50% they turn back on the insulin in less than 5 min. While two thirds of LGS events are during the day, LGS events lasting 2 h are mainly at night; however, these make up only 10% of all LGS events. Applying the LGS feature results in an increase of approximately 35 mg/dl/h with suspend and 2 h

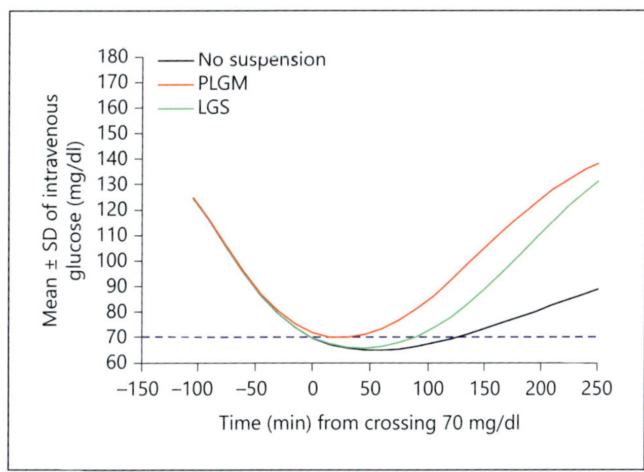

Fig. 6. Reduction of hypoglycemia with LGS and PLGM.

after with no increase in the hyperglycemia region (>180 mg/dl, 10 mmol/l). Thus, the LGS feature in SAP has been the first step towards a semiclosed loop in routine outpatient care.

Predictive Low Glucose Suspend

To further improve hypoglycemia prevention, there is an alternative to raising the LGS threshold. Implementing a predictive LGS when rapidly falling glucose values are predicted to reach the hypoglycemic range would trigger insulin suspension and could be even more effective in preventing low glucose [23]. Data for 50 virtual subjects ('in silico testing') were generated by using the University of Virginia/Padova type 1 diabetes simulator, quantifying the potential benefits of glucose prediction to reduce the number and duration of hypoglycemia epidsodes by using predicted rather than measured continuous glucose values [34]. Indeed, this allowed a 75% reduction of the number of hypoglycemic events and the time spent in hypoglycemic range, supporting the use of preventive hypoglycemic alerts on the basis of glucose prediction methods.

Currently under investigation is the 'Predictive Low Glucose Management (PLGM)' feature as the next iterative step after the success of the LGS system in the Paradigm Veo pump (fig. 6). To use this feature, the user will be required to select a predictive horizon (e.g. 30 min) when a predictive sensor low glucose suspension threshold (e.g. 80 mg/dl) would trigger the PLGM feature. When this feature is selected, if the sensor glucose prediction reaches a level equal to or lower than the programmed threshold, the user receives an alert and the pump suspends. The subject then has the option to continue suspending the pump or resume insulin delivery. Once the prediction horizon is safely above the threshold or after 120 min have elapsed (or if the user does not cancel suspend within 2 h), the pump will automatically resume insulin delivery at the previously programmed basal rate. The intended use of the PLGM system is to work as a supervisory system that monitors glucose levels and advises when and for how long a suspension of basal delivery is warranted. Initial research of the PILGRIM (Predictive Low Glucose Management in Real-Time Sensing Insulin Pump Therapy) study in adolescents and young adults with type 1 diabetes with exercise-induced hypoglycemia indicates that this approach may be a further stepping stone in the development of a commercially available closed-loop system.

References

1 The DCCT Research Group: Epidemiology of severe hypoglycemia in the Diabetes Control and Complications Trial. Am J Med 1991;90:450–459.

2 Amin R, Ross K, Acerini CL, Edge JA, Warner J, Dunger DB: Hypoglycemia prevalence in prepubertal children with type 1 diabetes on standard insulin regimen: use of continuous glucose monitoring system. Diabetes Care 2003;26:662–667.

3 Ryan EA, Germsheid J: Use of continuous glucose monitoring system in the management of severe hypoglycemia. Diabetes Technol Ther 2009;11:635–639.

4 Tattersall RB, Gill GV: Unexplained deaths of type 1, diabetic patients. Diabet Med 1991;8:49–58.

5 Thordarson H, Sovik O: Dead in bed syndrome in young diabetic patients in Norway. Diabet Med 1995;12:782–787.

6 Sartor G, Dahlquist G: Short-term mortality in childhood onset insulin-dependent diabetes mellitus: a high frequency of unexpected deaths in bed. Diabet Med 1995;12:607–611.

7 Gill GV, Woodward A, Casson IF, Weston PJ: Cardiac arrhythmia and nocturnal hypoglycaemia in type 1 diabetes – the 'dead in bed' syndrome revisited. Diabetologia 2009;52:42–45.

8 Suys B, Heuten S, De Wolf D, Verherstraeten M, de Beeck LO, Matthys D, Vrints C, Rooman R: Glycemia and corrected QT interval prolongation in young type 1 diabetic patients. What is the relation? Diabetes Care 2006;29:427–429.

9 Buckingham B, Wilson DM, Lecher T, Hanas R, Kaiserman K, Cameron F: Duration of nocturnal hypoglycemia before seizures. Diabetes Care 2008;31: 2110–2112.

10 O'Connell MA, Donath S, O'Nel DN, Colman PG, Ambler GR, Jones TW, Davis EA, Cameron FJ: Glycaemic impact of patient-led use of sensor guided pump therapy in type 1 diabetes: a randomised controlled trial. Diabetologia 2009;52:1365–1372.

11 Kordonouri O, Pankowska E, Rami B, Kapellen T, Coutant R, Hartmann R, Lange K, Knip M, Danne T: Sensor augmented pump therapy from the diagnosis of childhood type 1 diabetes: results of the Paediatric Onset Study (ONSET) after 12 months of treatment. Diabetologia 2010;53:2487–2495.

12 Raccah D, Sulmont V, Reznik Y, Guerci B, Renard E, Hanaire H, Jeandidier N, Nicolino M: Incremental value of continuous glucose monitoring when starting pump therapy in patients with poorly controlled type 1 diabetes. Diabetes Care 2009;32:2245–2250.

13 Bergenstal RM, Tamborlane WV, Ahmann A, Buse JB, Dailey G, Davis SN, Joyce C, Peoples T, Bruce-MA, Perkins A, Welsh JB, Willi SM, Wood MA; STAR 3 Study Group: Effectiveness of sensor-augmented insulin-pump therapy in Type 1 diabetes. N Engl J Med 2010;363:311–320.

14 Bode BW, Gross K, Rikalo N, Schwartz S, Wahl T, Page C, Gross T, Mastrototaro J: Alarms based on real-time sensor glucose values alert patients to hypo- and hyperglycemia: the Guardian Continuous Monitoring System. Diabetes Technol Ther 2004;6: 105–113.

15 Danne T, Lange K, Kordonouri O: Real-time glucose sensors in children and adolescents with type-1 diabetes. Horm Res 2008;70:193–202.

16 Juvenile Diabetes Research Foundation Continuous Glucose Monitoring Study Group, Beck RW, Hirsch IB, Laffel L, Tamborlane WV, Bode BW, Buckingham B, Chase P, Clemons R, Fiallo-Scharer R, Fox LA, Gilliam LK, Huang ES, Kollman C, Kowalski AJ, Lawrence JM, Lee J, Mauras N, O'Grady M, Ruedy KJ, Tansey M, Tsalikian E, Weinzimer SA, Wilson DM, Wolpert H, Wysocki T, Xing D: The effect of continuous glucose monitoring in well-controlled type 1 diabetes. Diabetes Care 2009;32:1378–1383.

17 El-Khatib FH, Russell SJ, Nathan DM, Sutherlin RG, Damiano ER: A bihormonal closed-loop artificial pancreas for type 1 diabetes. Sci Transl Med 2010;2: 27ra27.

18 Steil GM, Rebrin K, Darwin C, Hariri F, Saad MF: Feasibility of automating insulin delivery for the treatment of type 1 diabetes. Diabetes 2006;55:3344–3350.

19 Hovorka R, Allen JM, Elleri D, Chassin LJ, Harris J, Xing D, Kollman C, Hovorka T, Larsen AMF, Nodale M, De Palma A, Wilinska ME, Acerini CL, Dunger DB: Manual closed loop insulin delivery in children and adolescents with type 1 diabetes: a phase 2 randomised crossover trial. Lancet 2010;375: 743–751.

20 Dassau E, Cameron F, Lee H, Bequette BW, Zisser H, Jovanovic L, Chase P, Wilson DM, Buckingham BA, Doyle FJ III: Real-time hypoglycemia prediction suite using continuous glucose monitoring: a safety net for the artificial pancreas. Diabetes Care 2010;33: 1249–1254.

21 Atlas E, Nimri R, Miller S, Grunberg EA, Phillip M: MD-Logic artificial pancreas system: a pilot study in adults with type 1 diabetes. Diabetes Care 2010;33: 1072–1076.

22 Perez-Gandia C, Facchinetti A, Sparacino G, Cobelli C, Gomez EJ, Rigla M, de Leiva A, Hernando ME: Artificial neural network algorithm for online glucose prediction from continuous glucose monitoring. Diabetes Technol Ther 2010;12:81–88.

23 Buckingham B, Cobry E, Clinton P, Gage V, Caswell K, Kunselman E, Cameron F, Chase HP: Preventing hypoglycemia using predictive alarm algorithms and insulin pump suspension. Diabetes Technol Ther 2009;11:93–97.

24 Brazg RL, Bailey TS, Garg S, Buckingham BA, Slover RH, Klonoff DC, Nguyen X, Shin J, Welsh JB, Lee SW: The ASPIRE study: design and methods of an in-clinic crossover trial on the efficacy of automatic insulin pump suspension in exercise-induced hypoglycemia. J Diabetes Sci Technol 2011;5:1466–1471.

25 Garg S, Brazg RL, Bailey TS, Buckingham BA, Slover RH, Klonoff DC, Shin J, Welsh JB, Kaufman FR: Reduction in duration of hypoglycemia by automatic suspension of insulin delivery: the in-clinic ASPIRE study. Diabetes Technol Ther 2012;14:205–209.

26 Attia N, Jones TW, Holcombe J, Tamborlane WV: Comparison of human regular and lispro insulins after interruption of continuous subcutaneous insulin infusion and in the treatment of acutely decompensated IDDM. Diabetes Care 1998;21:817–821.

27 Danne T, Kordonouri O, Holder M, Haberland H, Golembowski S, Remus K, Bläsig S, Wadien T, Zierow S, Hartmann R, Thomas A: Prevention of hypoglycemia by using low glucose suspend function in sensor-augmented pump therapy. Diabetes Technol Ther 2011;13:1129–1134.

28 Bugler J: An estimation of the amount of data required to measure glycaemic variability (abstract). 1st ATTD Meet Proceed, Prague, 2008. www.kenes.com/attd2008/program/ViewAbstract.asp.

29 Xing D, Kollman C, Beck RW, Tamborlane WV, Laffel L, Buckingham BA, Wilson DM, Weinzimer S, Fiallo-Scharer R, Ruedy KJ; Juvenile Diabetes Research Foundation Continuous Glucose Monitoring Study Group: Optimal sampling intervals to assess long-term glycemic control using continuous glucose monitoring. Diabetes Technol Ther 2011;13: 351–358.

30 Cryer PE, Davis SN, Shamoon H: Hypoglycemia in diabetes. Diabetes Care 2003;26:1902–1912.

31 Choudhary P, Evans ML, Hammond PJ, Shaw JA, Pickup JC, Amiel SA: Insulin pump therapy with automated insulin suspension in response to hypoglycemia. Diabetes Care 2011;34:2023–2025.

32 Agrawal P, Welsh JB, Kannard B, Askari S, Yang Q, Kaufman FR: Usage and effectiveness of the low glucose suspend feature of the Medtronic Paradigm Veo insulin pump. J Diabetes Sci Technol 2011;5:1137–1141.

33 Ly TT, Nicholas JA, Retterath A, Davis EA, Jones TW: Analysis of glucose responses to automated insulin suspension with sensor-augmented pump therapy. Diabetes Care 2012;35:1462–1465.

34 Zecchin C, Facchinetti A, Sparacino G, Cobelli C: Reduction of number and duration of hypoglycemic events by glucose prediction methods: a proof-of-concept in silico study. Diabetes Technol Ther 2013; 15:66–77.

Thomas Danne, MD
Diabetes Center for Children and Adolescents
Auf der Bult Kinder- und Jugendkrankenhaus
Janusz-Korczak-Allee 12, DE–30173 Hannover (Germany)
E-Mail danne@hka.de

Bruttomesso D, Grassi G (eds): Technological Advances in the Treatment of Type 1 Diabetes.
Front Diabetes. Basel, Karger, 2015, vol 24, pp 166–189 (DOI: 10.1159/000363512)

Artificial Pancreas: A Review of Fundamentals and Inpatient and Outpatient Studies

Simone Del Favero[a] · Daniela Bruttomesso[b] · Claudio Cobelli[a]

Departments of [a]Information Engineering and [b]Internal Medicine, Unit of Metabolic Diseases, University of Padova, Padova, Italy

Abstract

The artificial pancreas (AP) is a device for automated modulation of insulin infusion that aims to maintain blood glucose in a nearly normal range. The core of the AP is the control algorithm, which is in charge of computing an effective insulin dose on the basis of continuous glucose monitoring readings. In the last 6 years, AP prototypes based on subcutaneous glucose sensing and subcutaneous insulin delivery have been extensively studied in clinical trials first on hospitalized patients and, more recently, in an outpatient setting. In this chapter we review the state of the art of the field, starting with a description of the various AP system components. In particular, we focus on the control techniques employed in the AP and on the principles on which they are based. We then move to AP testing: the preclinical stage (mostly done in silico), the inpatient clinical studies, and finally the outpatient studies. We also discuss the technological requirements for an ambulatory AP.

Although type 1 diabetes is associated with increased morbidity and decreased life expectancy, strong evidence indicates that good metabolic control decreases diabetes complications [1–3]. Tight glucose control, however, increases the risk of hypoglycemia. To make diabetes control easier, new insulin analogues have been developed and infusion devices have been improved. Glucose monitoring has improved, too, with the introduction of devices for continuous glucose monitoring (CGM) which detect in real time the rate and direction of glucose changes. More recently, pumps and CGM devices have been connected to form an integrated system, the so-called 'artificial pancreas' (AP), whose scope is to ensure better glycemic control by frequently changing the insulin infusion rate on the basis of past, present, and forecasted glucose readings, as computed by a suitable control algorithm (fig. 1).

The pathway that led to the present models of AP started with the development of the first portable insulin pump by Kadish [4] in 1964. Prototypes of the AP with intravascular sensing and delivery, devised in the 1970s by Albisser et al. [5], Pfeiffer et al. [6], and Mirouze et al. [7] paved the way for the first commercial closed-loop bedside device, the Biostator (Miles Laboratories, Elkhart, Ind., USA) [8], which combined minute-by-minute glucose monitoring from whole blood via a glucose-oxidase sensor and intravenous infusion of insulin and dextrose. Drawbacks included risk of infection and thrombosis, wastage of blood, and sampling port occlusion. The following years witnessed attempts to miniaturize the Biostator, the introduction of new devices for insulin administration and glucose sensing, and the exploration of new routes of insulin delivery, in particular the intraperitoneal and the subcutaneous routes.

In this chapter we review closed-loop insulin delivery systems and comment on recent results obtained with the AP in inpatient and outpatient settings. It should be noted that the picture has rapidly evolved thus far and only a few outpatient studies have been published, but a number of groups have reported at conferences the completion of their outpatient studies.

Components of the Artificial Pancreas

Glucose Sensor

CGM systems are minimally invasive devices that provide frequent (every 1–5 min) measurements of glucose concentration in the interstitial fluid. Measurements are obtained, in most of the recent models, via a glucose-oxidase reaction on a needle usually inserted in the abdominal tissue. It is now well documented that the sustained use of CGM improves metabolic control in young and adult patients with type 1 diabetes both when CGM is used in conjunction with continuous subcutaneous insulin infusion (CSII) and with multiple daily injections [9, 10]. Moreover, providing frequent glucose concentration measurement without requiring venous access, CGM overcomes the portability limitations of the Biostator. An extensive review of this technology can be found in other chapters of this book [11–14]. Here we simply review aspects relevant for an AP.

Although greatly improved, CGM still has a number of limitations. First, depending on the device, the sensor usually needs to be calibrated twice a day according to the glucose values obtained with a glucometer. To be accurate, calibrations should be performed during periods of stable glucose levels and in the normoglycemic range. Even with this precaution, due to uncertainties affecting the calibration process, blood-interstitium delay, and transduction sensitivity drifts, the CGM reading might present bias with respect to true blood glucose concentration. In addition, random noise corrupts CGM readings. As a consequence, sensors currently on the market show mean relative absolute deviation around 13–15%.

These limitations of the CGM readings reliability affect the AP performance, and extensive research is underway to improve sensor accuracy and precision. This is being done both by improving the sensing chemical technology [13] and by using signal processing techniques that intelligently enhance sensor performance (the Smart Sensor Concept, see [14, 15]).

Moreover, the sensor is prone to dislodgement and to temporary failures related to biomechanical issues of the sensor-tissue interface [16]. For instance, pressure application on the sensor (e.g. by rolling on the sensor while sleeping), can alter the glucose-diffusion process in the insertion region and, hence, the sensitivity of the sensor, producing a systematic underestimation of glucose concentration for several minutes. Algorithms attempting to detect these events are being developed (see [17] and references therein).

Insulin Administration

In principle, insulin can be delivered intraperitoneally (closely resembling the healthy subject physiology), intravenously as was done with the Biostator, or subcutaneously.

Intraperitoneal insulin administration has many favorable aspects, including predominant and reproducible absorption through the portal venous system, a quick time to peak and return to baseline plasma insulin levels, and efficacy in disposing a portal glucose load comparable to that observed after intravenous insulin administration. Feasibility of its use for an AP has been shown by Renard et al. [18]. Negative aspects of intraperitoneal insulin administration are the necessity of implantation, the costs associated with the technology, and the necessity of an hospital stay both to refill the reservoir (every 40 days) and to implement procedures to prevent aggregation of the concentrated insulin solutions (400 U/ml). A further complication of the intraperitoneal route is the production of anti-insulin antibodies. Although the use of an implantable port (DiaPort R) connected to an intraperitoneal catheter and to an external insulin pump may improve patient autonomy, at present the intraperitoneal route is certainly less employed in the AP prototypes with respect to the subcutaneous route.

Intravenous administration is easily tunable, has no absorption delay, and thus has a rapid action. The major shortcoming of this route is the formation of clots at the catheter tip when pumps with pulsatile infusion regimen are used and, in spite of its effectiveness in glucose control, an AP for home use based on intravenous insulin administration is not a real option at present. However, this approach has proven its strength in the treatment of brittle diabetes in intensive care units, often employing proportional derivative algorithms.

The subcutaneous route seems today the most practical for the AP in spite of the delay of insulin absorption since great experience with SCII has accumulated and there has been tremendous pump improvement in terms of safety, dimension, comfort, and mode of administration. Furthermore, the advent of short-acting insulins has contributed to the improvement of pump performance by allowing precise insulin dosing at meals and fine modulation of basal insulin infusion during physical activity, stress events, infections, pregnancy, and parturition. The cons are the unavoidable delay in insulin adsorption and action after subcutaneous administration (around 100 min). The delays associated with the subcutaneous route are a major challenge for control algorithms and limit the possibility to achieve tight glycemic control, especially after meals, since meal effects are usually faster than insulin action, leading to glucose levels well above the normal range. Moreover, residual insulin activity remaining after disposal of meal components can lead to postprandial hypoglycemia.

Patients in the Loop

To mitigate postprandial excursions caused by intrinsic delays in the subcutaneous route, a practical option is to require that the patient announce an upcoming meal. The information to be announced to the controller might go from the timing of the meal, which is used to trigger a priming bolus, to the specification of timing and carbohydrate content of the meal. Intermediate solutions require the specification of the meal timing and a gross estimate of the meal size, selected among some predefined options, e.g. small, medium, or large. Although more burdensome for the patient, meal announcement can significantly improve meal control with respect to unannounced meal schemes, as illustrated by Weinzimer et al. [19], and is therefore employed in a number of AP prototypes currently being tested.

Other Hormones

Glucagon Infusion

Dual-hormone AP is a closed-loop system in which, in addition to insulin, the controller can also inject glucagon to prevent hypoglycemia without requiring external carbohydrate administration [20]. This is an appealing opportunity since the use of glucagon significantly eases the control problem as in these systems the controller can steer blood glucose concentration both up and down, injecting either glucagon or insulin, in contrast to single-hormone AP where the controller can only decrease blood glucose concentration through insulin administration. Limitations are glucagon chemical instability, a tendency to form amyloid fibrils in solution, potential inefficacy once glycogen depots in the liver have been depleted [20, 21], and side effects such as nausea related to its sustained infusion.

Pramlintide Infusion

An alternative approach to limit postprandial glucose excursions is to delay gastric emptying with preprandial injections of pramlintide, an analogue of amylin. Reduced glucose peaks can be achieved thanks to a better match between carbohydrate and insulin absorption [22].

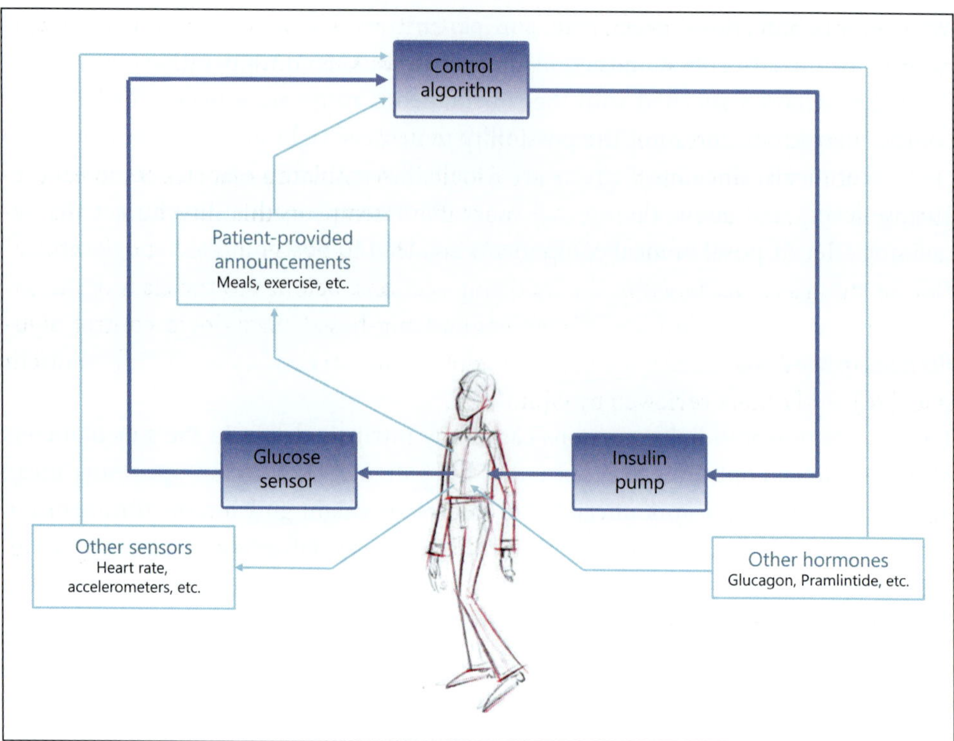

Fig. 1. The AP: a device for automated insulin-infusion based on patient glycemia. Essential components are the insulin pump (responsible for insulin delivery), the CGM glucose sensor (provides quasicontinuous glucose concentration measurements), and the control algorithm (the intelligence of the system) that is in charge of computing the insulin dose to be injected. Ancillary modules can be added to achieve better glycemic control, especially in response to challenging events such as meals and exercise. The patient might be requested to announce to the controller an upcoming meal/exercise event. In addition to insulin, other hormones can be infused, like glucagon or amylin analogues. Finally, additional patient vital signals (e.g. heart rate) can be measured by other sensors to detect glycemia-impacting events such as physical exercise.

Sensing Other Signals

Other sensors, such as accelerometers, heart rate monitors, and sweat sensors can be included in the loop. Their signals can be used by the controller to detect unannounced physical exercise and to distinguish it from other glycemia-impacting events such as emotional stress [23].

Control Algorithm

The control algorithm plays a pivotal role in the AP by regulating insulin infusion on the basis of glucose levels (past, present, and projected), patient data, and built-in principles based on diabetes pathophysiology, noise analysis, and error identification. Over time, several types of algorithms have been developed.

Clinical Practice-Inspired and 'Fuzzy-Logic' Controllers

One possibility for the design of a control logic is to emulate a diabetes specialist reasoning in an automated fashion. A remarkable attempt in this direction is the so-called 'Medical Doctor Logic (MD-Logic)' [24]. This controller, tested in a number of clinical studies as discussed in the following sections, belongs to the class of the so-called 'fuzzy-logic' algorithms. Other engineering-based fuzzy-logic control algorithms for an AP have been developed, notably by Ibbini and Masadeh [25], Mauseth et al. [26], and others reviewed by Grant [27].

Physiology Inspired

Recently, Herrero et al. [28] proposed a physiology-inspired controller that is based on a subcellular mathematical model of β-cell insulin secretion in response to glucose, equipped with the so-called 'insulin feedback' [29], which allows the effect of the delays inherent in the subcutaneous route to be mitigated.

Proportional-Integrative-Derivative Control

Proportional-integral-derivative control (PID) is a highly consolidated control technique used in industrial applications. PID was the technique of choice in the early prototypes of intravenous AP.

PID algorithms increase insulin delivery when the difference between measured and target glucose increases (proportional component), when the glucose rate of change increases (derivative component), and when the area of the difference between the actual and target glucose profile increases. The integral component can be seen as a slow basal adjustment, while the derivative and proportional actions in response to a meal resemble the biphasic insulin secretion of β-cells – the dynamic phase being mostly provided by the derivative component and the static phase delivery mostly by the proportional component. In view of this PID, the controller can also be considered physiology inspired. The PID controller proposed by Steil et al. [30] was further refined by equipping it with insulin feedback, which allows the insulin delivery rate to be decreased in response to rising plasma insulin levels, similarly to what happens to the β-cells [31, 32]. Insulin feedback mitigates the effects of the delays associated with the subcutaneous insulin administration.

Model Predictive Control

In contrast to PID algorithms, which can only react to past glycemic values, model predictive control (MPC) algorithms are proactive and attempt to determine the optimal insulin infusion to be delivered by considering its predicted effects on future glycemic levels. More specifically, the control algorithm is allowed to perform a control move, i.e. to increase/decrease basal insulin at each control step (5–15 min). The

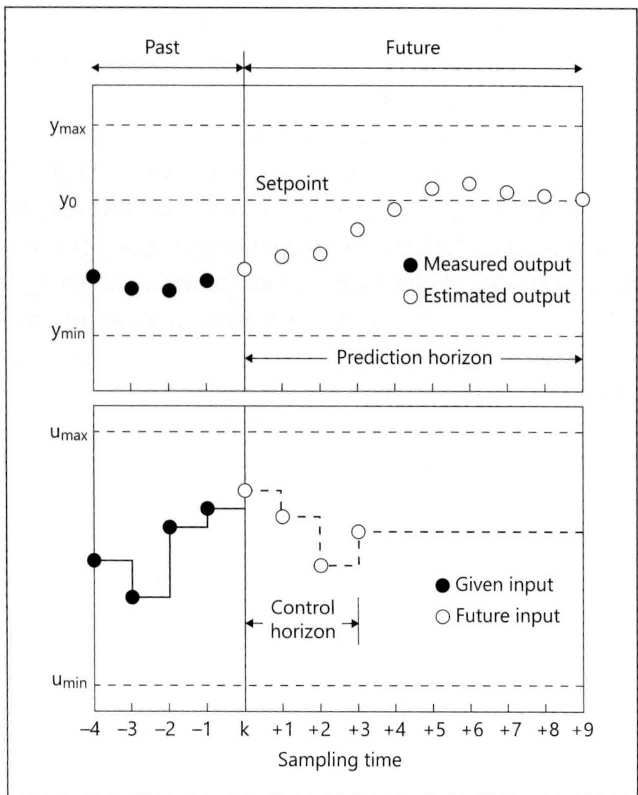

Fig. 2. Illustration of MPC reasoning.

control algorithm considers all the possible sequences of control moves applicable in the future and chooses the sequence that is predicted to better bring glycemic levels to the desired target and maintain it there. Since the prediction is affected by errors, only the first move in the sequence is applied and, after 5–15 min, the previously computed optimal sequence of control actions is updated based on the new measurements that become available. A pictorial representation of this reasoning method is reported in figure 2.

MPC is somewhat similar to a chess player who considers the sequences of possible future moves and chooses the most effective one, based on its predicted effect on the game. Then, the chess player applies the first moves of the sequence he planned and waits for the opponent move. If the opponent's move was not considered in the player's prediction, he will recompute the sequence of optimal moves, taking into account the new information, apply the first move of the sequence, wait for the opponent move, and so on.

Prediction in MPC is formulated on the basis of a mathematical model that can be based on a priori knowledge (physiological, clinical, and experimental) or can be learned from the observed behavior. The model can be either linear, as in Magni et al. [33], or nonlinear, as in Hovorka et al. [34].

The decision of the best sequence of moves is performed by assigning to each sequence a cost and choosing the cheapest one. For example, in Magni et al. [33] the cost is proportional to the area between predicted glycemia and target vale. Moreover, large deviations of insulin infusion from the current basal values are also penalized with an extra cost. An interesting concept is the zone penalty [35]: the chosen control action has a cost only if it leads to a predicted value outside the nearly normal range (e.g. 70–180 mg/dl during the day), while all predicted values in the safe zone are equally cheap, regardless how close they are to the target. This strategy, known as 'zone MPC' has the advantage of making the controller more robust to sensor fluctuation due to noise.

Finally, at difference with the PID strategy, MPC can actively take into account that there are unfeasible control actions, such as infusing a negative amount of insulin, and exclude them.

Other MPC algorithms have also been proposed in the literature [36–38].

Multimodular Control

Given the complexity of the glycemic control and the need to guarantee safety, a number of study groups have equipped their AP prototypes with a safety module (e.g. [28, 39, 40]), i.e. algorithms to reduce or stop insulin infusion if hypoglycemia is foreseen [41, 42] by employing different reasoning and different models with respect to the control algorithm.

Integration and parallel development of safety and control algorithms was studied by Kovatchev et al. [43], who proposed a modular architecture for AP, and was further refined by Patek et al. [40]. The architecture (fig. 3) solves integration hurdles, decoupling functionalities among modules and hence allowing independent development and deployment. The bottom module (Safety Supervision Module) contains the safety algorithm and is authorized to override upper-layer commands to reduce proposed insulin infusion if patient safety is predicted at risk. The intermediate module, called the 'Range Control Module', modulates insulin injection to maximize time in the nearly-normal range. Two implementations of this module have been proposed: the Hyperglycemia Mitigation Module, which is heuristic, and a MPC module.

The Hyperglycemia Mitigation Module ensures, by design, conservative insulin injection to avoid hypoglycemic episodes induced by overtreatment. A less conservative implementation of the Range Control Module is based on a MPC regulator [33, 44, 45]. In this case, a control action aims to enforce tight glycemic control. The controller is informed by the individual's conventional therapy, but every 15 min the controller is allowed to deviate from CSII therapy if the optimal infusion computed with MPC techniques also deviates. This formulation implies that preprandial boluses are triggered by patient announcement and employs an estimate of the meal's carbohydrate content. For the MPC regulator, controller aggressiveness is individualized for each subject by the upper module (Initialization Module) based on readily available patient characteristics, e.g. body weight, insulin-to-carbohydrate ratio, and basal insulin delivery [44, 45].

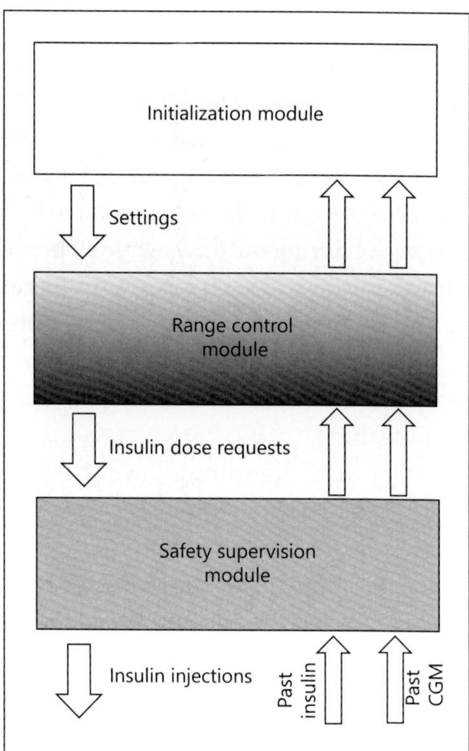

Fig. 3. Modular architecture proposed by Patek et al. [40] and Kovatchev et al. [43].

Preclinical Testing: In Silico Studies

In the last decade, the development, tuning, and testing of AP control algorithms has been accelerated by the availability of accurate computer simulators of a type 1 diabetic patient, allowing fast and cheap simulation studies known as in silico studies.

The first example of an in silico designed AP was used in the ADICOL project [46], and was based on the Cambridge simulator [47]. The Cambridge simulator includes interpatient variability by allowing tests on 18 virtual subjects, each described by a different model parameter vector. A subset of the virtual subjects' parameters were estimated from experimental data collected in subjects with type 1 diabetes mellitus, and the remaining parameters were drawn from informed probability distributions. Further details on the simulator can be found in Wilinska et al. [48] and the references therein.

Another simulator, known as the UVA/PADOVA Type 1 Diabetes Simulator, was proposed by Kovatchev et al. [49]. In 2008, this simulator was accepted by the FDA as a substitute for preclinical trials of certain insulin treatments, including closed-loop algorithms [49], leading to a true paradigm change in the AP field: the UVA/PADOVA Simulator has been successfully used by 32 research groups in academia, as well as by companies active in the field of type 1 diabetes mellitus. The simulator recreates meal

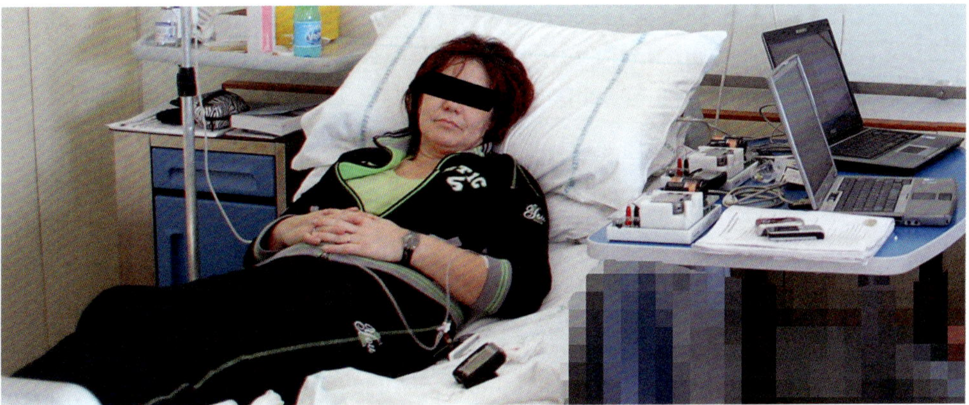

Fig. 4. Inpatient study during the exercise test [51]. Note the double catheters allowing frequent venous access. Running the APS system on a laptop, a number of wired connections were still present.

challenges and includes a population of 300 in silico subjects (100 adults, 100 adolescents, 100 children). Each virtual subject is described by a model parameter vector, which is randomly extracted from an appropriate joint parameter distribution. With respect to the 2008 version [49], a new version has recently been released [50], including counterregulation modeling and an improved description of the hypoglycemic region.

Inpatient Studies

Platform

To guarantee the safety and correct functioning of the devices, the collection of frequent blood samples was usually a mandatory requirement during inpatient studies. For example, Breton et al. [51] collected at least one blood sample every 30 min and measured blood glucose with the YSI2300 STAT Plus analyzer (Yellow Spring Instrument, Farnborough, UK). Sampling was more frequent during exercise (every 5 min) and meals (every 10 min). The need for an open intravenous access for frequent blood sampling strongly limited patient freedom (fig. 4, 5). Given this constraint, technological requirements for inpatient AP prototypes were rather limited. In some cases (e.g. the trial by Hovorka et al. [52]), a manual closed-loop system was employed, which meant that a human operator was manually inserting on a laptop the sensor reading at each control step (usually 15 min); based on the reading, the control algorithm suggested insulin infusion that if deemed safe by the attending physician, was manually programmed on the pump.

Other studies employed a laptop, an important example being the APS system [53], a Matlab-based platform that allowed communication with a number of different sensors and pumps so that the sensor-controller and controller-pump communications did not require study team intervention. The APS system, by enabling automated data transfer, has been used in many inpatient studies (e.g. [51]).

Results

The last 7 years have seen extensive testing and constant improvements of AP prototypes, so that it can now be stated that this constantly evolving technology represents an exciting new opportunity for patients with diabetes.

Steil et al. [30] first demonstrated that it was possible to reach all-day glucose control with a subcutaneous closed-loop system based on a PID algorithm. In a group of 10 adult patients in a closed-loop regimen for 29 h, they found that glucose levels stayed on target longer than during CSII (75 vs. 63% of time). However, postprandial glucose changes were not fully satisfactory and the risk of late hypoglycemia was not improved. Using the same algorithm on a group of adolescents followed for 34 h, Weinzimer et al. [19] compared the effects of a fully closed-loop versus a closed-loop which included an insulin bolus administered 10–15 min before meals and covering 25–50% of the meal insulin requirement. Considering glucose values after meals, they found that both systems were superior to CSII, and a hybrid closed-loop system was better than a fully closed-loop system. Subsequently, the PID algorithm was modified to include a feedback insulin model [31]. A trial of this system in 8 adults, with the administration of 2 units of insulin immediately before meals obtained good control of high glucose levels immediately after meals, but there was a still a certain incidence of hypoglycemic episodes [32].

Recently, Weinzimer et al. [22] tested a PID controller with insulin feedback and pramlintide coadministration at mealtime on 8 adolescents and young adults (15–28 years of age). They were controlled for 24 h (3 meals) without pramlintide, while in the other 24 h, pramlintide was coadministered. No meal announcement was provided to the control algorithm. The authors reported a significantly delayed postprandial peak excursion.

The MD-Logic control algorithm has been tested in inpatient settings [24, 54, 55]. The study by Atlas et al. [24] was a prospective pilot study on 7 adults admitted twice for 8 h, in a fasting and meal-challenge condition. Two of them additionally underwent a 24-hour closed-loop admission with encouraging results. Nimri et al. [54] tested the controller during dinner and overnight on 3 adolescents and 4 adults. In 1 of the 2 admissions, dinner was scheduled after physical exercise. The authors showed safe control in both cases. CGM data collected at home with standard care were presented for qualitative comparison. Nimri et al. [55] reported a randomized cross-over, multicenter study with 12 patients (children, adolescents, and adults) studied overnight, showing a significant increase of time spent in the near normal range of 63–140 mg/dl, reduced average glucose, and reduced glucose variability when compared with the CSII nights.

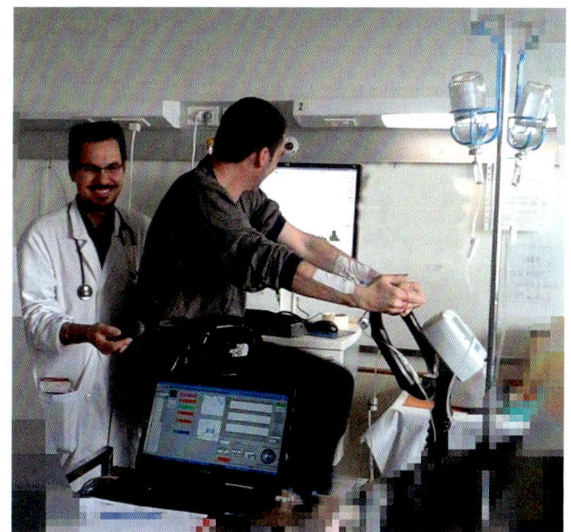

Fig. 5. Inpatient study [58].

A clinical test on a small number of subjects (10 enrolled, 7 completed) of another fuzzy-logic control algorithm employing meal announcement is reported in Mauseth et al. [56]. In the paper by Capel et al. [57], a rule-based control algorithm was tested in 10 subjects overnight and challenged at breakfast. The authors showed improvements of overnight control, with an increased time in target and reduced time in hypoglycemia with respect to standard CSII. The breakfast control was not different with respect to open loop.

MPC-based control algorithms have been extensively tested. A first version of the modular controller has been tested overnight and at breakfast [58–60]. The studies involved 20 adults and was performed in 3 centers, showing that the MPC-based modular controller improved time-in-target and had less hypoglycemic episodes overnight, although breakfast control was still unsatisfactory. An improved version of the same controller was successively tested on 12 patients in a randomized 22-hour study [51], starting after lunch, prescribing moderate physical exercise and facing the challenge of dinner and breakfast. The study showed that the overall percent time in near-normoglycemia (70–180 mg/dl) increased significantly and that the percent time in tight control (80–140 mg/dl) increased significantly overnight, while improvements in tight control on the overall study time were not statistically significant, due to the effect of meal perturbation. Moreover, overnight average plasma glucose was significantly reduced as was the dispersion around the average (i.e. standard deviation, measured intrasubject). Improved glucose control was achieved without a significant increase in the risk of hypoglycemia and with a significant decrease in the overall average plasma glucose. Using the same protocol, Breton et al. [51] tested a more conservative algorithm (H2MS [40]) on 15 adults and 11 adolescents. This controller allowed time spent in near-normoglycemia to improve significantly with respect to traditional therapy, with a maximal effect overnight. As expected by design, the time spent in the tight glycemic range did not differ between the two admissions overnight. Improved glycemic control was achieved with simultaneous significant reduction of hypoglycemia. Breton et al. [51] also made a comparison among the two controllers, restricting the analysis to the adult population only and suitably compensating for the difference in the baseline standard therapy of the two populations. Results show that both MPC and H2MS similarly increased time spent in near-normoglycemia, while MPC increased overnight time spent in tight glycemic control further in comparison to H2MS. The comparison of the occurrence of hypoglycemia in H2MS and MPC was not conclusive.

A relevant contribution in this field comes from studies that tested an MPC-based algorithm in adults, adolescents, and children, and during pregnancy [52, 61–65]. For adults, similarly to the modular MPC controller mentioned above, the algorithm was first assessed overnight in a randomized study [61]. Twelve patients were tested after consuming a medium-size dinner (60 g of carbohydrates, eating-in scenario), whereas 12 were tested after a later large evening meal (100 g of carbohydrates) accompanied by white wine (eating-out scenario). Time in the near-normoglycemic range increased significantly in both scenarios and was more pronounced in the eating-out one. Improved glycemic control was achieved together with a significant reduction of overnight time spent in hypoglycemia (plasma glucose ≤70 mg/dl).

Nineteen adolescents and children were studied overnight by Hovorka et al. [52], where closed-loop insulin delivery was challenged with a standard, rapid, and slow absorption meal and with physical exercise. They consistently found that the closed-loop system increased the time spent on glucose target and halved the time spent with a low glucose reading. Elleri et al. [62, 63] assessed in hospital settings a portable ambulatory prototype for an overnight closed-loop regimen on 8 children and 8 young adolescents, respectively. The study proved that the closed-loop regimen implemented on the portable platform was reliable and safe. Early initiation of the closed-loop regimen (18:00 instead of 21:00) led to a significantly higher time in the 71–145 mg/dl range in the adolescents, while there were no significant differences in children. More recently, Elleri et al. [64] tested the same controller in 12 adolescents in a randomized 36-hour study involving physical exercise. The authors showed a significant increase in time spent in target and a significant reduction of average blood glucose.

This MPC-based controller has also been tested in pregnancy. Murphy et al. [65] studied 10 women at 28 and 32 weeks of gestation without finding any significant difference in the control achieved by the MPC algorithm, while in another study Murphy et al. [66] reported a randomized cross-over study on 12 women comparing closed-loop insulin delivery with CSII. The study was repeated twice, 1–6 weeks apart. Closed-loop insulin delivery was found to be as effective as conventional CSII, with less time spent in extreme hypoglycemia.

Recently, the two MPC-based controllers mentioned above were used in a large multicenter study within the AP@home European Project, where they were compared with standard CSII therapy and against each other [67]. Six centers and 47 patients were involved in this randomized 3-arm trial, where each admission lasted about 22 h including meal and exercise. Both algorithms were detuned in this trial to guarantee higher safety and avoid hypoglycemia. An almost threefold reduction of time in hypoglycemia in both closed-loop algorithms with respect to open-loop was achieved at the expense of an higher average glucose level. There were no significant differences in outcomes between algorithms.

Recently, an adaptive, multivariable MPC controller algorithm also measuring additional signals such as energy expenditure and galvanic skin response was tested on 3 patients with encouraging results [23]: closed-loop control was performed for 32 and 60 h without any patient announcement of physical activity and meal. In a study by Dassau et al. [68], a different individualized MPC-based controller, designed for a fully automated closed-loop system (no meal announcement), was tested in 22 and 17 subjects with positive results. Finally, another MPC-based controller was tested overnight in 6 patients [38].

Important work has also been done to test dual-hormone approaches by exploiting glucagon infusion. A dual-hormone fuzzy-logic AP was recently tested by Haidar et al. [69] in 15 adults during a 15-hour visit including exercise, dinner, a bedtime snack, and an overnight stay. The study showed a statistically significant improvement in time spent in the target range and a significant reduction of time in hypoglycemia (both below 72 and 54 mg/dl). A bihormonal proportional-derivative controller was tested by van Bon et al. [70, 71] in 6 patients for 3 days and in 10 patients for 8 h, where it was challenged by meal and exercise, although in this case the number of hypoglycemic episodes were larger in closed-loop systems than in open-loop systems.

A different bihormonal proportional-derivative controller controller, called the 'fading memory proportional derivative' was proposed and tested by Castle et al. [72]. Thirteen subjects were studied in a closed-loop system using insulin plus placebo versus plus glucagon: 7 subjects received glucagon boluses while 6 subjects received glucagon as a square wave. The admissions lasted 22 h and an open-loop preprandial bolus was also delivered. Bolus glucagon delivery significantly reduced the frequency of hypoglycemic events and the need for carbohydrate treatment, while the results were not statistically significant for square wave glucagon infusion. Interestingly, glucagon was not completely effective at preventing hypoglycemia. A refined adaptive version of this algorithm was tested by El Youssef et al. [73] in 14 subjects and compared to the nonadaptive version. An interesting feature of the protocol included the administration of oral hydrocortisol every 4 h to simulate insulin sensitivity changes induced by medical and emotional stress. The adaptive controller proved capable of following insulin sensitivity changes and achieved better performance versus the nonadaptive version.

El-Khatib et al. [74] recently introduced a bihormonal system in which insulin is administered under the control of an MPC algorithm and glucagon is administered

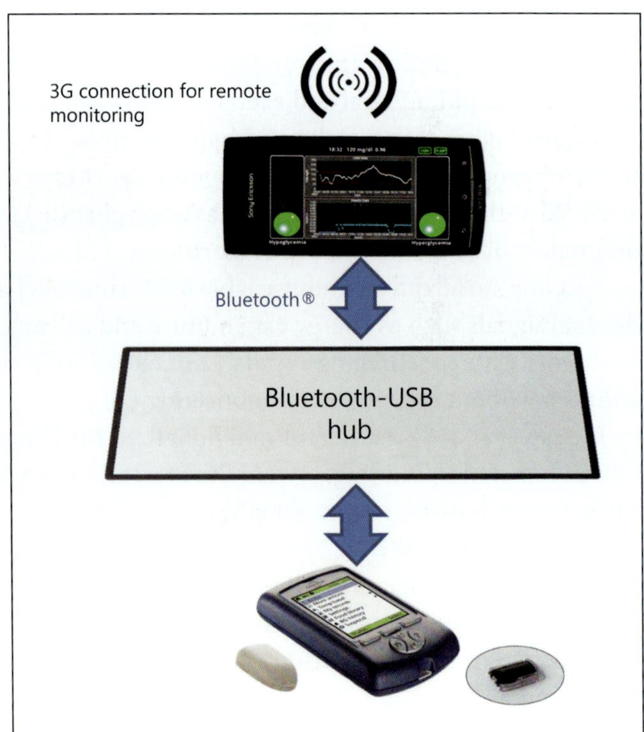

Fig. 6. The DiAs System [77] when used with the OmniPod insulin pump and the Dexcom Seven Plus Sensor as in [85–87].

by a PID control algorithm. A study by these authors in 11 adult patients followed for 27 h showed that the system is capable of preventing hypoglycemia. The same controller was subsequently tested in a 6-patient study lasting 2 days with patients exercising for 30 min/day and eating a high carbohydrate diet: results confirmed that a bihormonal system with priming insulin bolus at mealtime (based only on subject weight and not meal carbohydrates content) allows good glucose control and low risk of hypoglycemia [75].

Outpatient Studies

Technology

The outpatient use of laptop-based platforms such as the APS is limited by the many wired connections among the components. Nonetheless, nonportable laptop-based platforms have been used bedside in outpatient studies for overnight closed-loop control only [76]. Recently, an important step forward for the implementation of an ambulatory AP has been proposed at the University of Virginia [77] (fig. 6). The system, called 'Diabetes Assistant (DiAs)', is capable of connecting with pumps and sensors and to command either open-loop insulin delivery or closed-loop control by

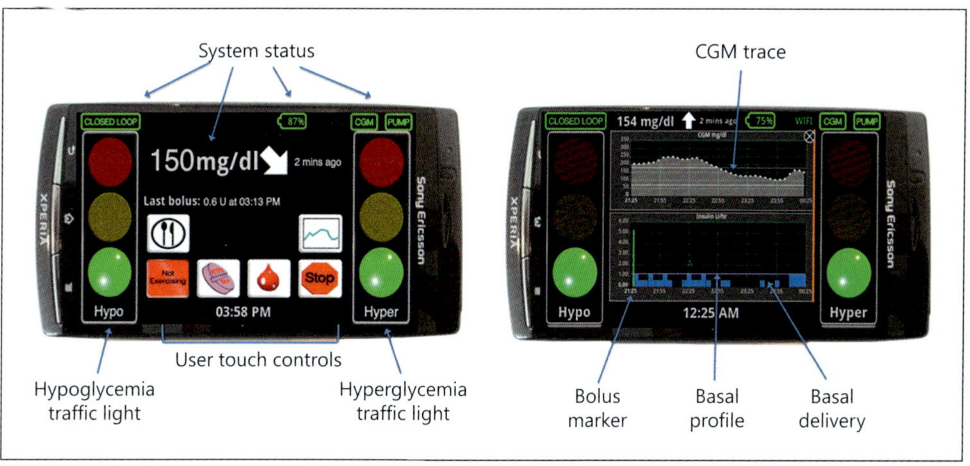

Fig. 7. The DiAs User Interface System [77].

running a control algorithm. Both modes of operation include the fully automated transfer of data from the sensor to DiAs and commands from DiAs to the insulin pump.

The central component of the DiAs system is an off-the-shelf smartphone running the Android® operating system. To ensure the operation of the smartphone as a medical device, its operating system was modified to disable processes not related to clinical operation and to include self-checks of system integrity. The communications between DiAs and the peripherals (pump and sensor) were wireless, giving the patient the freedom to be fully detached from the DiAs controller. In case a Bluetooth® communication port is not available on the pump or sensor, the system components worn by the patient have to include a relay system, processing the accessible signals on the pump and sensor and converting them to Bluetooth.

User-DiAs interaction takes place using a graphical user interface (fig. 7), allowing sensor calibrations, insertion of meal carbohydrate content, preprandial capillary glucose level, and other information the subject wishes to provide (e.g. exercise or hypoglycemia treatment). Moreover, the interface can display CGM traces and insulin delivery graphs. Finally, the user interface can be used to initialize the system with his/her average daily insulin dose, basal rate, carbohydrate ratio, and correction factor. User interaction is also required when the system signals imminent risk for hypo- or hyperglycemia, prompted to the user attention by the traffic lights visible in figure 7.

Other examples of portable platforms are the Medtronic platform based on a BlackBerry Storm smartphone [78] and the Florence Platform (mentioned earlier) in collaboration with Abbot Diabetes Care (Alameda, Calif., USA). The Florence Platform is based on a slightly bigger but still portable computer running Windows, and has been employed in an inpatient setting [63].

Telemedicine

One of the critical issues in moving from inpatient to outpatient trials is to guarantee the highest possible level of safety for the patient, a mandatory prerequisite to gain approval from regulatory bodies. Obviously, the inpatient risk-mitigation solution, i.e. having attending personnel directly watching the patient, cannot be proposed in an outpatient setting as it would interfere with the study, especially overnight, and limit the patients in their activities. To guarantee patient safety in an outpatient setting, the DiAs streams patient and system data in real-time to a telemonitoring website, exploiting the smartphone 3G connectivity. By accessing to the website via an ordinary PC, the study team can monitor from a remote location the status of several patients and check the correct functioning of the system throughout the trial, without interfering/interacting with the experiment. Two examples of telemedicine websites, which have been used by the authors and their collaborators in their outpatient trials are described by Place et al. [79] and Lanzola et al. [80].

The usefulness, necessity, and feasibility of telemonitoring in view of upcoming studies and in the market stage of the AP is a matter of debate. Since 24/7 monitoring will hardly be sustainable, Web-based remote alarm systems, possibly sending e-mail messages to patients, caregivers, and the study teams are currently under review.

Assessment of Clinical Outcomes

During hospital trials, accurate blood glucose measurements are collected by means of dedicated instruments, e.g. YSI or HemoCue® (Angelholm, Sweden), whose accuracy and precision are comparable to gold-standard laboratory measurements. All these techniques are invasive as they require either a blood drop from a fingerprick or venous blood sampling, so that frequent measurements are possible only in an inpatient setting and for a short time. Straightforward employment of CGM traces for a clinical trial assessment may be a suboptimal choice, as recently shown in Hovorka et al. [81] since CGM sensor accuracy and precision limit the possibility to realistically assess the glycemic control achieved. The issue holds for both closed-loop and open-loop systems.

Three contributions have explicitly dealt with the problem of using CGM for a clinical trial assessment. The first one, proposed by Kovatchev and Breton is discussed in a paper by Beck et al. [82]. In the second contribution, Hovorka et al. [81] proposed two algorithms for CGM-based trial assessment. The first is based on an off-line retrospective CGM adjustment, and the second, rather than attempting to reduce CGM error, aims to reduce the bias in the CGM-based estimation of time in target, time below target, and time above target by probabilistically accounting for the possibility that the true blood glucose could be in a different range with respect to that of CGM. The third contribution comes from Del Favero et al. [83], where the problem of blood glucose profile reconstruction from CGM traces is faced with a constrained semiblind deconvolution algorithm that exploits the high accuracy of (possibly sparse) the blood glucose reference measurements collected. The authors of the three methods have validated them with clinical data showing their effectiveness in reducing the error when assessing a clinical trial with respect to the use of CGM data only. At present, a comparison of the three methods on the same dataset has not been made.

Results

The next step in the AP development is testing the safety and efficacy of AP prototypes in a real-life scenario, i.e. outside the hospital environment and free of strict protocol prescriptions. At the time this chapter was written, a few outpatient studies had completed the peer-review process and been published, but a number of groups working in the field have reported at conferences the completion of their outpatient studies. Published results are available for the MD-Logic control algorithm, the multimodular controller proposed by the authors' team, and the PID controller coinfusing glucagon.

The overnight safety and efficacy of a MD-Logic AP was tested in an outpatient setting in a large randomized study [76] involving 54 young patients (10–18 years of age) attending a diabetes camp and showing significant reduction of time spent in hypoglycemia. Since the focus was on overnight control, the closed loop system was not active during the day and the algorithm was implemented on a nonportable bedside platform. Significant reduction of time spent in hypoglycemia and a significant improvement of hypoglycemia-related outcomes was also shown in the study by Nimri et al. [84], who reported the interim analysis of a randomized outpatient trial involving 15 patients (children, adolescents, and adults) studied for 4 consecutive nights at their home.

The authors' group tested two control algorithms of increasing complexity in an outpatient setting: the H2MS and the modular MPC controller, both of which were previously tested and compared in an inpatient setting [51]. H2MS implemented on the DiAs portable platform was employed in the first pilot study [85], which involved 2 centers, with 1 patient each. The study was held in hotel near the local hospital and lasted about 42 h with the platform active for the whole time and the patient allowed to move freely in the facility and in its immediate vicinities. The study started at 18:00 and the first 14 h (until breakfast) were in an open-loop mode, delivered through the platform. Upon regulatory body request, the first 8 h after closed-loop activation were spent in the hospital, but with the patient free to move. Figure 8 shows how the portable platform allows patients to move freely during the study and to test the system in a daily-life scenario. With an identical protocol but improved technology, the study was repeated in 4 centers on 20 patients [86]. Only 2 out of the 4 centers were requested to have the subjects spend the first hours after closed-loop activation in the hospital and the other 2 performed the study on a fully outpatient basis. The DiAs platform worked for 97.7% of the time, showing the feasibility of the outpatient portable closed-loop system.

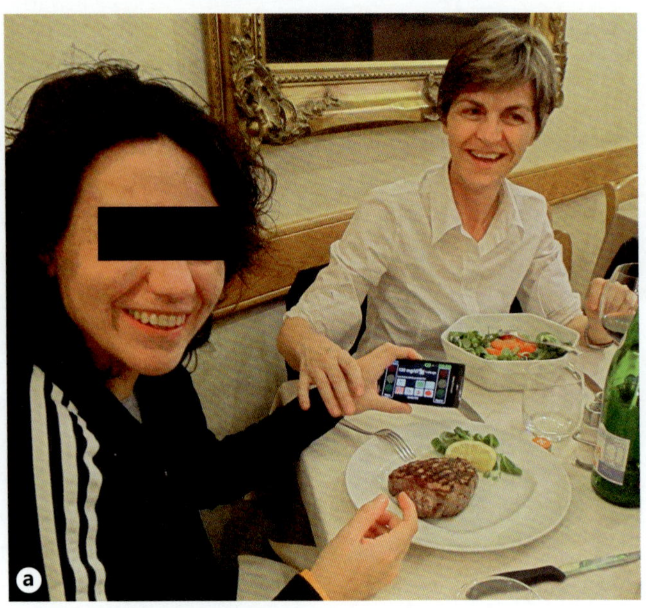

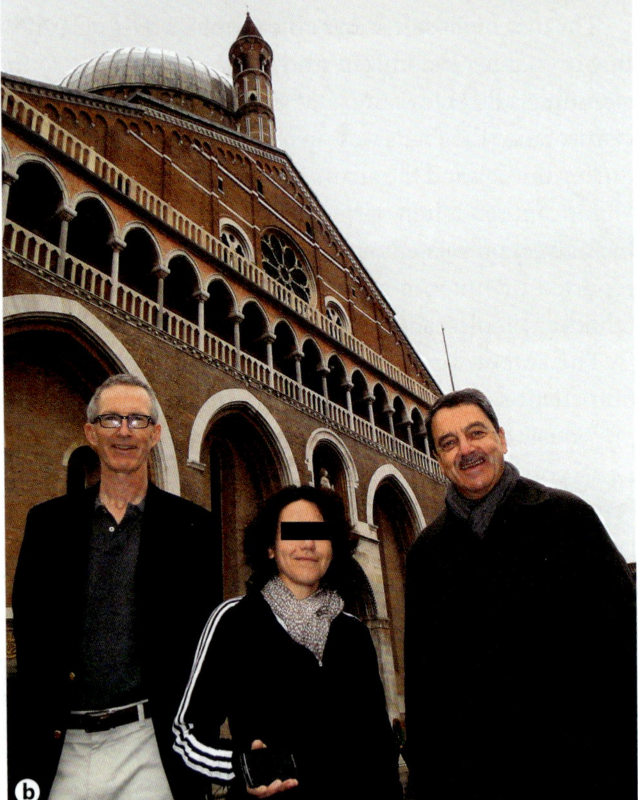

Fig. 8. Two outpatient studies [85, 86]. **a** Dinner at a local restaurant. **b** Walk downtown with the study team. The portable platform allows the patient to move freely during the study.

The MPC controller was tested with the same protocol in 5 patients in one center [87] and in a larger randomized study involving 4 centers and 20 subjects [88], showing significant reduction in the number of hypoglycemic episodes and on the rescue carbohydrate treatment assumed for hypoglycemia treatment with respect to CSII therapy, at the expense of slightly but statistically significant higher average blood glucose (152.1 vs. 161.13 mg/dl, p = 0.042)

Finally, van Bon et al. [89] reported a nonrandomized feasibility study of a portable bihormonal AP in home settings under free-living conditions for 48 h in 16 patients. Of the 11 patients analyzed, significantly lower median glucose levels were found on day 2 in the closed-loop mode with respect to the open-loop mode, at the expense of more time in hypoglycemia.

Conclusions

In this chapter we illustrated the components of an AP with special focus on the control algorithm and reviewed the results of inpatient and outpatient clinical studies. Inpatient validation has consistently shown that closed-loop control is an exciting opportunity for diabetes therapy. Published outpatient studies are still of limited durations (days), but the picture is rapidly evolving with many groups running outpatient studies that are scheduled to last weeks and even months.

References

1 Klein BE, Klein R, McBride PE, Cruickshonks KJ, Polta M, Knutson MD, Moss SE, Reinke JO: Cardiovascular disease, mortality, and retinal microvascular characteristics in type 1 diabetes: Wisconsin epidemiologic study of diabetic retinopathy. Arch Intern Med 2004;164:1917–1924.

2 Nathan DM, Cleary PA, Backlund JY, Genuth SM, Lachin JM, Orchard TJ, Raskin P, Zinman B; Diabetes Control and Complications Trial/Epidemiology of Diabetes Interventions and Complications (DCCT/EDIC) Study Research Group: Intensive diabetes treatment and cardiovascular disease in patients with type 1 diabetes. N Engl J Med 2005;353: 2643–2653.

3 White NH, Sun W, Cleary PA, Danis RP, Davis MD, Hinsworth DP, Hubbard LD, Lachin JM, Nathan DM: Prolonged effect of intensive therapy on the risk of retinopathy complications in patients with type 1 diabetes mellitus: 10 years after the Diabetes Control and Complications Trial. Arch Ophthalmol 2008; 126:1707–1715.

4 Kadish AH: Automation control of blood sugar a servomechanism for glucose monitoring and control. Trans Am Soc Artif Intern Organs 1963;9:363–367.

5 Albisser AM, Leibel BS, Ewart TG, Davidovac Z, Botz CK, Zingg W: An artificial endocrine pancreas. Diabetes 1974;23:389–396.

6 Pfeiffer EF, Thum C, Clemens AH: The artificial beta cell – a continuous control of blood sugar by external regulation of insulin infusion (glucose controlled insulin infusion system). Horm Metab Res 1974;6: 339–342.

7 Mirouze J, Selam JL, Pham TC, Cavadore D: Evaluation of exogenous insulin homoeostasis by the artificial pancreas in insulin-dependent diabetes. Diabetologia 1977;13:273–278.

8 Clemens AH, Chang PH, Myers RW: The development of Biostator, a Glucose Controlled Insulin Infusion System (GCIIS). Horm Metab Res 1977;(Suppl 7):23–33.

9 Bergenstal RM, Tamborlane WV, Ahmann A, Buse JB, Dailey G, Davis SN, Joyce C, Peoples T, Perkins BA, Welsh JB, Willi SM, Wood MA; STAR 3 Study Group: Effectiveness of sensor-augmented insulin-pump therapy in type 1 diabetes. N Engl J Med 2010; 363:311–320.

10 Diabetes Research in Children Network (DirecNet) Study Group, Buckingham B, Beck RW, Tamborlane WV, Xing D, Kollman C, Fiallo-Scharer R, Mauras N, Ruedy KJ, Tansey M, Weinzimer SA, Wysocki T: Continuous glucose monitoring in children with type 1 diabetes. J Pediatr 2007;151:388–393.e1–2.

11 Bode BW, Battelino T: Continuous glucose monitoring in 2012. Diabetes Technol Ther 2013;(Suppl 1): S13–S23.

12 Kumareswaran K, Evans ML, Hovorka R: Closed-loop insulin delivery: towards improved diabetes care. Discov Med 2012;13:159–170.

13 Girardin CM, Huot C, Gonthier M, Delvin E: Continuous glucose monitoring: a review of biochemical perspectives and clinical use in type 1 diabetes. Clin Biochem 2009;42:136–142.

14 Sparacino G, Facchinetti A, Cobelli C: 'Smart' continuous glucose monitoring sensors: on-line signal processing issues. Sensors (Basel) 2010;10:6751–6772.

15 Facchinetti A, Sparacino G, Guerra S, Luijf YM, DeVries JH, Mader JK, Ellmerer M, Benesch C, Heinemann L, Bruttomesso D, Avogaro A, Cobelli C; AP@home Consortium: Real-time improvement of continuous glucose monitoring accuracy: the smart sensor concept. Diabetes Care 2013;36:793–800.

16 Helton KL, Ratner BD, Wisniewski NA: Biomechanics of the sensor-tissue interface-effects of motion, pressure, and design on sensor performance and foreign body response-part II: examples and application. J Diabetes Sci Technol 2011;5:647–656.

17 Facchinetti A, Del Favero S, Sparacino G, Cobelli C: On online failure detection method of the glucose sensor-insulin pump system: improved overnight safety of type-1 diabetic subjects. IEEE Trans Biomed Eng 2013;60:406–416.

18 Renard E, Place J, Cantwell M, Chevassus H, Palerm CC: Closed-loop insulin delivery using a subcutaneous glucose sensor and intraperitoneal insulin delivery: feasibility study testing a new model for the artificial pancreas. Diabetes Care 2010;33:121–127.

19 Weinzimer SA, Steil GM, Swan KL, Dziura J, Kurtz N, Tamborlane WV: Fully automated closed-loop insulin delivery versus semiautomated hybrid control in pediatric patients with type 1 diabetes using an artificial pancreas. Diabetes Care 2008;31:934–939.

20 Bakhtiani PA, Zhao LM, El Youssef J, Castle JR, Ward WK: A review of artificial pancreas technologies with an emphasis on bi-hormonal therapy. Diabetes Obes Metab 2013;15:1065–1070.

21 Pedersen JS: The nature of amyloid-like glucagon fibrils. J Diabetes Sci Technol 2010;4:1357–1367.

22 Weinzimer SA, Sherr JL, Cengiz E, Kim G, Ruiz JL, Carria L, Voskanyan G, Roy A, Tamborlane WV: Effect of pramlintide on prandial glycemic excursions during closed-loop control in adolescents and young adults with type 1 diabetes. Diabetes Care 2012;35: 1994–1999.

23 Turksoy K, Bayrak ES, Quinn L, Littlejohn E, Cinar A: Multivariable adaptive closed-loop control of an artificial pancreas without meal and activity announcement. Diabetes Technol Ther 2013;15:386–400.

24 Atlas E, Nimri R, Miller S, Grunberg EA, Phillip M: MD-Logic artificial pancreas system: a pilot study in adults with type 1 diabetes. Diabetes Care 2010;33: 1072–1076.

25 Ibbini MS, Masadeh MA: A fuzzy logic based closed-loop control system for blood glucose level regulation in diabetics. J Med Eng Technol 2005; 29:64–69.

26 Mauseth R, Hirsch IB, Bollyky J, Kircher R, Matheson D, Sanda S, Greenbaum C: Use of a 'fuzzy logic' controller in a closed-loop artificial pancreas. Diabetes Technol Ther 2013;15:628–633.

27 Grant P: A new approach to diabetic control: fuzzy logic and insulin pump technology. Med Eng Phys 2007;29:824–827.

28 Herrero P, Georgiou P, Oliver N, Johnston DG, Toumazou C: A bio-inspired glucose controller based on pancreatic β-cell physiology. J Diabetes Sci Technol 2012;6:606–616.

29 Palerm CC: Physiologic insulin delivery with insulin feedback: a control systems perspective. Comput Methods Programs Biomed 2011;102:130–137.

30 Steil GM, Rebrin K, Darwin C, Hariri F, Saad MF: Feasibility of automating insulin delivery for the treatment of type 1 diabetes. Diabetes 2006;55:3344–3350.

31 Steil GM, Panteleon AE, Rebrin K: Closed-loop insulin delivery-the path to physiological glucose control. Adv Drug Deliv Rev 2004;56:125–144.

32 Steil GM, Palerm CC, Kurtz N, Voskanyan G, Roy A, Paz S, Kandeel FR: The effect of insulin feedback on closed-loop glucose control. J Clin Endocrinol Metab 2011;96:1402–1408.

33 Magni L, Raimondo DM, Bossi L, Dalla Man C, De Nicolao G, Kovatchev B, Cobelli C: Model predictive control of type 1 diabetes: an in silico trial. J Diabetes Sci Technol 2007;1:804–812.

34 Hovorka R, Canonico V, Chassin LJ, Haueter U, Massi-Benedetti M, Orsini Federici M, Pieber TR, Schaller HC, Schaupp L, Vering T, Wilinska ME: Nonlinear model predictive control of glucose concentration in subjects with type 1 diabetes. Physiol Meas 2004;25:905–920.

35 Grosman B, Dassau E, Zisser HC, Jovanovic L, Doyle FJ 3rd: Zone model predictive control: a strategy to minimize hyper- and hypoglycemic events. J Diabetes Sci Technol 2010;4:961–975.

36 Lee H, Buckingham BA, Wilson DM, Bequette BW: A closed-loop artificial pancreas using model predictive control and a sliding meal size estimator. J Diabetes Sci Technol 2009;3:1082–1090.

37 Cameron F, Bequette BW, Wilson DM, Buckingham BA, Lee H, Niemeyer G: A closed-loop artificial pancreas based on risk management. J Diabetes Sci Technol 2011;5:368–379.

38 Schmidt S, Boiroux D, Duun-Henriksen AK, Frøssing L, Skyggebjerg O, Jørgensen JB, Poulsen NK, Madsen H, Madsbad S, Nørgaard K: Model-based closed-loop glucose control in type 1 diabetes: the DiaCon experience. J Diabetes Sci Technol 2013;7:1255–1264.

39 Elleri D, Allen JM, Nodale M, Wilinska ME, Acerini CL, Dunger DB, Hovorka R: Suspended insulin infusion during overnight closed-loop glucose control in children and adolescents with type 1 diabetes. Diabet Med 2010;27:480–484.

40 Patek SD, Magni L, Dassau E, Karvetski C, Toffanin C, De Nicolao G, Del Favero S, Breton M, Man CD, Renard E, Zisser H, Doyle FJ 3rd, Cobelli C, Kovatchev BP; International Artificial Pancreas (iAP) Study Group: Modular closed-loop control of diabetes. IEEE Trans Biomed Eng 2012;59:2986–2999.

41 Hughes CS, Patek SD, Breton MD, Kovatchev BP: Hypoglycemia prevention via pump attenuation and red-yellow-green 'traffic' lights using continuous glucose monitoring and insulin pump data. J Diabetes Sci Technol 2010;4:1146–1155.

42 Dassau E, Cameron F, Lee H, Bequette BW, Zisser H, Jovanovic L, Chase HP, Wilson DM, Buckingham BA, Doyle FJ 3rd: Real-time hypoglycemia prediction suite using continuous glucose monitoring: a safety net for the artificial pancreas. Diabetes Care 2010;33:1249–1254.

43 Kovatchev B, Patek S, Dassau E, Doyle FJ, Magni L, De Nicolao G, Cobelli C; Juvenile Diabetes Research Foundation Artificial Pancreas Consortium: Control to range for diabetes: functionality and modular architecture. J Diabetes Sci Technol 2009;3:1058–1065.

44 Soru P, De Nicolao G, Toffanin C, Dalla Man C, Cobelli C, Magni L; AP@home consortium: MPC based artificial pancreas: strategies for individualization and meal compensation. Ann Rev Control 2012;36:118–128.

45 Toffanin C, Messori M, Di Palma F, De Nicolao G, Cobelli C, Magni L: Artificial pancreas: MPC design from clinical experience. J Diabetes Sci Technol 2013;7:1470–1483.

46 Hovorka R, Chassin LJ, Wilinska ME, Canonico V, Akwi JA, Federici MO, Massi-Benedetti M, Hutzli I, Zaugg C, Kaufmann H, Both M, Vering T, Schaller HC, Schaupp L, Bodenlenz M, Pieber TR: Closing the loop: the ADICOL experience. Diabetes Technol Ther 2004;3:307–318.

47 Chassin LJ, Wilinska ME, Hovorka R: Evaluation of glucose controllers in virtual environment: methodology and sample application. Artif Intell Med 2004;32:171–181.

48 Wilinska ME, Budiman ES, Taub MB, Elleri D, Allen JM, Acerini CL, Dunger DB, Hovorka R: Overnight closed-loop insulin delivery with model predictive control: assessment of hypoglycemia and hyperglycemia risk using simulation studies. J Diabetes Sci Technol 2009;3:1109–1120.

49 Kovatchev BP, Breton M, Dalla Man C, Cobelli C: In silico preclinical trials: a proof of concept in closed-loop control of type 1 diabetes. J Diabetes Sci Technol 2009;3:44–55.

50 Dalla Man C, Micheletto F, Lv D, Breton M, Kovatchev B, Cobelli C: The UVA/PADOVA Type 1 Diabetes Simulator: new features. J Diabetes Sci Technol 2014;8:26–34.

51 Breton M, Farret A, Bruttomesso D, Anderson S, Magni L, Patek C, Dalla Man C, Place J, Demartini S, Del Favero S, Toffanin C, Hughes C, Dassau E, Zisser H, Doyle FJ III, De Nicolao G, Avogaro A, Cobelli C, Renard E, Kovatchev B; International Artificial Pancreas Study Group: Fully integrated artificial pancreas in type 1 diabetes: modular closed-loop glucose control maintains near-normoglycemia. Diabetes 2012;61:2230–2237.

52 Hovorka R, Allen JM, Elleri D, Chassin LJ, Harris J, Xing D, Kollman C, Hovorka T, Larsen AM, Nodale M, De Palma A, Wilinska ME, Acerini CL, Dunger DB: Manual closed-loop insulin delivery in children and adolescents with type 1 diabetes: a phase 2 randomized crossover trial. Lancet 2010;375:743–751.

53 Dassau E, Zisser H, Palerm C, Buckingham B, Jovanovic L, Doyle FJ 3rd: Modular artificial beta-cell system: a prototype for clinical research. J Diabetes Sci Technol 2008;2:863–872.

54 Nimri R, Atlas E, Ajzensztejn M, Miller S, Oron T, Phillip M: Feasibility study of automated overnight closed-loop glucose control under MD-Logic artificial pancreas in patients with type 1 diabetes: the DREAM Project. Diabetes Technol Ther 2012;14:728–735.

55 Nimri R, Danne T, Kordonouri O, Atlas E, Bratina N, Biester T, Avbelj M, Miller S, Muller I, Phillip M, Battelino T: The 'Glucositter' overnight automated closed-loop system for type 1 diabetes: a randomized crossover trial. Pediatr Diabetes 2013;14:159–167.

56 Mauseth R, Hirsch IB, Bollyky J, Kircher R, Matheson D, Sanda S, Greenbaum C: Use of a 'fuzzy logic' controller in a closed-loop artificial pancreas. Diabetes Technol Ther 2013;15:628–633.

57 Capel I, Rigla M, García-Sáez G, Rodríguez-Herrero A, Pons B, Subías D, García-García F, Gallach M, Aguilar M, Pérez-Gandía C, Gómez EJ, Caixàs A, Hernando ME: Artificial pancreas using a personalized rule-based controller achieves overnight normoglycemia in patients with type 1 diabetes. Diabetes Technol Ther 2013;16:172–179.

58 Bruttomesso D, Farret A, Costa S, Marescotti MC, Vettore M, Avogaro A, Tiengo A, Dalla Man C, Place J, Facchinetti A, Guerra S, Magni L, De Nicolao G, Cobelli C, Renard E, Maran A: Closed-loop artificial pancreas using subcutaneous glucose sensing and insulin delivery and a model predictive control algorithm: preliminary studies in Padova and Montpellier. J Diabetes Sci Technol 2009;3:1014–1021.

59 Clarke WL, Anderson S, Breton M, Patek S, Kashmer L, Kovatchev B: Closed-loop artificial pancreas using subcutaneous glucose sensing and insulin delivery and a model predictive control algorithm: the Virginia experience. J Diabetes Sci Technol 2009;3: 1031–1038.

60 Kovatchev B, Cobelli C, Renard E, Anderson S, Breton M, Patek S, Clarke W, Bruttomesso D, Maran A, Costa S, Avogaro A, Dalla Man C, Facchinetti A, Magni L, De Nicolao G, Place J, Farret A: Multinational study of subcutaneous model-predictive closed-loop control in type 1 diabetes mellitus: summary of the results. J Diabetes Sci Technol 2010;4: 1374–1381.

61 Hovorka R, Kumareswaran K, Harris J, Allen JM, Elleri D, Xing D, Kollman C, Nodale M, Murphy HR, Dunger DB, Amiel SA, Heller SR, Wilinska ME, Evans ML: Overnight closed-loop insulin delivery (artificial pancreas) in adults with type 1 diabetes: crossover randomised controlled studies. BMJ 2011;342: d1855.

62 Elleri D, Allen JM, Nodale M, Wilinska ME, Mangat JS, Larsen AM, Acerini CL, Dunger DB, Hovorka R: Automated overnight closed-loop glucose control in young children with type 1 diabetes. Diabetes Technol Ther 2011;13:419–424.

63 Elleri D, Allen JM, Biagioni M, Kumareswaran K, Leelarathna L, Caldwell K, Nodale M, Wilinska ME, Acerini CL, Dunger DB, Hovorka R: Evaluation of a portable ambulatory prototype for automated overnight closed-loop insulin delivery in young people with type 1 diabetes. Pediatr Diabetes 2012;13:449–453.

64 Elleri D, Allen JM, Kumareswaran K, Leelarathna L, Nodale M, Caldwell K, Cheng P, Kollman C, Haidar A, Murphy HR, Wilinska ME, Acerini CL, Dunger DB, Hovorka R: Closed-loop basal insulin delivery over 36 hours in adolescents with type 1 diabetes: randomized clinical trial. Diabetes Care 2013;36: 838–844.

65 Murphy HR, Elleri D, Allen JM: Closed-loop insulin delivery during pregnancy complicated by type 1 diabetes. Diabetes Care 2011;34:406–411.

66 Murphy HR, Kumareswaran K, Elleri D, Allen JM, Caldwell K, Biagioni M, Simmons D, Dunger DB, Nodale M, Wilinska ME, Amiel SA, Hovorka R: Safety and efficacy of 24-h closed-loop insulin delivery in well-controlled pregnant women with type 1 diabetes: a randomized crossover case series. Diabetes Care 2011;34:2527–2539.

67 Luijf YM, DeVries JH, Zwinderman K, Leelarathna L, Nodale M, Caldwell K, Kumareswaran K, Elleri D, Allen JM, Wilinska ME, Evans ML, Hovorka R, Doll W, Ellmerer M, Mader JK, Renard E, Place J, Farret A, Cobelli C, Del Favero S, Dalla Man C, Avogaro A, Bruttomesso D, Filippi A, Scotton R, Magni L, Lanzola G, Di Palma F, Soru P, Toffanin C, De Nicolao G, Arnolds S, Benesch C, Heinemann L; AP@home Consortium: Day and night closed-loop control in adults with type 1 diabetes: a comparison of two closed-loop algorithms driving continuous subcutaneous insulin infusion versus patient self-management. Diabetes Care 2013;36:3882–3887.

68 Dassau E, Zisser H, Harvey RA, Percival MW, Grosman B, Bevier W, Atlas E, Miller S, Nimri R, Jovanovic L, Doyle FJ 3rd: Clinical evaluation of a personalized artificial pancreas. Diabetes Care 2013;36: 801–809.

69 Haidar A, Legault L, Dallaire M, Alkhateeb A, Coriati A, Messier V, Cheng P, Millette M, Boulet B, Rabasa-Lhoret R: Glucose-responsive insulin and glucagon delivery (dual-hormone artificial pancreas) in adults with type 1 diabetes: a randomized crossover controlled trial. CMAJ 2013;185:297–305.

70 van Bon AC, Hermanides J, Koops R, Hoekstra JB, DeVries JH: Postprandial glycemic excursions with the use of a closed-loop platform in subjects with type 1 diabetes: a pilot study. J Diabetes Sci Technol 2010;4:923–928.

71 van Bon AC, Jonker LD, Koebrugge R, Koops R, Hoekstra JB, DeVries JH: Feasibility of a bihormonal closed-loop system to control postexercise and postprandial glucose excursions. J Diabetes Sci Technol 2012;6:1114–1122.

72 Castle JR, Engle JM, El Youssef J, Massoud RG, Yuen KC, Kagan R, Ward WK: Novel use of glucagon in a closed-loop system for prevention of hypoglycemia in type 1 diabetes. Diabetes Care 2010;33:1282–1287.

73 El Youssef J, Castle JR, Branigan DL, Massoud RG, Breen ME, Jacobs PG, Bequette BW, Ward WK: A controlled study of the effectiveness of an adaptive closed-loop algorithm to minimize corticosteroid-induced stress hyperglycemia in type 1 diabetes. J Diabetes Sci Technol 2011;5:1312–1326.

74 El-Khatib FH, Russell SJ, Nathan DM, Sutherlin RG, Damiano ER: A bihormonal closed-loop artificial for type 1 diabetes. Sci Transl Med 2010;2:27ra27.

75 Russel SJ, El-Khatib FHE, Nathan DM, Magyar KL, Jiang J, Damiano ER: Blood glucose control in type 1 diabetes with a bihormonal bionic endocrine pancreas. Diabetes Care 2012;35:2148–2155.

76 Phillip M, Battelino T, Atlas E, Kordonouri O, Bratina N, Miller S, Biester T, Stefanija MA, Muller I, Nimri R, Danne T: Nocturnal glucose control with an artificial pancreas at a diabetes camp. N Engl J Med 2013;368:824–833.

77 Keith-Hynes P, Guerlain S, Mize B, Hughes-Karvetski C, Khan M, McElwee-Malloy M, Kovatchev BP: DiAs user interface: a patient-centric interface for mobile artificial pancreas systems. J Diabetes Sci Technol 2013;7:1416–1426.

78 O'Grady MJ, Retterath AJ, Keenan DB, Kurtz N, Cantwell M, Spital G, Kremliovsky MN, Roy A, Davis EA, Jones TW, Ly TT: The use of an automated, portable glucose control system for overnight glucose control in adolescents and young adults with type 1 diabetes. Diabetes Care 2012;35:2182–2187.

79 Place J, Robert A, Ben Brahim N, Keith-Hynes P, Farret A, Pelletier A, Buckingham B, Breton M, Kovatchev B, Renard E: DiAs web monitoring: a real-time remote monitoring system designed for artificial pancreas outpatient trials. J Diabetes Sci Technol 2013;7:1427–1435.

80 Lanzola G, Scarpellini S, Di Palma F, Toffanin C, Del Favero S, Magni L, Bellazzi R; on behalf of the AP@home Consortium: Monitoring artificial pancreas trials through agent-based technologies: a case report. J Diabetes Sci Technol 2014;8:216–224.

81 Hovorka R, Nodale M, Haidar A, Wilinska ME: Assessing performance of closed-loop insulin delivery systems by continuous glucose monitoring: drawbacks and way forward. Diabetes Technol Ther 2013; 15:4–12.

82 Beck RW, Calhoun P, Kollman C: Challenges for outpatient closed-loop studies: how to assess efficacy. Diabetes Technol Ther 2013;15:1–3.

83 Del Favero S, Facchinetti A, Sparacino G, Cobelli C: Improving accuracy and precision of glucose sensor profiles: retrospective fitting by constrained deconvolution. IEEE Trans Biomed 2014;61:1044–1053.

84 Nimri R, Muller I, Atlas E, Miller S, Kordonouri O, Bratina N, Tsioli C, Stefanija MA, Danne T, Battelino T, Phillip M: Night glucose control with MD-Logic artificial pancreas in home setting: a single blind, randomized crossover trial-interim analysis. Pediatr Diabetes 2014;15:91–99.

85 Cobelli C, Renard E, Kovatchev BP, Keith-Hynes P, Ben Brahim N, Place J, Del Favero S, Breton M, Farret A, Bruttomesso D, Dassau E, Zisser H, Doyle FJ 3rd, Patek SD, Avogaro A: Pilot studies of wearable outpatient artificial pancreas in type 1 diabetes. Diabetes Care 2012;35:65–66.

86 Kovatchev BP, Renard E, Cobelli C, Zisser HC, Keith-Hynes P, Anderson SM, Brown SA, Chernavvsky DR, Breton MD, Farret A, Pelletier MJ, Place J, Bruttomesso D, Del Favero S, Visentin R, Filippi A, Scotton R, Avogaro A, Doyle FJ 3rd: Feasibility of outpatient fully integrated closed-loop control: first studies of wearable artificial pancreas. Diabetes Care 2013;36:1851–1858.

87 Del Favero S, Bruttomesso D, Di Palma F, Lanzola G, Visentin R, Filippi A, Scotton R, Toffanin C, Messori M, Scarpellini S, Keith-Hynes P, Kovatchev BP, DeVries JH, Renard E, Magni L, Avogaro A, Cobelli C; AP@home Consortium: First use of model predictive control in outpatient wearable artificial pancreas. Diabetes Care 2014;37:1212–1215.

88 Kovatchev BP, Renard E, Cobelli C, Zisser HC, Keith-Hynes P, Anderson SM, Brown SA, Chernavvsky DR, Breton MD, Farret A, Place J, Bruttomesso D, Del Favero S, Boscari F, Galasso S, Avogaro A, Magni L, Doyle FJ 3rd: Safety of outpatient closed-loop control: first randomized cross-over trials of a wearable artificial pancreas. Diabetes Care 2014, E-pub ahead of print.

89 van Bon AC, Luijf YM, Koebrugge R, Koops R, Hoekstra JB, Devries JH: Feasibility of a portable bihormonal closed-loop system to control glucose excursions at home under free-living conditions for 48 hours. Diabetes Technol Ther 2013;16:131–136.

Claudio Cobelli, PhD
Department of Information Engineering, University of Padova
Via Gradenigo 6/A
IT–35131 Padova (Italy)
E-Mail cobelli@dei.unipd.it

Bruttomesso D, Grassi G (eds): Technological Advances in the Treatment of Type 1 Diabetes.
Front Diabetes. Basel, Karger, 2015, vol 24, pp 190–209 (DOI: 10.1159/000363513)

Continuous Intraperitoneal Insulin Infusion from Implantable Pumps

Eric Renard[a–c]

[a]Department of Endocrinology, Diabetes and Nutrition, Montpellier University Hospital, [b]INSERM CIC 1411 and [c]Institute of Functional Genomics, CNRS 5203/INSERM U661/University of Montpellier I and II, Montpellier, France

Abstract

Continuous intraperitoneal insulin infusion (CIPII) presents specific pharmacokinetics and pharmacodynamics which allow insulin replacement in a way closer to physiology than subcutaneous insulin delivery. Insulin absorption occurs faster, mainly in the hepatic venous portal system, which results in lower peripheral insulin levels. Insulin action on glucose levels is quicker, more reproducible, and shorter, which allows a more accurate and reactive tuning. CIPII was initially used in patients with brittle diabetes, via the percutaneous implantation of abdominal catheters to which portable pumps were connected. The development of fully implantable, programmable insulin pumps followed the availability of concentrated insulin preparations which were stable for weeks at body temperature. Clinical studies have documented the improved stability of blood glucose levels under CIPII, resulting in sustained near-normoglycemia combined with a dramatic reduction of hypoglycemic excursions in patients who were poorly controlled with subcutaneous insulin infusion. Episodes of underdelivery still affect CIPII from implanted pumps. Pump slowdowns occur periodically due to gradual depots of aggregated insulin in the pumping mechanism. Although fully reversible by NaOH rinsing of the pump insulin pathways, these recurrent reductions of insulin delivery remain a limitation of this technology. Recent trials have shown interest in CIPII in artificial pancreas models.

Although the concept of implantable insulin delivery systems for diabetes treatment started moving towards materialization more than 40 years ago, less than 500 patients worldwide are using such devices for insulin administration at the present time. Only one model of implantable insulin pump is commercially available in the European Union, but none in the USA. However, the project of implantable insulin pumps is motivated by three noble objectives: (1) to develop by continuous intraperitoneal insulin infusion (CIPII) a route of delivery more physiological than subcutaneous infusion, (2) to free patients of externally worn infusion devices, and (3) to finally steer towards an implantable artificial β-cell by the addition of a glucose sensor that would allow closed-loop insulin delivery.

As early as 1969, Perry Blackshear, Henry Buchwald, and co-workers [1] designed the first single-rate implantable pump for medication delivery at the University of Minnesota, which was developed further to infuse insulin by Infusaid (Norwood, Mass., USA). Insulin was infused continuously, using an intravenous route, from this device by a constant vapor pressure exerted on the reservoir by Freon gas. Although improvements in glucose control were obtained with this pump model in mostly type 2 diabetic patients, delivery problems occurred due to insulin aggregation in the system and variations of insulin flow rate related to altitude and body temperature that altered vapor pressure of the Freon gas [2]. Variable-rate implantable peristaltic insulin pumps were firstly designed at the beginning of the 1980s by Siemens AG (Erlangen, Germany) [3] and Sandia (Albuquerque, N.Mex., USA) [4]. Insulin aggregation in the pump or in the delivery catheter was still the main issue that limited clinical use of these devices [5]. Clinical trials with implantable insulin pumps could only start again in 1986 when the problem of insulin stability had been solved by the addition of polyethylene-polypropylene glycol (Genapol®; Hoechst AG, Frankfurt, Germany) to insulin preparations, resulting in U-100 and U-400 Hoe 21PH insulin formulations [6]. This surface-active agent was able to prevent interactions between insulin and pump flow pathways that promoted insulin aggregation. Three pump models were designed to use this Genapol-stabilized insulin: the Promedos ID1 pump by Siemens AG, PIMS (Programmable Implantable Medication System) by MiniMed Inc., and Model 1000 pump by Infusaid [7–9]. Whereas the Promedos ID1 and Infusaid Model 1000 were tested using intravenous and intraperitoneal routes, PIMS only used intraperitoneal delivery. Because of the early catheter occlusions with the intravenous route, intraperitoneal insulin delivery was then preferred. After promising feasibility trials (see section: Feasibility and Effectiveness of Implantable Pump Therapy), further improved pump models were designed by Siemens-Elema (Promedos ID3) and MiniMed Inc. (MIP2001). While Siemens-Elema and Infusaid-Pfizer stopped their research and development in this field in the 1990s, only MiniMed Inc., merging to Medtronic in August 2001, continued to develop implantable insulin delivery systems. Finally, the first combination of an implantable insulin pump (MIP2007) and a long-term intravenous glucose sensor, forming the Long-Term Sensor System (LTSS), was implanted in a patient with type 1 diabetes in 2000 [10]. A first short-term trial of closed-loop insulin delivery using LTSS was achieved in this patient in 2001 and has been reproduced [11]. The longevity of the implanted sensors, barely exceeding 6 months, led to the interruption of this project. More recent experiments have shown the feasibility of closed-loop insulin delivery by the combination of the MIP2007 and a subcutaneous glucose sensor [12].

The limited expansion of implantable insulin pumps as a way to use CIPII has led to the recent development of the DiaPort® by Roche Diagnostics (Mannheim, Germany) on the basis of former experiences with implanted abdominal catheters for CIPII.

Rationale for Intraperitoneal Insulin Delivery

The Diabetes Control and Complications Trial (DCCT) has clearly shown that near-normoglycemia must be the treatment goal of type 1 diabetes mellitus in order to reduce the incidence of diabetic complications [13]. Although intensive subcutaneous insulin treatment using multiple daily injections or continuous subcutaneous insulin infusion (CSII) could lead to sustained glycated hemoglobin (HbA_{1c}) levels close to 7%, the high incidence of severe hypoglycemia appeared as a significant side effect that limited the benefit of this route of insulin delivery. Poorly reproducible and predictable insulin effects with the subcutaneous route are the main causes of the variability of blood glucose levels and hence of hypoglycemic events [5]. Many factors are involved in this poor reliability of subcutaneous insulin delivery. Absorption of subcutaneous insulin may vary 20–30% in a single patient using the same dose of insulin, injected at the same site when looking at plasma insulin peaks or areas under the insulin-response curves, whether using regular or intermediate-acting insulin [14]. Moreover, insulin dose, injection site, depth of injection, environmental temperature, and exercise all influence the quickness and duration of insulin action. Although fast-acting insulin analogues reduce both the time of subcutaneous absorption and duration of insulin action, resulting in a more reactive insulin effect, the reduction of hypoglycemic events has been inconstantly significant in clinical trials when compared with regular insulin [15].

In order to overcome these problems, both intravenous and intraperitoneal insulin administrations have been considered as more physiological means of delivery. The intravenous route is more straightforward and has been used in first attempts of continuous insulin infusion using portable or implantable pumps [5]. Moreover, the first artificial pancreas models were made possible by intravenous insulin infusion, which has provided highly reproducible and reactive metabolic effects [16]. However, the development of pumps using a pulsatile way of infusion has been associated with an increased incidence of catheter obstructions that have favored the intraperitoneal route since 1985.

Pharmacokinetics and Pharmacodynamics of Intraperitoneal Insulin Infusion

Intraperitoneal insulin delivery was initially used in diabetic patients with renal failure treated by peritoneal dialysis and shown to be effective and convenient in these subjects [17]. Several studies have since been performed in animal models to assess the characteristics of peritoneal insulin absorption [18, 19]. Insulin absorption from the peritoneal space was shown to be dependent on volume, concentration, and time [18]. More interestingly, insulin was first distributed to the portal vein before entering the systemic circulation [19]. A positive gradient between portal and systemic blood insulin was further demonstrated by intraperitoneal insulin administration that differed from intramuscular insulin injection but mimicked endogenous insulin secretion. In humans, intraperitoneal insulin delivery has been shown to allow quicker insulin peaks than the subcutaneous route: 70 versus 120 min, with plasma insulin levels returning to baseline after 165 min as in normal subjects [20]. While the rate of systemic appearance of intraperitoneal infused insulin was lower than subcutaneous infused insulin at steady-state, the percent increase in the rate of systemic appearance after an increase of infusion rate was higher with the intraperitoneal route [21]. These data showed a quicker absorption of insulin from the peritoneum that prefigured a higher reactivity in clinical use, and suggested the likely role of the liver in modulating peripheral insulin delivery. As a result, lower peripheral insulinemia, close to physiological levels, was obtained in steady-state conditions with the intraperitoneal route in comparison to subcutaneous insulin delivery. However, the answer to the question of whether hepatic insulinization secondary to intraperitoneal insulin delivery controls hepatic glucose output better than systemic insulin delivery is still unclear. Since systemic insulin levels reduce the delivery of gluconeogenic substrates from peripheral tissues to the liver with respect to portal insulin, they may in fact also lower fasting hepatic glucose output [22]. Studies in animals and humans comparing the effects of intraperitoneal and intravenous insulin infusions have shown similar reductions of hepatic glucose output.

Clinical Experience of Intraperitoneal Insulin Infusion by Percutaneously Implanted Abdominal Catheters

Because of the clinical problems related to prolonged intravenous insulin infusion (limited venous access and tolerance, thrombosis), the experience with intraperitoneal insulin delivery has been wider. The first case reports of intraperitoneal insulin delivery from portable pumps and via a catheter that was indwelled into the peritoneal cavity through the abdominal wall indicated effectiveness of this therapeutic mode in brittle diabetes after failure to achieve glucose control with subcutaneous, intramuscular, and sometimes intravenous insulin [5]. Selam [23] reported a large experience with this technique, totaling 472 patient-months in 40 type 1 diabetic patients. Metabolic control was significantly improved with reduced insulin doses. The technique, however, was associated with frequent local infectious complications around the implantation site of the catheter. No overdelivery of insulin occurred, but underdeliveries related to pump failures or catheter obstructions were reported, resulting in the 1-year survival rates of the pump and catheter being 46 and 70%, respectively. Fibrin nodes at the catheter tip or omental encapsulation of the catheter were shown to explain catheter obstructions in a further report.

To overcome these problems, specific ports were implanted in the abdominal wall through which the peritoneal catheter reached peritoneal space [24]. Using this technique, blocked catheters were expected to be more easily replaced. However, infections around the port frequently led to port removal, and catheter replacements in case of encapsulation remained sometimes hardly achievable. A new device (DiaPort) that might reduce the incidence of these complications is currently under investigation in Europe. In spite of the drawbacks of these externally worn devices, intraperitoneal insulin infusion has been shown to provide tighter glucose control than subcutaneous infusion or injections during the operating time. A crucial benefit was the combination of a similar HbA_{1c} or mean blood glucose, and a very low incidence of severe hypoglycemia, related to the pharmacokinetics of the intraperitoneal route [25].

Technological Requirements for Implantable Pumps

Requirements for implantable insulin pumps include physically and chemically stable insulin preparations, miniaturized and telemetry-controlled safe and reliable infusion systems, biocompatible materials for pumps and catheters, and a sustained power source for long-term infusion from the implanted pump. Easy access to the pump reservoir for insulin refills and to the peritoneal catheter in case of underdelivery are also mandatory.

Conditions for Insulin Preparations

The trend for insulin aggregation (i.e. physical instability) is a crucial phenomenon to overcome to allow safe and reliable artificial insulin delivery devices, as shown by the rapid failures of initial attempts to develop implantable pumps. The two main mechanisms involved in insulin aggregation are isoelectric precipitation and noncovalent polymerization (or fibrillation) [26]. Insulin precipitation is promoted by pH fall and metal ions. This process can be overcome by stabilizing solution pH by using buffer, preventing CO_2 diffusion into the insulin solution by an appropriate choice of catheter components, and avoiding metal ion liberation from the pump materials. The formation of insoluble insulin fibrils is promoted in artificial insulin delivery devices by a combination of heat, movement, and hydrophobic interactions. Interactions between insulin and hydrophobic surfaces have been pointed out as key determinants of the aggregating process. Conformational changes of the tertiary structure of insulin at liquid-solid and liquid-air interfaces have been suspected of inducing insulin noncovalent polymerization by promoting interactions between hydrophobic nonpolar side chains of insulin molecules. Hence, the pump fluid system should be inert, airtight, and with a hydrophilic minimal inner surface. The elaboration of Genapol, a surface-active agent able to prevent hydrophobic interactions of insulin with surface materials of pump reservoirs and tubings by providing hydrophilicity, allowed con-

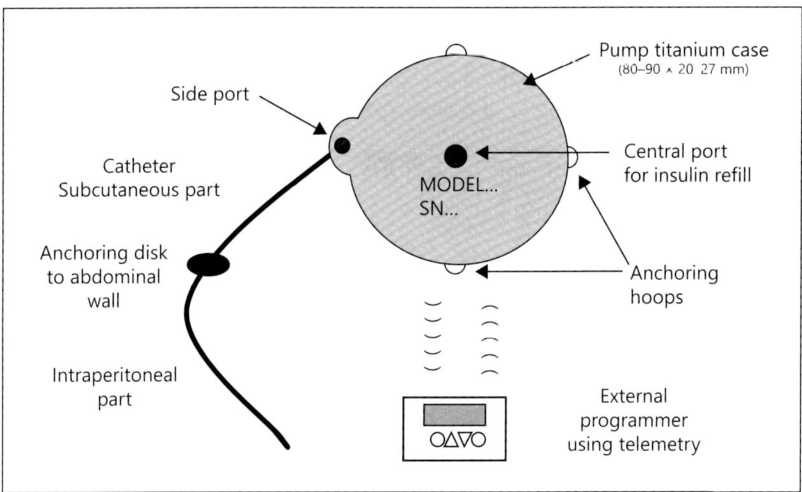

Fig. 1. Scheme of an implantable insulin pump.

siderable improvements in the physical stability of insulin preparation for implantable systems [6].

During the last years, a similar preparation of insulin for implantable pumps has been developed by Sanofi (Paris, France) by replacing semisynthetic human insulin with recombinant human insulin. U-400 solution of this insulin is currently investigated in MIP2007.

Conditions for Implantable Pumps

Required components of an implantable insulin pump include an insulin reservoir, a pump and valves, a motor and a battery to supply the power, a clock, a computer, and a radio transmitter and receiver. All these elements are enclosed in a titanium case that comprises a connecting outlet for catheter attachment (fig. 1). An external programmer is used to modulate insulin delivery according to patient needs.

The insulin reservoir must be easily accessible for refills through a subcutaneous port, and large enough to cover insulin requirements over at least 1 month. Subcutaneous implantations in the lower quadrants of the abdomen have been chosen to allow easy access to the pump. The reservoir may be under positive or negative pressure according to the pumping principle. Among the three pump models that were developed around 1990, two had a reservoir under negative pressure (MiniMed Implantable Pump Model 2001 and Promedos ID 3) and one had a reservoir under positive pressure (Infusaid Model 1000) (table 1). The advantage of negative pressure is the prevention of insulin refills outside the reservoir since insulin passively enters the reservoir. However, while air bubbles in insulin solution may be expelled from the reservoir and through the pump and catheter in case of positive pressure, they will expand in reservoirs under negative pressure and may lead to air-locks of the pump.

Table 1. Main characteristics of programmable implantable insulin pumps investigated in diabetic patients since 1985

Model	Pump mechanism	Pressure in reservoir	Reservoir capacity, ml	Insulin concentration	Stroke volume, µl	Programmable basal rates, n/day	Bolus range, IU	Weight, g (filled with insulin)	Size, mm[a]
Siemens ID1	peristaltic	negative	10	U-100	NC	1	0–14	180	85×60×22
Siemens ID3	piston	negative	20	U-100	1	6	NC	165	80×21
Infusaid M1000	accumulator valve	positive	25	U-100	1	6	0–99.9	300	90×27
MiniMed PIMS	diaphragm	negative	10	U-400	2	24	1–31	215	81×23
MiniMed MIP 2001	piston	negative	15	U-400	0.5	2	0.2–32	162	81×20
Medtronic-MiniMed MIP 2007	piston	negative	15	U-400	0.5	48	0–35	146	81×20

NC = Not communicated. [a] Length × width × thickness for Siemens ID1; diameter × thickness for other pumps.

Because the reservoir capacity is hardly reducible, implantable pumps are difficult to miniaturize under a certain limit.

Pulsatile pumps have been favored over peristaltic pumps since 1985. The main advantages of pulsatile pumps are the reduction in energy demand and the minimized stress to infused insulin [5]. Pump strokes are programmed by the use of an external telemetry programmer that orders pump cycles according to desired insulin delivery. The clock allows programming of several basal rates throughout the day. Implantable infusing systems have been designed to stop insulin delivery and provide a corresponding warning sign to the patient on the programmer screen in case of suspected electronic or mechanic malfunction of the device. Moreover, the physician can set a maximum limit of insulin dose that can be programmed per hour to prevent excessive insulin delivery following an erroneous order.

The power supply for the motor and the computer are provided by an internal battery that needs a life span of several years. The three models mentioned above had an expected battery life around 3 years, whereas the battery of the recent model MIP2007 made by Medtronic-MiniMed may provide energy for 7–10 years.

Conditions for Peritoneal Catheters

The major anticipated event related to the peritoneal catheter is its occlusion, as shown by previous experiences with intraperitoneal infusion from external pumps [23, 24]. Several mechanisms of catheter obstruction have been described: (1) precipitation of insulin, (2) tip occlusion by fibrin nodes, and (3) encapsulation of the catheter tip by fibrous and/or omental tissue [5]. Bowel perforation, although only reported in rare cases, can be prevented by a smooth catheter tip. In order to prevent CO_2 diffusion inside the catheter that would promote insulin precipitation, polyethylene is used as an interior component of the catheter. To avoid visceral or peritoneal trauma, a silicone coating is used on the external side of the catheter. The tip is exclusively composed of silicone, except for the Promedos ID3 system in which the cath-

Table 2. Key studies for the assessment of feasibility and effectiveness of implantable insulin pumps for the treatment of type 1 diabetes mellitus

Authors (pump model, manufacturer)	Reference	Cumulative experience, p-y	HbA_{1c}, %			Severe hypoglycemia, n/p-y	Local events, n/p-y	Catheter obstructions, n/p-y
			initial	final	p			
Point Study Group (Promedos ID 1, Siemens AG)	[7]	18.2	7.6 (5.9–9.1)	7.0 (5.7–8.3)	<0.05	0.22	0.55	0.27
Saudek et al. (PIMS, MiniMed Inc.)	[8]	28	9.2±0.4	8.2±0.4		0.00	0.04	0.14
Selam et al.[a], (Model 1000, Infusaid)	[9]	73	7.4±1.2	7.1±1.0		0.05	0.03	0.29
Hanaire-Broutin for EVADIAC (MIP 2001, MiniMed Inc., Model 1000, Infusaid, Promedos ID 3, Siemens Elema)	[31]	353	7.4±1.8	6.8±1.0	<0.001	0.025	0.08	0.13

p-y = Patient-year. [a] Intravenous and intraperitoneal catheters.

eter tip is covered by a titanium cap. The catheter is left free in the peritoneal cavity and made visible on X-ray by a specific index along its entire length. Various catheter lengths have been used in intraperitoneal insulin delivery. Short catheters with their tip lying in the upper or middle part of the peritoneal cavity allow quicker insulin peaks, but do not significantly influence average metabolic control [20]. Whether the length of the catheter plays a role in the risk of occlusion is controversial, but long catheters in short patients may generate subcostal or pelvic pain likely due to irritations of the diaphragm or the Douglas cul-de-sac, respectively. The causal mechanisms of catheter obstructions have so far remained speculative (see section: Adverse Events with Implantable Pumps and Preventive Solutions) and no preventive measures in the design of catheters can be clearly established.

The availability of a side port at the pump outlet or at the proximal part of the catheter appears as a very useful tool to manage underdelivery events [9]. This port must be accessible by percutaneous puncture for diagnostic or therapeutic procedures.

Feasibility and Effectiveness of Implantable Pump Therapy

We will only consider here studies that were designed and achieved from the availability of Hoe 21PH. These experiments were performed with programmable, variable-rate devices (table 2).

Pilot Feasibility Studies

The first trial using Hoe 21PH insulin tested the peristaltic pump Promedos ID1 designed by Siemens. Twenty pumps were implanted into type 1 diabetic patients in four

European centers (Milano, Vienna, Munich-Schwabing, and Munich-Bogenhausen), known as the Point Study Group, for a 1-year feasibility study [7]. Five pumps were implanted in the infraclavicular fossa and used the intravenous route via the subclavian vein, while the other 15 systems were implanted in a lower quadrant of the abdomen and infused insulin intraperitoneal. The pump was a roller-pump that infused Hoe 21GH insulin, 14% polygeline being added to the U-100 Genapol-stabilized insulin preparation. The pump was housed in a titanium-covered, square-angled case weighing 180 g with a refilling port but no side port. Over 18.2 patient-years of experience, three pumps were prematurely explanted because of pump failure (n = 1), severe infection of the pump-pocket (n = 1), and skin necrosis over the implant (n = 1). Complications at the implantation site dominated this trial, including infections, skin atrophy, hematomas or seromas, and pain, with some of these events requiring surgical revisions or premature explantations. The shape of the pump was likely responsible for these problems, with the square edges likely causing skin trauma. Five catheter occlusions were also reported due to thrombotic or fibrotic material, but no blockage primarily related to insulin precipitation occurred. Metabolic control was similar with intravenous and intraperitoneal routes and significantly improved with a reduction of HbA_{1c} from 7.6 to 7% ($p < 0.05$). Severe hypoglycemia was uncommon (0.22 per patient-year).

Successful in vitro and animal studies assessing Hoe 21PH stability in the PIMS designed by MiniMed allowed a human feasibility study that was performed in two US centers (Baltimore, Md., and Irvine, Calif.) [8]. Eighteen type 1 diabetic patients received PIMS-delivered intraperitoneal insulin for 4–25 months, with a cumulated experience of 28 patient-years. PIMS was composed of a disk-shaped titanium-covered unit weighing 220 g that was implanted in a lower quadrant of the abdomen and an external programmer using telemetry. Infused insulin was U-400 Hoe 21PH and pump refills were made every 2 months. PIMS was a pulsatile pump with a reservoir under negative pressure and a battery with an expected life of 5 years, allowing basal and bolus insulin delivery. During the whole experience, only one pump presented a malfunction due to premature battery depletion and only one pump-pocket complication was reported. No incident of insulin aggregation occurred, thus confirming previous nonhuman experiments. Four catheters were blocked by omental encapsulations, two of them being freed using laparoscopy with a rapid recurrence in 1 case. Metabolic control improved when compared with data obtained with previous subcutaneous insulin treatment using portable pumps or multiple daily injections for the 3 months preceding the implantations: HbA_{1c} dropped from 9.2 ± 0.4 to $8.2 \pm 0.4\%$ after 18 months, and the standard deviation of mean blood glucose levels significantly decreased ($p < 0.01$). No severe hypoglycemia or ketoacidosis occurred.

A few years later, results of a multicenter clinical trial with Infusaid Model 1000 pumps were reported [9]. Fifty-six type 1 diabetic patients were enrolled in this study that investigated the safety, feasibility, and efficacy of these implantable pumps from a cumulative experience of 73 patient-years. U-100 Hoe 21PH was delivered by the pumps with monthly refills, using the intravenous route in 18 cases and the intraperitoneal route in 38 cases. No pump overdelivery or stopping occurred during the investigation that lasted up to 1.7 year. Local tolerance at the implantation site was excellent with only one instance of skin ulceration and one of pump dislodgment. Underdeliveries were the most common events that were reported. Pump flow slowdowns occurred in 50 pumps after 10 ± 3 months, which were resolved by alkaline lavages of pump reservoir and flow pathway, and likely related to insulin aggregates. Catheter obstructions occurred in 52% of the intravenous catheters and in 21% of the intraperitoneal ones. All but 2 cases (1 intravenous, 1 intraperitoneal) were resolved by catheter flushing through the side port. Six events of intravenous catheter migrations due to a lack of anchoring at the subclavian site and two episodes of subclavian vein thrombosis that required explantations, combined with the overall 1-year survival rate of 64% for intravenous catheters before requiring a new surgery (vs. 94% for intraperitoneal catheters), raised doubt about the safety of prolonged intravenous infusion. Metabolic results showed a noticeable reduction of severe hypoglycemic events from 0.47 to 0.05 per patient-year, whereas HbA_{1c} was not significantly improved. No difference was identified between intravenous and intraperitoneal infusion in terms of efficacy. Patient satisfaction significantly improved according to the DQOL (DCCT questionnaire for the analysis of diabetes-related quality of life), while data of impact and worry scales were unchanged. The disclosure of serious alterations of the membrane located at the refill port after repeated punctures during bench tests prompted the cessation of insulin refills of pumps that were implanted in humans. Infusaid, which later merged to Pfizer, decided to stop the development of this implantable pump model.

The Vienna group reported in abstract form the first data obtained with the Promedos ID3, a new pulsatile pump model infusing U-100 Hoe 21PH from a reservoir under negative pressure [27]. Specific pump failures required 3 premature explantations and 25 programmer dysfunctions were reported. Among 5 catheter occlusions detected by the specific built-in pressure sensor, 4 could be resolved by flushing the catheter through the side port. Although interesting by its specific characteristics, this pump model was not further developed by Siemens-Elema.

The largest experience with the three available pump models at the beginning of 1990s was reported by the EVADIAC study group, which collected data generated by 7 French centers in a central registry [28]. The whole experience represented 224 type 1 diabetic patients in whom 260 pumps were implanted (205 MIP 2001, 48 Infusaid Model 1000, and 7 Promedos ID3) followed up for 353 patient-years. The EVADIAC experience was the first to point out the metabolic benefits of implantable pumps using an intraperitoneal route. While HbA_{1c} fell from 7.4 ± 1.8 to 6.8 ± 1.0%, with a sustained improvement over 30 months, the incidence of severe hypoglycemic events dramatically decreased from 15.2 to 2.5 per 100 patient-years ($p < 0.001$). Interestingly, severe hypoglycemia was reported to recur in a subset of patients who went back to multiple daily injections or CSII after leaving the implantable pump trial, while HbA_{1c} also went back to higher levels.

Nathan et al. [29] addressed the question of the mechanism of this reduction of severe hypoglycemic events. Attempts to induce hypoglycemia were performed in 8 patients using subcutaneous or intraperitoneal/intravenous insulin administration at 2 different doses, the higher one being 1.75 times the normally used dose to cover a meal intake. The explanation for the higher occurrence of hypoglycemia with subcutaneous insulin came from the measurements of plasma insulin levels that were significantly higher at 180 and 240 min after subcutaneous insulin administration for both doses. The area under the curve for insulin was also higher: between 120 and 240 min for both doses after subcutaneous insulin. These data documented the reduced risk of hypoglycemia with implantable pumps using the intraperitoneal or intravenous route by showing the physiological profiles of obtained postprandial insulin levels. In addition, Oskarsson et al. [30] demonstrated that the glucagon response to induced hypoglycemia by intravenous insulin was improved after a prolonged intraperitoneal insulin infusion from implantable pumps when compared with the response obtained when the same patients were treated with CSII. The glucagon response to exercise was similarly improved after prolonged intraperitoneal insulin treatment using implantable pumps. Both more physiological insulin kinetics and improved counterregulatory capacity may thus be involved in the metabolic benefits obtained with implantable pumps.

Besides improved effectiveness in blood glucose control with implantable pumps, the EVADIAC study group also reported the broadest assessment of adverse effects that might occur with these devices [31]. While pump failures were uncommon (2.5 events per 100 patient-years), pump-pocket complications and catheter-related problems occurred with higher incidences, 8 and 13.5 events per 100 patient-years, respectively. Gradual slowdowns of insulin delivery, reversible after alkaline infusion through the system that can dissolve insulin aggregates, were reported with all Infusaid pumps after an average of 10 months. Similar events also occurred in 8 MiniMed pumps and in 1 Promedos device. Although 36 out of 260 pumps required explantations for local or technical problems and 90 surgical reinterventions were needed during the overall reported experience, only 11 out of 224 patients were advised to abandon pump therapy.

To address the potential usefulness of implantable pumps in type 2 diabetes mellitus, seven Veterans Affairs medical centers in the USA performed a randomized clinical trial to determine the effectiveness and the acceptability of this therapy in insulin-treated type 2 diabetic patients [32]. One hundred and twenty-one male type 2 diabetic patients treated by at least 1 insulin injection per day with an HbA_{1c} level of 8% or above were randomly treated and followed-up for 1 year with multiple daily injections or a MiniMed implantable pump model 2001. Mean blood glucose levels and HbA_{1c} were improved in both groups with no significant difference. However, blood glucose fluctuations, incidence of mild clinical hypoglycemia, and weight gain were significantly lower with implantable pumps. Although 25% of subjects experienced underdeliveries due to insulin aggregates with these devices, impact of the disease and the total DQOL score were rated significantly better by the patients treated by implanted pumps.

Studies Assessing Specific Benefits of Continuous Intraperitoneal Insulin Infusion
The availability of fast-acting insulin analogues for CSII led the EVADIAC Group to assess whether previously shown benefits of intraperitoneal insulin versus CSII using regular insulin on blood glucose control remained consistent versus lispro insulin used for CSII. A comparative short-term study was performed in 14 type 1 diabetic patients who moved from CSII using lispro insulin to implantable pumps. Reported data show that intraperitoneal insulin treatment led to significantly lower blood glucose levels, noticeably concerning preprandial values. HbA_{1c} and blood glucose stability were also significantly improved by implantable pumps [33].

The EVADIAC group also reported various cases of failures of glucose control with subcutaneous insulin delivery due to unreliable insulin absorption, resulting in subcutaneous insulin resistance or Buschke scleredema [34]. CIPII led to dramatic improvements of glucose control in these uncommon situations for which intravenous insulin infusion was previously the only choice for glucose control.

Another interesting experience was published by Dutch investigators concerning implantable insulin pumps in patients with brittle diabetes. The patients they investigated showed poor metabolic control and related frequent hospital admissions when recruited. Although the long-term metabolic control achieved with implantable pumps was still far from near-normoglycemia, a significant sustained reduction of HbA_{1c} was obtained from 10.0 ± 2.3 to 9.0 ± 1.6% ($p = 0.023$), and the average yearly hospital stay dramatically reduced from 45 to 13 days ($p = 0.005$) [35].

The Zwolle Group more specifically addressed the question of the benefits of CIPII versus CSII in a randomized control trial [36]. In this crossover study including 24 patients with type 1 diabetes, CIPII from implanted insulin pumps improved HbA_{1c} levels by 0.76% versus CSII and significantly increased time spent in the 4.6–17.3 mmol/l glucose range according to continuous glucose recordings, while hypoglycemic events were similar. Quality of life was also significantly improved with CIPII.

Recently, the EVADIAC group reported sustained improvement of glucose control for up to 5 years with implantable pumps with HbA_{1c} levels in the 7.5–7.6% range, with no simultaneous changes in body weight and diabetic complications [37].

Adverse Events with Implantable Pumps and Preventive Solutions

Although the studies reported above supported the long-term feasibility of implantable pump therapy in type 1 diabetic patients and pointed out specific benefits on blood glucose control, most of them also reported adverse events that raised questions about the risk/benefit ratio of this technique.

Complications at the Implantation Site
Renard et al. [38] first reported a significant incidence of these complications that were responsible for pump explantations in a series of 40 type 1 diabetic patients treated by MiniMed Model 2001 pumps. During 58.5 patient-years of cumulative experience with these implanted pumps, 7 patients presented severe pump-pocket complications that resulted in 5 explantations and 9 other surgical interventions that finally failed in saving the pump. Lesions in fluid accumulation around the pump led to skin retraction or atrophy, and finally to skin erosion in 5 cases. Four complications occurred in the first 6 months following implantation in patients who performed strenuous physical activity, sometimes in the immediate weeks following surgery. Three other events occurred after more than 1 year of follow-up, without any identified traumatic factor. In these cases, coagulase-negative staphylococcus and granulocytes were identified in the seroma surrounding the pump, suggesting an infectious origin. In a further report, the same authors could better document the outcomes of 10 other pump-pocket seromas [39]. Five seromas with no indication of infection resolved with rest. In the other cases, staphylococcus epidermidis was identified in the fluid accumulation and explantation could not be avoided, except for 1 case treated by long-term antibiotics. Interestingly, isolated strains of staphylococcus in 3 seromas could be compared to strains that had been previously isolated in skin samples from the same patients before the occurrence of the events. The genetic analysis of the respective strains demonstrated that the ones isolated in seromas were identical or closely related to those previously identified in skin flora. These data suggested that a likely seeding from skin flora was responsible for the infected seromas with poor outcome. Antibiotic cover for each puncture of the pump-pocket was proposed as a prophylactic measure to avoid these complications.

The Infusaid Multicenter Implantable Insulin Pump Study Group cited 23 complications at the implantation site that occurred in 19 patients during a cumulative experience of 435 patient-years, resulting from 117 Model 1000 pumps implanted at 16 centers [9]. Although the overall incidence of pump-pocket complications appeared much lower than in the preceding report (5.3/100 vs. 24/100 patient-years), the percentage of affected individuals was very similar: 16.2 vs. 17.5%. However, outcomes were less severe since only 7 pumps (36.8% of pumps with local complications vs. 100%) had to be explanted and 3 of them could be replaced at a different site with success. In the largest cumulated multicenter experience ever published (1,180 patient-years), the EVADIAC Study Group reported that 84 out of 352 patients (24%) were affected by complications at the implantation site [40]. Sixty-four percent of these patients required pump explantations. Lesions included local inflammatory reactions, skin atrophy or erosion, chronic seromas, and infections. No risk factor could be identified, but complications seemed to occur more frequently in centers with a limited number of implants, suggesting the role of a lack of experience in the occurrence of these events.

Underdelivery Problems
Acute underdeliveries related to pump failure (electronic or mechanical) that rapidly lead to hyperglycemia and ketosis are very uncommon events [31]. Premature battery depletions have now and then been reported, but also remain anecdotic events [8, 31]. Only 5 such events were reported in the EVADIAC experience, which gathered data from 260 pumps implanted between September 1989 and January 1993 in France [31]. These rare incidents can be easily diagnosed by a warning sign on the programmer screen.

The two main causes of insulin underdelivery are catheter occlusions and insulin precipitates in pumps. Most incidents develop progressively and are suggested by a necessary increase of insulin dose programming to maintain glucose control. Because of the frequent time delay between starting underdelivery and adaptation of insulin dose by the patients, impaired glucose control due to an unknown reason is the common indicator of delivery problems [41]. Since a systematic comparison is performed at pump refills between expected insulin volume remaining in reservoir, which is calculated from programmed orders kept in memory, and actual remaining insulin quantity drawn from the reservoir, a suspected underdelivery can be confirmed in most cases by the observed discrepancy between these two values. When this calculated '% error' exceeds 10–20, depending on investigators, further investigations are indicated to explore the mechanism of underdelivery and find a remedy. Cases of sudden catheter blockages are characterized by acute hyperglycemia rapidly associated with ketosis and complicated by ketoacidosis if no compensatory administration of insulin is performed by subcutaneous injections.

The primary investigation of the peritoneal catheter is the most effective way to discriminate between a catheter obstruction and a pump slowdown due to insulin aggregation. Injecting an X-ray-visible soluble dye through the side port can help visualize a catheter obstruction or encapsulation in most cases. A laparoscopic approach of the peritoneal cavity will then allow the cleaning of the catheter. If the catheter looks free on X-ray examination, a rinsing procedure will be scheduled to dissolve likely insulin precipitates in the pump ejection chamber. An alternative option reverses the order of procedures, starting by a systematic NaOH rinsing. Catheter visualization by X-ray investigation is performed only if NaOH rinsing fails.

Reported incidences of intraperitoneal catheter obstructions extend between 7.8 and 57.3 per 100 patient-years [7–9, 31, 42]. The Montpellier group pointed out that patients who had previously used intraperitoneal insulin delivery with portable pumps accounted for the high incidence of intraperitoneal catheter obstructions they reported, while patients with more than 21 years of diabetes duration also experienced more frequent catheter obstructions [42]. In a further report, these authors showed that according to used insulin batches that differed in their preparation process, the incidence of catheter obstructions could vary from 9 to 79 per 100 patient-years [41]. Two types of obstructions have been described: (1) tip obstructions by fibrin clots, and (2) encapsulations forming a more or less extended sock around the peritoneal catheter

[7, 8, 42]. Renard et al. [42] first reported that amyloid deposits showing a positive staining by anti-insulin antibodies were present in encapsulation tissue and surrounded by a granulomatous inflammatory reaction involving giant cells and fibrous tissue. This observation is in good accordance with that of a variable incidence of catheter obstructions according to the insulin batch used [41] and with the previously described formation of modified insulin resulting from Hoe 21PH residence in reservoir [6].

Flow slowdowns related to insulin aggregates in the accumulation chamber of the Infusaid Model 1000 affected 86% of investigated pumps after an average postimplantation time of 10 months in the initial feasibility trial [9], and 100% of 48 pumps in EVADIAC experience after a similar postimplantation period [31]. All of these events were solved by NaOH rinsing of pumps. Both the design of the accumulation chamber and the lower concentration of insulin used (U-100 vs. U-400 in MiniMed pumps), which reduces the physical stability of insulin solution, have been suspected as promoters of this frequent insulin aggregation. Such incidents were uncommon with MIP2001 until 1992 when a modification in the preparation procedure of Hoe 21PH insulin batches aiming at increasing chemical stability resulted in high rates of underdeliveries related to insulin aggregation in pumps [41]. According to used insulin batches, the incidence of these events extended between 27.1 and 121 per 100 patient-years. Investigations showed that insulin aggregation occurred on the titanium ferrule of the ejection chamber that was in contact with the silicon rubber part of the pump piston, resulting in a backflow of insulin towards the reservoir that is under negative pressure in MiniMed pumps. Although these incidents were solved in most cases by NaOH rinsing, their frequent occurrence tended to impair metabolic control and made the management of the therapy more difficult. A revision of insulin preparation process then provided improved physical stability of insulin batches and could decrease the incidence of backflows from 113 to 6 per 100 patient-years [43]. Meanwhile, the compliance of the catheter side port was also improved to allow a better outflow of insulin. An EVADIAC trial reported an overall dramatic reduction of underdeliveries in 40 MIP2001 that were equipped with this modified side port and infused stabilized Hoe 21PH ETP insulin: after a cumulated experience of 49.3 patient-years, reported incidences of catheter obstructions and backflows were 4 and 12.1 per 100 patient-years, respectively. Further cumulative follow-up of 106 patient-years showed a stable incidence of 4 catheter obstructions per 100 patient-years, but backflows still occurred with an incidence of 33.7 per 100 patient-years [44].

Anti-Insulin Antibody Production

The immunogenicity of peritoneal insulin delivery has been shown in animal studies as well as in humans treated by intraperitoneal insulin from external pumps. The Montpellier Group mentioned an average two- to threefold increase of circulating anti-insulin antibodies detected by a radioimmunoelectrophoretic method after 6–84 months of intraperitoneal insulin delivery from external pumps according to the use of U-40 acidic porcine insulin or U-100 neutral porcine insulin, respectively [45]. However, patient response was heterogeneous, including a subset of nonresponders. Clinical consequences of high anti-insulin antibody titers appeared rather beneficial in this report since they were associated with reduced insulin requirements and improved metabolic control.

A first report on anti-insulin antibodies in patients treated by implantable insulin pumps using an intraperitoneal route was published by the Irvine Group [46]. Using a radioimmunoassay technique, they identified 2 groups of patients among a series of 25 type 1 diabetic subjects treated for 3–6 years: responders and nonresponders, with the responders representing 11% of the total. The increase of antibodies in responders was slow over an average duration of 22 months, and was followed by a spontaneous decrease of titers regardless of whether intraperitoneal therapy went on or not. Among the 11 responders, 4 subjects had clinical syndromes that consisted of increasing daily insulin requirements contrasting with nocturnal hypoglycemia despite minimal basal infusion rates. Although these patients associated the clinical syndromes with high antibody titers, other patients with similarly high titers had no clinical symptoms. The causal relationship was thus not fully established, although altered pharmacokinetics of insulin had been previously described in patients treated by a subcutaneous route with high anti-insulin antibody levels. Shortly afterwards, the Strasbourg Group similarly reported an increase of anti-insulin antibodies in about half of the cases of a series of 62 type 1 diabetic patients treated by intraperitoneal insulin from several pump models [47]. In 2 cases, daytime insulin resistance also contrasted with nocturnal hypoglycemia despite nighttime pump stop.

The Marseilles Group also reported increased anti-insulin antibody levels, detected by both radioimmunoassay and ELISA methods, in a series of 17 type 1 diabetic patients treated by implantable pumps using the intraperitoneal route [48]. Although no distinction was made between responders and nonresponders, the standard deviation of antibody titers was broad. No clinical manifestations were associated with high antibody levels.

It has been speculated that conformational modifications of the insulin molecule in implantable pumps might account for the production of specific anti-insulin antibodies, maybe in relationship with the formation of insulin aggregates. Whether the affinity to insulin of these antibodies could be lower and consequently promote alterations of insulin pharmacokinetics responsible for clinical syndromes has not been explored.

Since the Strasbourg study, as well as clinical experience, shows that an anti-insulin antibody response is more likely to occur in patients who present high antibody levels before moving to intraperitoneal delivery, CIPII must be thoroughly debated, if not banned, in such cases due to the risk of inducing deleterious glucose disturbances related to anti-insulin antibody increase.

Current Indications for Implantable Pumps and Perspectives

Both the results of the feasibility studies detailed above and the data provided by recent clinical reports allow some proposals of indications for implantable pumps in type 1 diabetes mellitus. The EVADIAC Group published a recent position statement on this topic [49].

The first proposal is that implantable pumps should be used in 'last resort' conditions when diabetic patients absolutely fail to achieve blood glucose control with any other means of insulin therapy, but may be reasonably improved by CIPII. These relatively uncommon situations include alterations of subcutaneous absorption of insulin, that extend from rare cases of subcutaneous insulin resistance to local skin reactions to insulin injections, e.g. lipodystrophies, or to CSII catheters, or brittle diabetes of unknown origin.

The second orientation towards CIPII from implantable pumps takes into account the documented improvements that this therapy may provide when compared with CSII using regular insulin or fast-acting analogues, i.e. better blood glucose stability, reduction of severe hypoglycemia, and lowered HbA_{1c} in some studies. According to this proposal, any type 1 diabetic patient who cannot achieve tight metabolic control with optimized subcutaneous insulin therapy could be eligible for an implantable pump if no contraindication is present. Patients who experience recurrent severe hypoglycemia under intensive subcutaneous insulin therapy would represent first rank indications for implantable pumps. A nonexhaustive list of contraindications may include:

- Conditions when the patient is unable to manage safely intensive insulin therapy because of lack of compliance to blood glucose monitoring, chronic psychiatric disorders or addictions, or eating disorders
- Situations in which pump use may be hazardous or prone to complications because of living conditions: work exposed to strong magnetic fields, very high temperatures, low atmospheric pressure (extended stays at an altitude higher or equal to 2,500 m), or high atmospheric pressure (underwater diving exceeding 8.50 m)
- Patients with serious associated disease, severe debilitating diabetic complications, or expected short life expectancy
- Proliferative or preproliferative retinopathy that represents only a temporary contraindication before laser therapy

It may, however, be argued against this more liberal attitude that the cost-effectiveness of this technique has been poorly investigated.

Several perspectives could hopefully influence this debate in favor of implantable pumps. First, the expected improvements in pump technology and insulin manufacturing process should be able to reduce the incidence of adverse events that still spoil the metabolic effectiveness of this therapy [44]. Second, the ultimate goal of implantable pump therapy is the availability of an artificial β-cell. After a long period of stagnation in the development of glucose sensors, major steps forward have been made in recent years [16]. After the pioneering LTSS trial that allowed closed-loop insulin delivery from implantable pumps connected to implanted intravenous sensors, Renard et al. [10–12] reported the effectiveness of an artificial pancreas model combining subcutaneous glucose sensors to CIPII from implanted pumps.

The recently reinitiated development of the DiaPort, a port implanted in the abdominal wall allowing the insertion of an intraperitoneal catheter which can be connected to a portable insulin pump, may represent an alternative to implanted insulin pumps to get the metabolic benefits of CIPII with reduced burdens and at a lower cost. The association of this insulin delivery system with a continuous glucose monitoring system might also represent an interesting option for the development of a wearable artificial pancreas.

References

1 Blackshear PH, Dorman FD, Blackshear PL Jr, Varco RL, Buchwald H: Permanently implantable self-recycling low-flow constant-rate multipurpose infusion pump of simple design. Surg Forum 1970;21: 136–137.

2 Blackshear PJ, Shulman GI, Roussell AM, Nathan DM, Minaker KL, Rowe AM, Robbins DC, Cohen AM: Metabolic response to three years of continuous, basal rate intravenous insulin infusion in type II diabetic patients. J Clin Endocrinol Metab 1985;61: 753–760.

3 Selam JL, Slingeneyer A, Chaptal PA, Franetzki M, Perstele K, Mirouze J: Total implantation of remotely controlled insulin minipump in a human insulin-dependent diabetic. Artif Organs 1982;6:315–319.

4 Shade DS, Eaton RP, Edwards WS: Programmable insulin delivery system: successful short-term implantation in man. JAMA 1982;247:1848–1853.

5 Selam JL, Charles MA: Devices for insulin administration. Diabetes Care 1990;13:955–979.

6 Grau U, Saudek CD: Stable insulin preparation for implanted insulin pumps. Laboratory and animal trials. Diabetes 1987;36:1453–1459.

7 One-year trial of a remote-controlled implantable insulin infusion system in type I diabetic patients. Point Study Group. Lancet 1988;2:866–869.

8 Saudek CD, Selam JL, Pitt HA, Waxman K, Rubio M, Jeandidier N, Turner D, Fishell RE, Charles MA: A preliminary trial of the programmable implantable medication system for insulin delivery. N Engl J Med 1989;321:574–579.

9 Selam JL, Micossi P, Dunn FL, Nathan DM: Clinical trial of programmable implantable insulin pumps for type 1 diabetes. Diabetes Care 1992;15:877–885.

10 Renard E: Implantable closed loop glucose-sensing and insulin delivery: the future for insulin pump therapy. Curr Opin Pharmacol 2002;2:708–716.

11 Renard E, Costalat G, Chevassus H, Bringer J: Artificial beta cell: clinical experience toward an implantable closed-loop insulin delivery system. Diabetes Metab 2006;32:497–502.

12 Renard E, Place J, Cantwell M, Chevassus H, Palerm CC: Closed-loop insulin delivery using a subcutaneous glucose sensor and intraperitoneal insulin delivery. Feasibility study testing a new model for the artificial pancreas. Diabetes Care 2010;33:121–127.

13 The Diabetes Control and Complications Trial Research Group: The effect of intensive treatment of diabetes on the development and progression of long-term complications in insulin-dependent diabetes mellitus. N Engl J Med 1993;329:977–986.

14 Zinman B: The physiologic replacement of insulin. An elusive goal. N Engl J Med 1989;321:363–370.

15 Zinman B, Tildesley H, Chiasson JL, Tsui E, Strack T: Insulin lispro in CSII: results of double-blind crossover study. Diabetes 1997;46:440–443.

16 Cobelli C, Renard E, Kovatchev B: Artificial pancreas: past, present, future. Diabetes 2011;60:2672–2682.

17 Diagnostic and therapeutic technology assessment: continuous peritoneal insulin infusion and implantable insulin infusion pumps for diabetic control. JAMA 1989;262:3195–3198.

18 Schade DS, Eaton RP, Davis T, Akiya F, Phinney E, Kubica R, Vaughn E, Pay PW: The kinetics of peritoneal insulin absorption. Metabolism 1981;30:149–155.

19 Nelson JA, Stephen R, Landau ST, Wilson DE, Tyler FH: Intraperitoneal insulin administration produces a positive portal-systemic blood insulin gradient in unanesthetized, unrestrained swine. Metabolism 1982;31:969–972.

20 Selam JL, Raymond M, Jacquemin JL, Orsetti A, Richard JL, Mirouze J: Pharmacokinetics of insulin infused intra-peritoneally via portable pumps. Diabete Metab 1985;11:170–173.

21 Giacca A, Caumo A, Galimberti G, Petrella G, Librenti MC, Scavini M, Pozza G, Micossi P: Peritoneal and subcutaneous absorption of insulin in type 1 diabetic subjects. J Clin Endocrinol Metab 1993;77:738–742.

22 Ader M, Bergman RN: Peripheral effects of insulin dominate suppression of fasting hepatic glucose production. Am J Physiol 1990;258:E1020–E1032.

23 Selam JL, Slingeneyer A, Saeidi S, Mirouze J: Experience with long-term peritoneal insulin infusion with portable pumps. Diabet Med 1985;2:41–44.

24 Wredling R, Adamson U, Lins PE, Backman L, Lundgren D: Experience of a long-term intraperitoneal insulin treatment using a new percutaneous access device. Diabet Med 1991;8:597–600.

25 Liebl A, Hoogma R, Renard E, Geelhoed-Duijvestijn PH, Klein E, Diglas J, Kessler L, Melki V, Diem P, Brun JM, Schaepelynck-Bélicar P, Frei T; European DiaPort Study Group: A reduction in severe hypoglycaemia in type 1 diabetes in a randomized crossover study of continuous intraperitoneal compared with subcutaneous insulin infusion. Diabetes Obes Metab 2009;11:1001–1008.

26 Brange J, Havelund S: Insulin pumps and insulin quality – requirements and problems. Acta Med Scand 1983;671:135–138.

27 Feinböck C, et al: Results and experiences with the programmable implanted insulin pump Siemens Promedos ID3. Horm Metab Res 1994;26:65.

28 Broussolle C, Jeandidier N, Hanaire-Broutin H for The Evadiac Study Group: French multicentre experience with implantable insulin pumps. Lancet 1994;343:514–515.

29 Nathan DM, Dunn FL, Bruch J, McKitrick C, Larkin M, Haggan C, Lavin-Tompkins J, Norman D, Simon D: Postprandial insulin profiles with implantable pump therapy may explain decreased frequency of severe hypoglycemia, compared with intensive subcutaneous regimens, in insulin-dependent diabetes mellitus patients. Am J Med 1996;100:412–417.

30 Oskarsson PR, Lins PE, Backman L, Adamson UC: Continuous intraperitoneal insulin infusion partly restores the glucagon response to hypoglycemia in type 1 diabetic patients. Diabetes Metab 2000;26:118–124.

31 Hanaire-Broutin H, Broussolle C, Jeandidier N, Renard E, Guerci B, Haardt MJ, Lassmann-Vague V; EVADIAC Study Group: Feasibility of intraperitoneal insulin therapy with programmable implantable pumps in IDDM: a multicenter study. Diabetes Care 1995;18:388–392.

32 Saudek CD, Duckworth WC, Giobbie-Hurder A, Henderson WG, Henry RR, Kelley DE, Edelman SV, Zieve FJ, Adler RA, Anderson JW, Anderson RJ, Hamilton BP, Donner TW, Kirkman MS, Morgan NA; Department of Veterans Affairs Implantable Insulin Pump Study Group: Implantable insulin pumps vs. multiple dose insulin for non-insulin-dependent diabetes mellitus: a randomized clinical trial. JAMA 1996;276:1322–1327.

33 Catargi B, Meyer L, Melki V, Renard E, Jeandidier N; EVADIAC Study Group: Comparison of blood glucose stability and HbA_{1c} between implantable insulin pumps using U400 HOE 21Ph insulin and external pumps using lispro in type 1 diabetic patients: a pilot study. Diabetes Metab 2002;28:133–137.

34 Baillot-Rudoni S, Apostol D, Vaillant G, Brun JM, Renard E; EVADIAC Study Group: Implantable pump therapy restores metabolic control and quality of life in type 1 diabetic patients with Buschke's non systemic scleroderma. Diabetes Care 2006;29:1710.

35 De Vries JH, Eskes SA, Snoek FJ, Pouwer F, Van Ballegooie E, Spijker AJ, Kostense PJ, Seubert M, Heine RJ: Continuous intraperitoneal insulin infusion in patients with 'brittle' diabetes: favourable effects on glycaemic control and hospital stay. Diabet Med 2002;19:496–501.

36 Logtenberg SJ, Kleepstra N, Houweling ST, Groenier KH, Gans RO, Van Ballegooie E, Bilo HJ: Improved glycemic control with intraperitoneal versus subcutaneous insulin in type 1 diabetes; a randomized controlled trial. Diabetes Care 2009;32:1372–1377.

37 Schaepelynck P, Renard E, Jeandidier N, Hanaire H, Fermon C, Rudoni S, Catargi B, Riveline JP, Guerci B, Millot L, Martin JF, Sola A; EVADIAC Group: A recent survey confirms the efficacy and the safety of implanted pumps during long-term use in poorly-controlled type 1 diabetes patients. Diabetes Technol Ther 2011;13:657–660.

38 Renard E, Bringer J, Jacques-Apostol D, Lauton D, Mestre C, Costalat G, Jaffiol C: Complications of the pump-pocket may represent a significant cause of incidents with implanted systems for intraperitoneal insulin delivery. Diabetes Care 1994;17:1064–1066.

39 Renard E, Rostane T, Carriere C, Marchandin H, Jacques-Apostol D, Lauton D, Gibert-Boulet F, Bringer J: Implantable insulin pumps: infections most likely due to seeding from skin flora determine severe outcomes of pump-pocket seromas. Diabetes Metab 2001;27:62–65.

40 Belicar P, Lassmann-Vague V; EVADIAC Study Group: Local adverse events associated with long-term treatment by implantable insulin pumps. Diabetes Care 1998;21:325–326.

41 Renard E, Bouteleau S, Jacques-Apostol D, Lauton D, Boulet-Gibert F, Costalat G, Bringer J, Jaffiol C: Insulin underdelivery from implanted pumps using peritoneal route: determinant role of insulin-pump compatibility. Diabetes Care 1996;19:812–817.

42 Renard E, Baldet P, Picot MC, Jacques-Apostol D, Lauton D, Costalat G, Bringer J, Jaffiol C: Catheter complications with implantable systems for peritoneal insulin delivery. An analysis of frequency, predisposing factors and obstructing materials. Diabetes Care 1995;18:300–306.
43 Renard E, Souche C, Jacques-Apostol D, Lauton D, Gibert-Boulet F, Costalat G, Bringer J, Jaffiol C: Improved stability of insulin delivery from implanted pumps using a new preparation process for infused insulin. Diabetes Care 1999;22:1371–1372.
44 Gin H, Renard E, Melki V, Boivin S, Schaepelinck-Belicar P, Guerci B, Selam JL, Brun JM, Riveline JP, Estour B, Catargi B; EVADIAC Study Group: Combined improvements in implantable pump technology and insulin stability allow safe and effective long term intraperitoneal insulin delivery in type 1 diabetic patients: the EVADIAC experience. Diabetes Metab 2003;29:602–607.
45 Bousquet-Rouaud R, Chante MA, Orsetti A, Mirouze J: Increase of anti-insulin antibody titer during continuous peritoneal insulin infusion. Artif Organs 1990;14(Suppl 3):241–243.
46 Olsen CL, Chan E, Turner DS, Iravani M, Nagy M, Selam JL, Wong ND, Waxman K, Charles MA: Insulin antibody responses after long-term intraperitoneal insulin administration via implantable programmable insulin delivery systems. Diabetes Care 1994;17:169–176.
47 Jeandidier N, Boivin S, Sapin R, Rosart-Ortega F, Uring-Lambert B, Reville P, Pinget M: Immunogenicity of intraperitoneal insulin infusion using programmable implantable devices. Diabetologia 1995;38:577–584.
48 Lassmann-Vague V, Belicar P, Raccah D, Vialettes B, Sodoyez JC, Vague P: Immunogenicity of long-term intraperitoneal insulin administration with implantable programmable pumps. Diabetes Care 1995;18:498–503.
49 Renard E, Schaepelynck-Belicar P; EVADIAC Group: Implantable insulin pumps: a position statement about their clinical use. Diabetes Metab 2007;33:158–166.

Prof. Eric Renard, MD, PhD
Department of Endocrinology, Diabetes and Nutrition
Lapeyronie University Hospital
FR–34295 Montpellier Cedex 5 (France)
E-Mail e-renard@chu-montpellier.fr

Bruttomesso D, Grassi G (eds): Technological Advances in the Treatment of Type 1 Diabetes.
Front Diabetes. Basel, Karger, 2015, vol 24, pp 210–225 (DOI: 10.1159/000363518)

Devices to Support Treatment Decisions in Type 1 Diabetes: The Diabeo System

S. Franc[a, b] · G. Charpentier[a, b]

[a]Centre d'Etudes et de Recherche pour l'Intensification du Traitement du Diabète (CERITD), Bioparc Génopole, Evry, and [b]Service de Diabétologie, Centre hospitalier Sud-Francilien, Corbeil-Essonnes, France

Abstract

Blood glucose control in type 1 diabetes has improved considerably since the DCCT due to general diffusion of 'physiological' basal-prandial therapeutic schedules, generalization of therapeutic educational programs, functional insulin therapy, insulin analogues, and insulin pumps. However, glycated hemoglobin (HbA_{1c}) averages 8% within various studies, which is still unsatisfactory. The creation of new technological tools could lead to new levels of success, as attested by the Diabeo system. This system comprises three programs. The first program automatically calculates basal and prandial insulin doses while taking account of blood glucose levels, carbohydrate intake, and physical activity, and is equipped with algorithms that allow automatic adjustment based on the results obtained. The entire system must first of all be configured by the doctor according to the patient's characteristics, and then it has to be downloaded to a smartphone from a secure website. All of the patient's results and data are then made available for consultation at all times by authorized caregivers, enabling remote monitoring to be performed. The second program analyzes the results and automatically generates coaching messages for the patient and messages for the caregiver in the event of underuse, unsatisfactory results, or inadequate operation of the system. The caregiver may then intervene in a timely fashion via a telephone consultation or modification of the patient's treatment profile. The third program optimizes the doctor's available time by delegating tasks and allowing action to be undertaken by a specialized telemedicine nurse working in conjunction with the responsible diabetologist. An initial version of the system, comprising only the first of these three programs, resulted in a mean reduction in HbA_{1c} of 0.9% at 6 months versus the control group in a population of patients with chronic glycemic control problems and treated with multiple injections or insulin pump. Analysis of individual patient data shows that the most compliant patients derived the greatest benefit from the dose calculation function, while less compliant patients benefited considerably from the telemonitoring function, which allowed short but repeated consultations at opportune moments. A large-scale national study is currently being initiated in France to confirm these favorable metabolic results at 1 year and to assess the medicoeconomic impact of this system after 2 years of use. Ultimately, the results may lead to granting of reimbursable status for the Diabeo system by the French national social security authorities, followed by widespread use of the system in France and international availability.

Since the DCCT, basal-prandial insulin regimens for the treatment of type 1 diabetes with frequent monitoring have been shown to be superior [1]. In the intervening period, the introduction of specific education programs regarding therapy, fast- and slow-acting insulin analogues, insulin pumps, and more recently continuous blood glucose (BG) monitoring, has resulted in a gradual improvement in glycemic control in this patient population. However, current results are still far from perfect, with only 25% of the 13,316 children and adolescents involved in the US T1D Exchange Clinic Registry achieving (HbA_{1c}) levels within the target range recommended by ISPAD, i.e. ≤7.5% [2]. Although the German and Austrian register, which collates data on 30,708 children and adolescents, has shown an improvement in glycemic control, with mean HbA_{1c} falling from 8.7 ± 1.8% in 1995 to 8.1 ± 1.5% in 2009, this is still far higher than the desired levels [3]. While the Australian register containing data on 1,683 children and adolescents showed a marked decrease in the incidence of episodes of severe hypoglycemia between 2000 and 2009, the mean HbA_{1c} level remained stable at around 8.3 ± 1.5% throughout the entire decade [4]. In France, the mean HbA_{1c} value in the subgroup of type 1 diabetes patients included in the national representative control sample of diabetic subjects (ENTRED) was 7.9% in 2007, with 38% of patients having HbA_{1c} >8%, or in other words, at high risk of subsequent development of diabetic complications [5].

Although functional insulin therapy is currently considered the reference treatment in type 1 diabetes and the one that best mimics physiological processes, it is difficult to maintain over time. In the DAFNE study, while patients assigned to functional insulin therapy initially showed a substantial decrease in HbA_{1c} from 9.4 to 8.4% at 6 months, this value subsequently increased over time [6]. In a further study of 111 patients with a mean HbA_{1c} reading of 8.6 ± 1.1% in 2002, this level was reduced to 8.1 ± 1.1% one year after the patients had undergone a structured DAFNE educational program. Seven years later, however, the mean level had risen again to 8.3 ± 1.2% [7].

This picture of inadequate glycemic control gives an idea of the difficulties facing patients as a result of the constraints associated with their disease. At every meal, patients must check their BG levels, count their carbohydrate intake, and accordingly adapt their insulin dose, while taking into consideration any possible physical activity that might warrant a dose reduction. The traditional paper notebooks used for self-monitoring of BG levels, in which data on glycemia and injected doses of insulin were recorded, are now obsolete as many subjects with type 1 diabetes simply neglect to fill them in. The glycemia data obtained during downloading of BG values from a glucose meter using specific software is difficult to use in practice as a basis for day-to-day adjustment of therapy. Could devices to support treatment decisions in type 1 diabetes possibly offer a solution to this problem? Several tools have been developed to facilitate the process of therapeutic decision-making for patients with type 1 diabetes, each offering different levels of functional support.

First Level: Electronic Diaries

There is growing evidence to suggest that regular assessment of BG levels might help insulin-treated patients achieve better glycemic control. Self-monitoring of BG has been shown to contribute to better adjustment of therapy and to help treat-to-treat goals be attained.

Since patients on basal-bolus treatment are often reluctant to use paper diaries, electronic equivalents have been developed to overcome these difficulties. These electronic diaries are more attractive than their paper counterparts and make it easier to control BG levels. BG values may either be entered manually or loaded directly into a smartphone. These systems can store data about BG values, insulin intake, food consumption, and physical activity and then transmit it to healthcare providers via e-mail. However, these electronic diaries do not propose suitable insulin doses and the practical value of such systems still needs to be assessed. It should be noted, however, that some patients are unable to interpret self-monitoring of BG data and translate it into appropriate therapeutic decisions for adjustment of their treatment. In such cases, a system that automatically proposes a suitable insulin dose, at least before meals, can be very useful.

Second Level: Automated Bolus Calculators

The question is whether built-in automated bolus calculators (ABCs) in insulin pumps or in BG meters represent added value in terms of patients' actual practice and their ability to make the right therapeutic decisions that will ensure improved metabolic control and quality of life.

ABCs have been developed for patients on basal-bolus insulin regimens. These systems, which calculate the doses of short-acting insulin required before meals, have been integrated into insulin pumps for over 10 years. They have recently been incorporated in BG meters and specifically designed for patients treated with multiple daily injections.

Patients on basal-bolus therapy, which includes carbohydrate counting, must perform complex preprandial calculations at least three times daily in order to determine the required preprandial dose of short-acting insulin. These calculations are based on current BG level, target BG, carbohydrate-to-insulin ratios, total grams of carbohydrates in meals, and insulin sensitivity factor. Another parameter integrated in the calculation is insulin on board, i.e. the amount of insulin theoretically active in the body, persisting from the previous dose and which must be subtracted from the prandial insulin dose in order to limit the risk of hypoglycemia. Although it would appear useful, this function has not been assessed per se.

ABCs have been shown to reduce the risk of miscalculation. In a recently published study [8] conducted in 205 insulin-treated patients comprising two distinct patient populations [carbohydrate counters ($n = 101$), who used a sophisticated formula, and noncarbohydrate counters, who used a simplified formula ($n = 104$)], 63% of the manually calculated doses were erroneous. This percentage was reduced to 6% when dose calculations were performed using an ABC ($p < 0.001$). The surveys showed that 83% of subjects felt more confident about using the ABC and that 87% preferred the meter over manual calculation. These results are consistent with those published by Gross et al. [9] for a population of 49 CSII-treated patients, showing that patients felt extremely confident about the insulin doses recommended by their pump.

Are Automated Bolus Calculators Useful in Improving Metabolic Control?
Studies have shown discordant results regarding improvement in metabolic control. In a small observational study ($n = 18$) of ABC users versus nonusers, although HbA_{1c} levels showed no improvement [10], ABC users exhibited lower mean postprandial BG levels than nonusers. However, the decision whether or not to use the ABC was at the patient's discretion, making the data difficult to interpret. Other studies have also reported better postprandial BG excursions with ABCs [9]. In a recent study conducted in Denmark in a population of patients treated with multiple daily injections, those randomized to the CarbCount ABC group, who were educated on functional insulin therapy and provided with an ABC, improved their HbA_{1c} levels after 16 weeks (CarbCount ABC group: −0.7% vs. baseline), as did those randomized to the CarbCount group not receiving an ABC. However, the difference between the two groups, which reflects the true efficacy of ABCs, was only 0.1% [11]. A recent prospective study in a population of 30 type 1 diabetes patients provided with an ABC showed a significant decrease in both HbA_{1c} ($p < 0.007$) and diurnal glucose variability ($p < 0.005$), as well as postprandial BG ($p < 0.05$) values [12]. Besides simplifying the bolus calculation and improving the parameters involved in metabolic control, ABCs were shown to reduce fear of hypoglycemia [13], thereby enhancing patient satisfaction and quality of life.

Although bolus calculators appear to be useful tools for insulin-treated patients, their potential to improve metabolic BG control is limited. First, they do not propose any adjustments to basal insulin, a key factor in metabolic control, and second, they do not incorporate any feedback to and from the healthcare provider since they function completely autonomously. Clearly these systems, which require further evaluation, can help patients, especially those with poor numeracy; however, they cannot overcome the more serious issue of acceptance by patients of their disease.

Third Level: Systems with Automated Feedback

The Diabetes Insulin Guidance System (DIGS) software (Hygieia Inc., Ann Arbor, Mich., USA), which automatically advises patients on adjustment of insulin dosage, was tested in a feasibility study conducted in three populations of patients with poor glycemic control (HbA_{1c} at baseline: $8.9 \pm 1.1\%$): (1) patients with type 1 diabetes, (2) patients with type 2 diabetes on basal-bolus therapy, and (3) patients with type 2 diabetes treated with twice-daily biphasic insulin [14]. During the 12-week intervention period, DIGS processed patients' glucose readings and provided insulin dosage adjustments on a weekly basis. If approved by the study team, the adjusted insulin dosage was communicated to the patients. The DIGS software recommended 1,734 insulin dosage adjustments, of which 1,731 (99.83%) were approved by the study team. The DIGS dosage adjustments resulted in a reduction in HbA_{1c} from 8.4 ± 0.8 to 7.9 ± 0.9% ($p < 0.05$), an improvement in mean glucose from 174.2 ± 36.7 mg/dl at baseline to 163.3 ± 35.1 ($p < 0.03$) and a 25.2% reduction in the incidence of hypoglycemia at 12 weeks.

Use of this type of system should not be restricted to subjects with type 1 diabetes since patients with type 2 diabetes also benefited from the decision-making program. Since the findings indicate that automatic advice on insulin dosage adjustment is both feasible and reliable, from a practical standpoint, the stage of systematic approval by the doctor should be skipped and the advice made immediately available to the patient.

Fourth Level: Decision-Support Systems

The future of devices to support treatment decisions in type 1 diabetes clearly rests on effective portable systems capable of responding to the key question permanently facing patients, namely the dose of insulin that must be injected. The dose of insulin must be calculated immediately by a powerful program carried everywhere by the patient, which requires no additional operations over and above the usual constraints of treatment and allows simple and frequent contact with the team of care providers. Among smartphones incorporating automated decision-making software [15], the Diabeo system alone has demonstrated real efficacy with regard to HbA_{1c} levels in type 1 diabetes.

This system, designed by CERITD with program development by Voluntis, incorporates three distinct programs. The first program calculates basal and prandial doses of insulin doses set by the treating doctor via a secure website in several steps. A medical prescription is in fact effectively delivered electronically:

- Definition of target fasting and postprandial BG levels and target HbA_{1c} values
- Prescription of basal insulin: doses of slow-acting insulin (1 or 2 injections), administration times and target BG levels required by the system for adjustment, or basal flow rates for pumps, and the 4 target glucose levels (bedtime, breakfast, lunch, and dinner) used for adjustment; the adjustment rules are then set for these doses (table 1)
- Prescription of the prandial dose, either functional insulin treatment (or carbohydrate counting) or fixed dietary plan; in both cases, the doctor must set either the insulin units per portion or grams of carbohydrates or the dose of insulin required for all meals (usually 3), and then set the adjustment rules for the various doses (table 2)

Table 1. Autoadjustment of basal insulin

Rule 1: Hypoglycemia: active
If at least one episode of hypoglycemia declared in last day, reduce dose by 0.1 U/h
Rule 2: Mean BG too low: active
If mean value of last 3 BG readings is <0.80 g/l, reduce dose by 0.1 U/h
Rule 3: BG too low: active
If at least 2 fasting BG readings in the last 3 days are <0.65 g/l, reduce dose by 0.1 U/h
Rule 4: Mean BG too high: active
If mean value of last 5 BG readings is >1.20 g/l and none are <0.80 g/l, increase dose by 0.1 U/l

The 4 rules (3 for dose reduction and 1 for dose increase) are used to adapt basal flow (BF) rates for an insulin pump. Four different BF rates may thus be adjusted in accordance with the target BG results for their respective activity periodsn, namely nighttime BG for the first nocturnal BF, breakfast BG BF for the end-of-night BF, lunch time BG for the morning BF, and dinner BG for the afternoon BF. Additional BF rates may be programmed, but these will not be used for automatic adjustment proposals. All figures shown are default values, but all can be modified by the doctor in accordance with patient requirements. The same principles apply for adjustment of one or two slow-acting insulins.

Table 2. Autoadjustment of fast-acting insulin

BG reading used for autoadjustment rules: postprandial
Rule 1: Hypoglycemia: active
If at least one episode of hypoglycemia is declared in the last day, reduce dose by 0.50 U/portion
Rule 2: Mean BG too low: active
If mean value of last 3 BG readings is <1.20 g/l, reduce dose by 0.50 U/portion
Rule 3: Mean BG too high: active
If mean value of last 5 BG readings is >1.60 g/l and none are <1.20 g/l, increase dose by 0.5 U/portion

The 3 rules (2 for dose reduction and 1 for dose increase) used to adjust 'units per portion' or carbohydrate ratio. The target BG levels are the postprandial levels for the meals in question. All figures shown are default values, but all can be modified by the doctor in accordance with patient requirements.

- Prescription of the correction factor in the event of hyperglycemia and rules for its implementation (table 3)
- Setting of the dose reduction algorithm in the event of physical exercise, evaluated by the patient as moderate or intense (table 4)

For greater ease of use, all target values and adjustment rules are preset in accordance with standard values, but they may all be modified by the doctor for each center and/or each patient in accordance with local practice and patient requirements.

Table 3. Correction

Preprandial correction	Active
Type of correction	Proportional
Preprandial correction	
Parameters for proportional correction	Adding 3 U reduces BG by 1.00 g/l
Correction target	1.00 g/l
Inverse correction	Yes
Parameters for proportional correction	Adding 3 U increases BG by 1.00 g/l
Postprandial correction	
Postprandial correction	Similar to preprandial correction
Adjustment	–50%
Parameters for similar postprandial proportional correction	Adding 1.5 U reduces BG by 1.00 g/l
Correction target	1.40 g/l

Rules for proportional correction in the event of excessively high BG levels. All figures shown are default values, but all can be modified by the doctor in accordance with patient requirements. Stepwise correction may be selected.

Table 4. Physical activity

Physical activity	Active
Reduction in total dose of fast-acting insulin in the event of moderate physical activity	–30%
Reduction in total dose of fast-acting insulin in the event of intense physical activity	–50%

Rules for adjustment of the nearest prandial bolus in the event of physical activity: a reduction in prandial bolus of 30 or 50% is proposed by the system by default when patients have undertaken or plan to undertake physical activity considered by them as moderate or intense. These values can be modified by the doctor.

The patient must sign an agreement protocol at this point, after which he can download this software which is ready for use on his smartphone (it is fully compatible with IPhones 4 and 5, and with most Android smartphones; a list is available at http://www.sanofi-diabete.fr/web/telemedecine/smartphones), and begin using it as follows: he can enter in the electronic logbook her/his BG levels for the 7 available time periods, before and after the 3 meals, and at bedtime; he can also select the second option with two additional times corresponding to midmorning and midafternoon (fig. 1). BG recordings can be entered automatically if the patient has an iBGStar BG meter and an IPhone, or manually if he has a compatible Android smart phone. In the event of hypoglycemia or hyperglycemia, the patient can either enter an explanation selected from a pull-down menu or enter his own free text.

If the patient is about to have a meal and is on functional insulin therapy (or carbohydrate counting), the system prompts the patient to enter (1) the quantity of car-

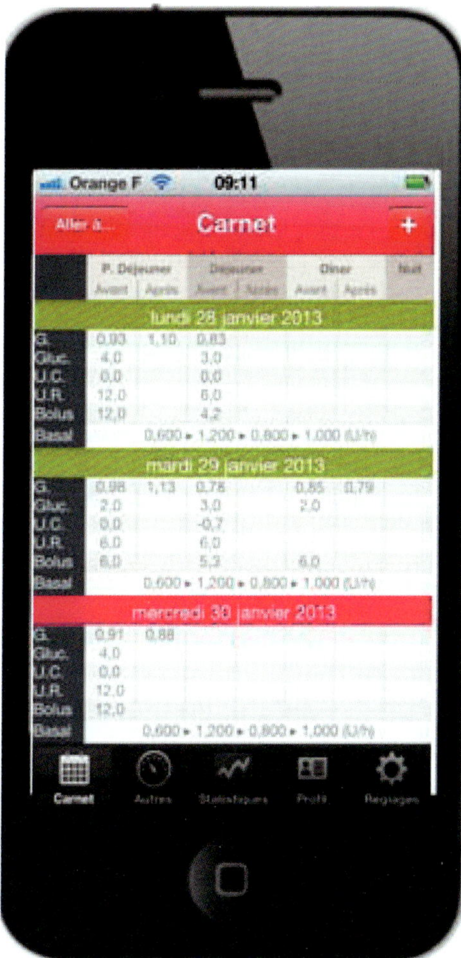

Fig. 1. The electronic logbook as it appears on the patient's smartphone (also shown on the website), with BG readings before and after each meal and at night (a 9-column format is available to allow a morning or afternoon snack to be included), carbohydrate intake for each meal and corresponding calculated insulin dose, any corrections based on preprandial glucose readings, total bolus that is automatically reduced in the event of physical activity, and basal insulin.

bohydrates to be ingested (number of grams or portion size depending on the initial selection made by the doctor), (2) whether any unscheduled moderate or intense physical activity is envisaged, and (3) the preprandial BG reading in order to calculate any necessary correction (fig. 2).

The system then proposes the prandial dose required based on the algorithms previously entered by the doctor for each of these three steps. The patient is free to accept or reject the suggested dose. The algorithms used to calculate 'units per portion' and 'compensation levels' have been adapted from the studies by Howorka et al. [16] and clinically validated [17]. The very simple algorithms used for adjustment to unscheduled physical activity were created by our team and clinically validated [18]. All values can be modified and adapted to individual patients by the treating doctor. For patients not practicing 'carbohydrate counting' but who are on a fixed diet, the doses are calculated on the basis of previously entered prandial doses for each meal, and can be

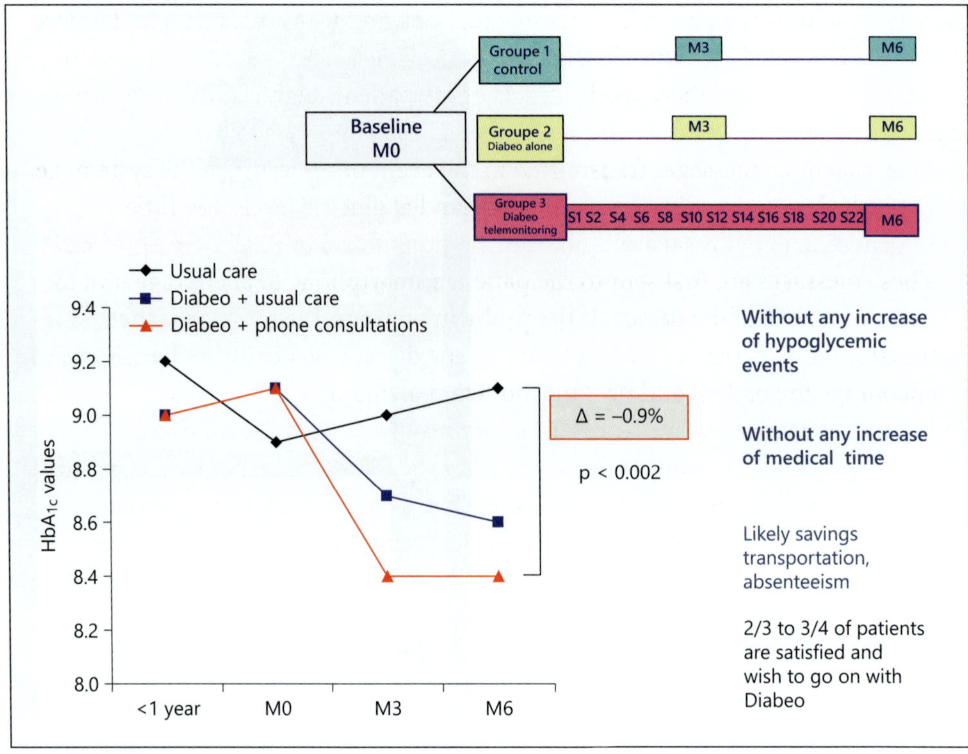

Fig. 2. Télédiab 1 study.

modified in accordance with a preset algorithm if the patient feels he has eaten more or less than normal. Allowance is also made for the preprandial BG level.

If the postprandial results do not lie within the target range, the system automatically proposes a modification of the setting for 'units per portion' or of the fixed insulin dose using the algorithm previously configured by the doctor (table 2); here again, the patient is free to accept or reject the proposed value.

Regarding basal insulin levels, the system may propose one or two basal insulin doses or four basal flow rates for a pump, which are then adapted in accordance with the target BG levels selected (breakfast, lunch, dinner, and bedtime) and with the adjustment algorithm configured by the doctor (table 1). The patient is free to accept or reject the new basal flow rates and doses proposed by the system.

All of the data are transmitted daily to a secure website, which authorized caregivers can access at all times. The data are transferred between the mobile application and the web server via an SSL protocol. All sensitive data used in the Diabeo system and uploaded to this server are fully secure; the data are encrypted and the server is hosted by a professional company specialized in medical data hosting.

The second program was developed to facilitate analysis of this plethora of data and to ensure optimal use of available care time. This program automatically analyses the data generated by the patient's electronic logbook and transmits alerts to designated caregivers in accordance with the algorithms previously configured by the doctor and the characteristics and therapeutic targets of the patient. Eighteen different automatic analytical messages have been configured:

- Five 'coaching' messages transmitted in the event of underuse of the system, i.e. too little data concerning pre- and postprandial glucose levels, too little information about meals, and no transmission of data or recent HbA_{1c} levels. These messages are first sent to the patient's smartphone to encourage him to make more use of the device. If the problem worsens, the message is then transmitted to caregivers, who can intervene directly, generally by telephone, to encourage the patient and prevent him from giving up on the system.
- Eight messages concerning unsatisfactory results: occurrence of severe hyperglycemia or episodes of moderate but excessively frequent hyperglycemia, occurrence of severe hypoglycemia or episodes of moderate but excessively frequent hypoglycemia, mean fasting and postprandial glucose readings or HbA_{1c} levels outside the target range, and excessive variation in glucose readings. These messages are shown in the patient's Web dossier and the caregiver is alerted by e-mail. The treatment profile can then be modified by the caregiver and may be downloaded to the patient's mobile telephone. However, after being informed, the patient is free to accept or reject any modification proposed by the caregiver.
- Five messages concerning inadequate functioning or utilisation of the system by the patient: excessive autoadjustment of a proposed insulin dose (<50 or >150%), autoadjustment of a parameter rejected by the patient on several successive occasions, new treatment profile proposed by the caregiver but rejected by the patient or awaiting acceptance for several days, excessively frequent modifications by the patient of his treatment. These alerts allow caregivers to intervene immediately, as required, generally by means of a telephone call.

The third program was developed to help and define tasks for nurses to whom work has been entrusted by the doctor, within the context of a 'personalized training plan'. This program has already undergone preliminary assessment [19].

The metabolic improvement provided by the first version of the Diabeo system, which comprised only the program used to calculate basal and prandial doses, was assessed in patients with chronic glucose control problems in the multicenter Télédiab 1 study.

Results of the Télédiab 1 Study

This study included 180 patients presenting chronically poorly controlled type 1 diabetes, with HbA_{1c} >8.0% over a period of several months despite basal-bolus therapy either by multiple injections or insulin pump (37%); mean baseline HbA_{1c}

was 9.07 ± 1.07%. The patients, who were followed up at 17 study centers in France, were randomized to 1 of 3 groups: a control group (G1), a group provided with a communicating smartphone equipped with the software but without remote follow-up (G2), or a group receiving a smartphone equipped with the software and with remote follow-up (G3). Patients in G1 and G2 underwent 3-monthly follow-up at a hospital by means of a standard face-to-face consultation, whereas patients in G3 did not attend the hospital but were followed up by means of short telephone consultations every 2 or 3 weeks. After 6 months, the patients in G3 experienced a 0.9% reduction in HbA_{1c} (0.60; 1.21; $p < 0.001$) versus the control group; an intermediate reduction in HbA_{1c} was seen in G2, for whom no remote follow-up was given: 0.7% (0.35; 0.99) versus the control group ($p < 0.001$) [20] (fig. 2). This improvement in HbA_{1c} was achieved without any change in the incidence of hypoglycemia, whether mild or severe. The daily frequency of self-monitoring of BG levels increased very slightly over the course of the study (3.29 ± 1.44 at baseline vs. 3.57 ± 1.35 at the end), but since it occurred in identical fashion in the three groups ('study effect'), it could not account for the improvement seen in HbA_{1c}. It thus appears that for equal frequency of self-monitoring of BG levels, Diabeo allowed patients to utilize their BG readings more successfully and calculate their insulin requirements more accurately. Incidentally, it should be noted that the insulin dose calculator was widely used by patients in G2 and G3 who were given the Diabeo system since the mean number of meals entered for which the calculator was used was 67% throughout the 6-month study.

In operational terms, the Diabeo system comprises two components: (1) a sophisticated technical system for calculating and adapting basal and prandial insulin doses, allowing optimization of data entered by the patient (capillary BG readings, ingested carbohydrate, and any physical activity), and (2) a remote follow-up system allowing motivational support to be given to patients and ensuring optimal use of caregivers' time, allowing short but repeated interventions at appropriate times upon worsening of BG values or when the patient's motivation to use the system declines.

The purely technical aspect appears important in this study; although used alone in G2, it resulted in a 0.7% improvement in HbA_{1c} while the addition of the second component in G3 resulted in a more modest improvement of 0.2%. However, it was not possible to evaluate the use of the latter component alone in a fourth group.

Another approach to this question is to examine whether such a system is really suited to all patients, or whether in fact only certain patients will benefit more from the technical component while others benefit more from the remote motivational and coaching aspects. To this end we carried out an analysis of individual day-to-day patient data and we compared patients in G2 and G3 according to whether they were 'high users' (i.e. use of the system to calculate insulin dose for more than 67% of meals) or 'low users' (use of the system for fewer than 67% of meals).

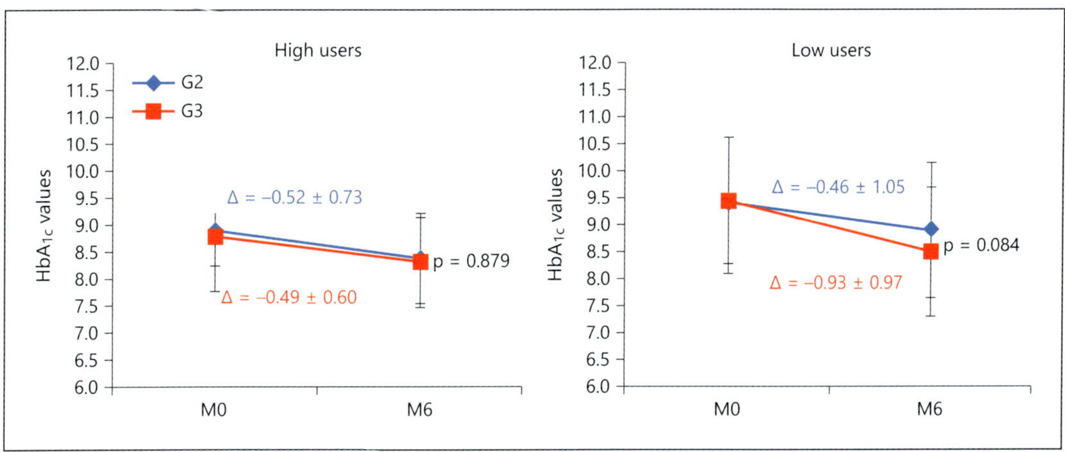

Fig. 3. High users of the system, showing identical improvement in HbA_{1c}, whether randomised (G3) or not (G2) to receive remote monitoring and teleconsultations. Low users receiving remote monitoring and teleconsultations showed twice as much improvement in their HbA_{1c} readings (G3).

This comparison yielded interesting results. The 56 'high users' of the system [90% of meals entered (77.2; 96.1)] appeared to differ from the 57 'low users' [28.6% of meals entered (6.2; 50.2)]. The former 'high users' who were more compliant with regard to the Diabeo system were older, had diabetes of longer standing, were more often employed in managerial posts, and were on functional insulin therapy more often than 'low users'. Their baseline HbA_{1c} values were also lower than those of the 'low users' [8.7 (8.3; 9.2) versus 9.0 (8.5; 10.1), p = 0.008].

The 'high users' also appeared to derive benefit solely from the 'technical' features of the system, and their HbA_{1c} showed similar improvement regardless of whether they used the noncommunicating system alone (G2: $\Delta HbA_{1c} = 0.52 \pm 0.73\%$) or received remote coaching as well (G3: $\Delta HbA_{1c} = -0.49 \pm 0.60\%$, p = 0.879). In contrast, while 'low users' showed some improvement with the noncommunicating system (G2: $\Delta HbA_{1c} = -0.46 \pm 1.05\%$), improvements in this group were far greater where remote coaching and follow-up were also provided (G3: $\Delta HbA_{1c} = -0.93 \pm 0.97\%$, p = 0.084; fig. 3).

The Diabeo system thus proved useful not only for fairly compliant patients with moderate glucose imbalance who used the dose calculation feature and accordingly carried out their injections, but also for patients with poor BG control, with major compliance problems, and who appeared to benefit more from the motivational support provided regularly through frequent telephone consultations made possible by a smartphone linked to the website [21].

Over and above the metabolic benefits, the Diabeo system also appears to provide medicoeconomic benefits. While the total medical time used during the two face-to-face consultations over the 6-month period in G1 and G2 (70 ± 31 and 70 ± 22 min) was identical to that used in telephone consultations for G3 (8.7 ± 4.9 telephone consultations lasting an average 7.4 ± 3 min), time-saving for patients was very different. Patients in G1 and G2 had to spend almost 5 h attending their consultations (transport, administrative issues, waiting times, etc.) compared with zero time loss for patients in G3, who were required to take no time off work as a result. Furthermore, transportation costs were clearly considerably lower in G3. It should be noted that in France, the social security system reimburses diabetic patients for travel expenses incurred through hospital consultations. In 2007, the mean annual reimbursement rate was EUR 314, for total annual diabetes-related expenditure of EUR 6,927 [5]. By limiting travel for patients followed up remotely, telephone consultations should thus reduce transportation costs quite considerably. This is particularly true for patients living in remote regions with limited access to healthcare or with low doctor-to-patient ratios. Finally, it is important for the purposes of medicoeconomic analysis to bear in mind the longer-term benefits due to reduced BG levels with regard to diabetes-related morbidity and mortality. Note that for reductions in HbA_{1c} comparable to those achieved in G3, the authors of DCCT calculated a 39% reduction in progression of retinopathy and a 25% reduction in onset of microalbuminuria [1]. This reduction in morbidity should have a major bearing on cost reduction, however difficult it may be in practice to quantify such benefits.

Can Such a System Be Routinely Used in the Entire Population?

This is the question adumbrated in France by the Higher Health Authority (HAS) and to which the TELESAGE study must provide an answer before recommendation and reimbursable status can be issued for this new treatment method based on a smartphone converted to a communicating medical device (DMC). This study will be conducted in a larger population (700 patients) and over a longer period (2 years) in partnership with the Sanofi medical group, who is sponsoring it. The study is scheduled to begin in France in 2013 and will be proposed to patients with type 1 or 2 diabetes with chronically poor metabolic control (HbA_{1c} >8.0%) despite basal-bolus treatment via multiple injections or an insulin pump, and either owning or planning to acquire a compatible smartphone.

The study is designed to evaluate the Diabeo system with its program for automatic analysis of teletransmitted data, programmed to analyze utilization of the system by the patient and to detect abnormal results. This automatic analysis system should allow caregivers to rapidly identify subjects in difficulty and no longer feeling motivated to continue, as well as those with BG levels falling outside the target range, and enable them to rapidly provide remote assistance for these patients and help them manage their therapy.

The TELESAGE study will also examine the question of reorganization of provision of care. Against a backdrop of a shortage of specialized medical time, it is planned to provide doctors with hours of specialized nursing assistance for the task of remote follow-up of these patients. The recent French Health Ministry report [22] proposes that intervention by paramedical staff should be formally encompassed in a program governing interprofessional cooperation protocol. This program has in fact already been incorporated in the Diabeo system. This reorganization of healthcare based upon interprofessional cooperation between doctors and specialized nursing staff should enable doctors to free up more time to work with those patients specifically identified as having difficulties.

The centers involved in this study will be randomized to receive the Diabeo system alone or Diabeo together with time from nurses specializing in 'telemedicine' and trained in diabetes care. The third group will form the control group and will receive standard treatment. The hundred or so centers in which the study is to be conducted will include university hospitals, general hospitals, and private practices (independent diabetologists). The primary study criterion, namely improvement in HbA_{1c}, will be evaluated at 1 year. A medicoeconomic analysis will be carried out in parallel, and will involve the most accurate assessment possible of the direct and indirect costs associated with provision of this type of care.

On completion of the TELESAGE study, it will be possible to indicate the degree of metabolic improvement achieved in the midterm using the Diabeo telemedicine system, combining a smartphone with a dose adapter and a telemonitoring program, depending on whether it is used alone or in conjunction with reorganized provision of healthcare via specialized nurses within the ambit of a cooperation protocol. It will be possible to determine the feasibility of such reorganization of healthcare within different types of medical practice, both in hospitals and in private practice. The medicoeconomic evaluation will be a decisive factor. The quality of the data collected should allow the French authorities to determine whether this tool, which has already proven its value in terms of metabolic improvement, is suited for general use and how it is to be funded; it will also provide information about how this tool may be integrated into the global management program for diabetic patients by means of optimized insulin delivery, and about how healthcare may be organized around patients in order to optimize treatment. At the same time, there are also plans to adapt the Diabeo device to other healthcare systems, in both Europe and America, and to introduce it into these regions.

Disclosure Statement

S. Franc and G. Charpentier work for CERITD, a nonprofit research body that developed the Diabeo system in partnership with the Voluntis company. Sanofi Aventis is the sponsor of the TELESAGE study.

References

1 Reliability and validity of a diabetes quality-of-life measure for the Diabetes Control and Complications Trial (DCCT). The DCCT Research Group. Diabetes Care 1988;11:725–732.

2 Wood JR, Miller KM, Maahs DM, Beck RW, Dimeglio LA, Libman IM, Quinn M, Tamborlane WV, Woerner SE; T1D Exchange Clinic Network: Most youth with type 1 diabetes in the T1D Exchange Clinic Registry do not meet American Diabetes Association or International Society for Pediatric and Adolescent Diabetes clinical guidelines. Diabetes Care 2013;36:2035–2037.

3 Rosenbauer J, Dost A, Karges B, Hungele A, Stahl A, Bächle C, Gerstl EM, Kastendieck C, Hofer SE, Holl RW; DPV Initiative and the German BMBF Competence Network Diabetes Mellitus: Improved metabolic control in children and adolescents with type 1 diabetes: a trend analysis using prospective multicenter data from Germany and Austria. Diabetes Care 2012;35:80–86.

4 O'Connell SM, Cooper MN, Bulsara MK, Davis EA, Jones TW: Reducing rates of severe hypoglycemia in a population-based cohort of children and adolescents with type 1 diabetes over the decade 2000–2009. Diabetes Care 2011;34:2379–2380.

5 Ricci P, Chantry M, Detournay B, Poutignat N, Kusnik-Joinville O, Raimond V, Thammavong N, Weill A; Le Comité scientifique d'Entred: Characteristics, vascular risk and complications in people with diabetes, in metropolitan France: major improvements between ENTRED 2001 and ENTRED 2007 studies. Bull Epidemiol Hebdomadaire 2009;42–43:450–455.

6 DAFNE Study Group: Training in flexible, intensive insulin management to enable dietary freedom in people with type 1 diabetes: Dose Adjustment for Normal Eating (DAFNE) randomised controlled trial. BMJ 2002;325:746.

7 Gunn D, Mansell P: Glycaemic control and weight 7 years after Dose Adjustment for Normal Eating (DAFNE) structured education in type 1 diabetes. Diabet Med 2012;29:807–812.

8 Sussman A, Taylor EJ, Patel M, Ward J, Alva S, Lawrence A, Ng R: Performance of a glucose meter with a built-in automated bolus calculator versus manual bolus calculation in insulin-using subjects. J Diabetes Sci Technol 2012;6:339–344.

9 Gross TM, Kayne D, King A, Rother C, Juth S: A bolus calculator is an effective means of controlling postprandial glycemia in patients on insulin pump therapy. Diabetes Technol Ther 2003;5:365–369.

10 Klupa T, Benbenek-Klupa T, Malecki M, Szalecki M, Sieradzki J: Clinical usefulness of a bolus calculator in maintaining normoglycaemia in active professional patients with type 1 diabetes treated with continuous subcutaneous insulin infusion. J Int Med Res 2008;36:1112–1116.

11 Schmidt S, Meldgaard M, Serifovski N, Storm C, Christensen TM, Gade-Rasmussen B, Nørgaard K: Use of an automated bolus calculator in MDI-treated type 1 diabetes: the BolusCal Study, a randomized controlled pilot study. Diabetes Care 2012;35:984–990.

12 Lepore G, Dodesini AR, Nosari I, Scaranna C, Corsi A, Trevisan R: Bolus calculator improves long-term metabolic control and reduces glucose variability in pump-treated patients with type 1 diabetes. Nutr Metab Cardiovasc Dis 2012;22:e15–e16.

13 Barnard K, Parkin C, Young A, Ashraf M: Use of an automated bolus calculator reduces fear of hypoglycemia and improves confidence in dosage accuracy in patients with type 1 diabetes mellitus treated with multiple daily insulin injections. J Diabetes Sci Technol 2012;6:144–149.

14 Bergenstal RM, Bashan E, McShane M, Johnson M, Hodish I: Can a tool that automates insulin titration be a key to diabetes management? Diabetes Technol Ther 2012;14:675–682.

15 Rossi MC, Nicolucci A, Pellegrini F, Bruttomesso D, Bartolo PD, Marelli G, Dal Pos M, Galetta M, Horwitz D, Vespasiani G: Interactive logbook for diabetes: a useful and easy-to-use new telemedicine system to support the decision-making process in type 1 diabetes. Diabetes Technol Ther 2009;11:19–24.

16 Howorka K, Thoma H, Grillmayr H, Kitzler E: Phases of functional, near-normoglycaemic insulin substitution: what are computers good for in the rehabilitation process in type I (insulin-dependent) diabetes mellitus? Comput Methods Programs Biomed 1990;32:319–323.

17 Franc S, Dardari D, Boucherie B, Riveline JP, Biedzinski M, Petit C, Requeda E, Leurent P, Varroud-Vial M, Hochberg G, Charpentier G: Real-life application and validation of flexible intensive insulin-therapy algorithms in type 1 diabetes patients. Diabetes Metab 2009;35:463–468.

18 Franc S, Dardari D, Biedzinski M, Requeda E, Canipel L, Hochberg G, Boucherie B, Charpentier G: Type 1 diabetes: dealing with physical activity. Diabetes Metab 2012;38:466–469.

19 Franc S, Juy O, Chaillous L, Benhamou PY, Penfornis F, Sonnet E, Mounier S, Petit MH, Boscus O, Laroye H, Canipel L, Charpentier G: Télémédecine et coopération interprofessionnelle médecin/infirmier, qu'en est-il en pratique? Diabetes Metab 2013; 39(suppl 1):abstract.

20 Charpentier G, Benhamou PY, Dardari D, Borot S, Franc S, Schaepelynck-Belicar P, Catargi B, Melki V, Chaillous L, Farret A, Vigeral C, Leguerrier AM, Mosnier-Pudar H, Moreau F, Winiszewski P, Vambergue A, Guerci B, Reffet S, Millot L, Quesada JL, Clergeot A, Halimi S, Ronsin O, Fagour C, Hanaire H, Renard E, Kessler L, Thivolet C, Bosson JL, Penfornis A; TeleDiab Study Group: The Diabeo software enabling individualized insulin dose adjustments combined with telemedicine support improves HbA_{1c} in poorly controlled type 1 diabetic patients: a 6-month, randomised, open-label, parallel group, multicenter trial (TeleDiab 1 study). Diabetes Care 2011;34:533–539.

21 Franc S, Benhamou PY, Dardari D, Penformis A, Vigeral C, Leguerrier AM, Mosnier-Pudar H, Moreau F, Winiszewski P, Vambergue A, Quesada J, Guerci B, Reffet S, Millot L, Borot S, Halimi S, Ronsin O, Fagour C, Hanaire H, Renard E, Kessler L, Thivolet C, Charpentier G: Which profile for the users of a software enabling individualized insulin dose adjustments combined with telemedicine support, the Diabeo system (abstract A-417-0010-00296). ATTD, Paris, 2013.

22 Telemedicine and Legal Responsibilities (report of May 5, 2012). Paris, DGOS (Healthcare Provision Office of the French Health Ministry), 2012.

Dr. Sylvia Franc
Department of Diabetes, Sud-Francilien Hospital
116 Bd Jean Jaurès
FR–91100 Corbeil-Essonnes (France)
E-Mail sylvia.franc@free.fr

Bruttomesso D, Grassi G (eds): Technological Advances in the Treatment of Type 1 Diabetes.
Front Diabetes. Basel, Karger, 2015, vol 24, pp 226–235 (DOI: 10.1159/000363519)

Diabetes Interactive Diary: A Mobile Phone-Based Telemedicine System for Carbohydrate Counting and Bolus Calculator

Giacomo Vespasiani[a] · Maria Chiara Rossi[b]

[a]Diabetes Unit, Madonna del Soccorso Hospital, San Benedetto del Tronto, and [b]Department of Clinical Pharmacology and Epidemiology, Fondazione Mario Negri Sud, Santa Maria Imbaro, Italy

Abstract

A flexible therapy for type 1 diabetes based on carbohydrate counting and insulin dose adjustment can promote glycemic control and quality of life without worsening severe hypoglycemia or cardiovascular risk. The complexity of the standard education required by the flexible therapy can be managed with the 'Diabetes Interactive Diary (DID)', a carbohydrate/bolus calculator for mobile phones. It also works as a telemedicine system based on communication between patient and physician via text messages (SMS). The efficacy and safety of the DID have been tested in 3 main studies. The DID was demonstrated to be effective in improving metabolic control as well as standard education while ensuring several additional benefits. First, it halved the time dedicated to education and simplified the calculation of carbohydrates content and insulin doses, allowing more individuals with type 1 diabetes to adopt the flexible regimen. Second, the use of the DID was also associated with an 86% decrease in risk of grade 2 hypoglycemia. Additionally, several quality of life scales were significantly improved, suggesting that the use of telemedicine can increase the acceptance of insulin treatment and help patients cope with the disease. Currently, the DID is available as a free app for smartphones.

Nutritional management is recognized as one of the cornerstones of diabetes care [1]. In fact, a correct diet translates into the prevention of both acute complications (hypoglycemia and hyperglycemia) and micro- and macrovascular complications [2]. In this context, carbohydrate counting is an important strategy to ensure an adequate diet for patients. It is usually based on estimating the carbohydrate content of foods being eaten, without patients being constrained to eat a specific amount of carbohydrate at each meal; the insulin bolus is then adjusted to match the dietary carbohydrate at each meal [3]. Therefore, carbohydrate counting represents an effective strategy to promote dietary freedom, quality of life, and glycemic control without worsening severe hypoglycemia or cardiovascular risk [4–6].

Nevertheless, the widespread use of carbohydrate counting is limited by the complexity of the educational approach. In fact, patients need to be taught about different aspects of nutrition with increasing levels of complexity. Level 1, or basic, introduces patients to the concept of carbohydrate counting and focuses on carbohydrate consistency. Level 2, or intermediate, focuses on the relationships among food, diabetes medication, physical activity, and blood glucose levels, and introduces the steps needed to manage these variables based on patterns of blood glucose levels. Finally, level 3, or advanced, is designed to teach patients who are using multiple daily injections or insulin infusion pumps how to match short-acting insulin to carbohydrates using the carbohydrate-to-insulin ratio. Other issues to be learned are portion control, food exchange, and glycemic index [3, 7].

Telemedicine, which is represented by all the technologies that support data recording and transmission via internet, telephone, or text messages (SMS), is emerging as a possible solution to simplify training and support patients [8]. The underlying assumption is that systems providing continuous and more frequent contact between patient and educator, or the simple aid of software as a vehicle for educational messages and reminders, can provide more immediate feedback and motivate and support the patient in the management of diet and therapy. In particular, the use of mobile phones, technology fully integrated in the daily life of the vast majority of people, can represent valid support for patients to overcome difficulties linked to the complexity of the education and the chronic burden of the disease on daily life [9, 10].

Diabetes Interactive Diary

The 'Diabetes Interactive Diary (DID)' is a software package developed by MeTeDa srl that can be installed on a patient's mobile telephone that works as a carbohydrate/insulin bolus calculator (fig. 1). It supports patients in recording the self-monitoring of blood glucose (SMBG) measurements on the glycemic diary, and helps them in the management of carbohydrate counting. In fact, every patient can decide what to eat during the meal, choosing between all the foods listed in the software; the quantification of the total calories and carbohydrates consumed is facilitated by a list of pictures showing the specific food and the amount ingested. On the basis of the carbohydrate-to-insulin ratio and glycemic correction factor, identified and prescribed by the responsible healthcare professional, and of the data stored by the patient, the DID automatically calculates the most appropriate short-acting insulin dose to be injected at each meal.

All the recorded data are sent to the physician on average every 1–3 weeks (depending on the needs of the patient) via text message or internet and reviewed on a personal computer at the diabetes clinic. Any new therapeutic and behavioral prescrip-

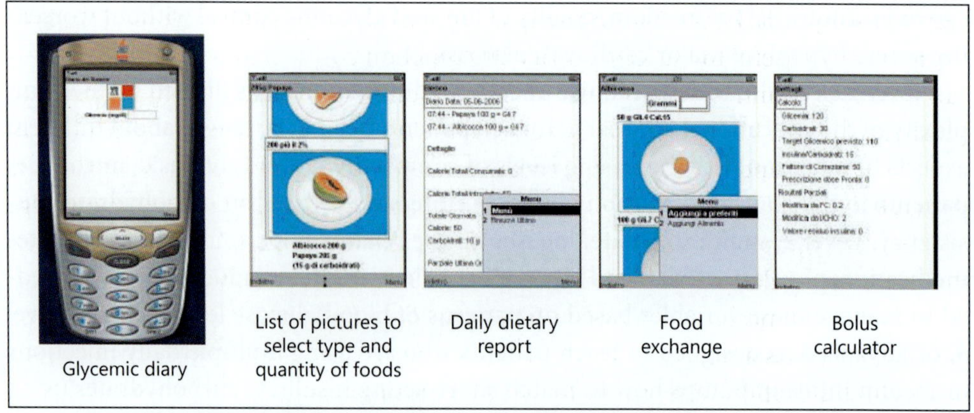

Fig. 1. The DID system: software for mobile phones containing an SMBG diary, food atlas, bolus calculator, and telemedicine system via text messages.

tion, i.e. a new correction factor or insulin sensitivity value, can be sent from the diabetes clinic's computer to the patient's mobile phone, ensuring regular and immediate feedback.

Clinical Research on Diabetes Interactive Diary

To avoid the methodological flaws found in previous studies on telemedicine systems [9–11], the DID underwent a process of evaluation not dissimilar to that usually adopted for pharmacological products. First, its feasibility, acceptability, and safety were investigated in a pilot study involving 50 patients [12]. Second, its effectiveness on metabolic control, weight loss, and quality of life and time devoted to education were preliminarily tested in the context of a randomized study [13]. Finally, a confirmatory randomized trial investigated the impact of the DID on risk of hypoglycemia and glycemic variability [14].

Diabetes Interactive Diary Study 1

In the first study on the DID system [12], 50 patients with type 1 diabetes were involved in a survey on their satisfaction with DID. Questionnaires were administered at baseline and after 12 weeks. Patients had a mean (±SD) age of 33.2 ± 8.9 years and a mean diabetes duration of 13.9 ± 9.5 years. Fifty-seven percent of the patients were treated with multiple injections of insulin and 43% with continuous subcutaneous insulin infusion. Mean levels of glycated hemoglobin (HbA_{1c}) were 7.2 ± 0.8%. Almost all the patients (91.7%) had received at least 13 years of school education (college degree).

On the questionnaire, the DID system was judged as 'excellent' or 'good' by 94% of the patients, 'extremely useful' or 'very useful' by 65%, and 'very easy' or 'somewhat easy' to use by 90%. Patients were also asked to rank the different functions of the DID from the most useful to the least useful. The function considered the most useful was carbohydrate counting (mean rank: 1.7 ± 1.0), followed by insulin bolus calculation (mean rank: 2.3 ± 1.5), food diary (mean rank: 2.7 ± 1.1), physical activity diary (mean rank: 3.7 ± 1.3), and food exchange (mean rank: 3.7 ± 1.4). Over 63% of the patients declared that the DID had changed their eating habits as a result of greater knowledge of the relationship between food, blood glucose, and insulin dose. During the study, the DID was regularly used by the participants. On average, information on carbohydrate content of meals was requested 3.1 ± 1.5 times a day, SMBG values were recorded 4.8 ± 2.3 times a day, and advice on insulin dose was requested 3.2 ± 1.3 times a day. Communication with the doctor via text message was rated as 'extremely effective' or 'very effective' by 85.5% of the patients. The main limitations of the system pointed out were the slowness of the software and the lack of some foods in the food atlas.

As for clinical aspects, no significant variations were shown between baseline and the end-of-study data in respect to HbA_{1c} (from 7.2 ± 0.8 to 7.2 ± 0.9%) and BMI (from 23.4 ± 3.2 to 23.6 ± 3.4). No patients reported serious hypoglycemic episodes requiring medical intervention during the study (fig. 1).

In conclusion, this study demonstrated that the DID was a feasible, safe, and easy-to-use tool to help diabetic patients manage nutrition and insulin therapy.

Diabetes Interactive Diary Study 2

The second study on the DID system [13] was an open-label, multicenter, randomized (1:1), parallel-group study involving 7 diabetes clinics from 4 countries (3 in Italy, 2 in England, and 2 in Spain). The study was designed to compare the use of the DID versus the standard carbohydrate counting education in improving glycemic control (HbA_{1c}) and whether it could do so in a shorter time period and more easily. Secondary endpoints were changes in fasting blood glucose (FBG) levels, bodyweight, lipid profile (serum total cholesterol, high-density lipoprotein cholesterol, low-density lipoprotein cholesterol, and triglycerides), and blood pressure. In addition, differences in time dedicated to educational activities, number of extra visits, and average cost of text messages were taken into consideration. Finally, changes in health-related quality of life were evaluated in the subgroup of Italian patients using generic [SF-36 Health Survey and World Health Organization (WHO) Well-Being Questionnaire] [15, 16] and diabetes-specific [WHO Diabetes Treatment Satisfaction Questionnaire (DTSQ)] measures [17].

Overall, 130 patients ≥18 years of age with type 1 diabetes not previously educated on carbohydrate counting and treated with multiple daily injections of short-acting and long-acting insulin analogues or with continuous subcutaneous insulin infusion were included. Furthermore, patients practiced SMBG at least 3 times a day. They were randomized to start the standard carbohydrate counting educational program or the DID educational program. Randomization was performed through a telephone call to the coordinating center. Random lists were stratified by the centers. To ensure equal allocation rates within centers, permuted block randomization was used.

Patients randomized to the experimental group attended a course on the use of the DID lasting up to 2 weeks. The course was provided as an outpatient program of 3 encounters with physician and/or dietician. Patients randomized to the control group received the standard educational approach adopted by the center to be ended within 3 months. Clinical data were collected at baseline, and after 3 and 6 months from randomization.

Patients in the DID arm and those in the standard group had a mean (±SD) age of 35.4 ± 9.5 and 36.1 ± 9.4 years ($p = 0.63$), respectively, while mean diabetes duration was 17.1 ± 10.3 and 17.1 ± 10.3 years in the two groups ($p = 0.37$). The other baseline clinical characteristics of patients randomized to the two study arms did not differ significantly.

Eleven patients withdrew from the study, 2 of whom were in the standard group (both patients were lost to follow-up) and 9 in the DID group (1 lost to follow-up and 8 for DID-related causes).

A significant reduction in HbA_{1c} levels of about 0.5% was documented in both groups after 3 months and was maintained to the end of study.

As for secondary study outcomes, after 6 months FBG decreased in the DID group (from 182.8 ± 85.6 to 162.9 ± 67.0 mg/dl) and increased in the standard group (from 176.9 ± 68.4 to 186.3 ± 79.1 mg/dl; $p = 0.13$). Increases in bodyweight were lower in the DID group (+0.7 ± 3.6 kg) than in the standard group (+1.5 ± 2.3 kg; $p = 0.22$), probably as a consequence of lower doses of insulin required. In fact, although we found no differences in mean daily doses of short-acting insulin between the two groups (DID group: 20.6 ± 8.2 UI/day; standard group: 20.1 ± 7.8 UI/day; $p = 0.92$), mean daily doses of long-acting insulin were lower in the DID group than in the standard group (DID group: 17.4 ± 7.4 UI/day; standard group: 21.4 ± 10.0 UI/day; $p = 0.12$). As for the other clinical parameters investigated, the DID group showed a significant decrease in triglyceride levels in comparison with the standard group. No other between-group changes were documented. Presumably, the reduction in the basal insulin dose could be due to a more correct titration made possible by more simple and frequent communication between patient and physician.

The improvement in metabolic control was obtained with a median of 6 h (2–15) to carbohydrate counting education in the DID group and a median of 12 h (2.5–25) in the standard group ($p = 0.07$). The median number of outpatient visits during 6 months was 4 (2–6) for the DID group and 3 (0–4) for the standard group ($p = 0.01$). The median (range) number of text messages sent by each patient during the study was 52 (6–75), and the median number of text messages sent by the physician was 39 (22–70). In other words, patients sent about 2 text messages per week to their physician, and the physician regularly replied to confirm the therapeutic scheme or to modify the parameters set in the DID (carbohydrate-to-insulin ratio, insulin sensitivity factor, and/or blood glucose goal). In terms of costs for the patient, assuming a cost of 10–15 cents per message and considering that, on average, each patient sent 52 text messages, the overall cost sustained did not exceed EUR 8.00.

Results of the quality of life evaluation performed on the subsample of 60 patients enrolled in the Italian centers show a statistically significant difference in favor of the DID group for the treatment satisfaction, as expressed by the DTSQ score. Similarly, the score testing the perceived frequency of hyperglycemic episodes significantly decreased after 3 months in the DID group, but not in the control group. Several SF-36 subscales (role physical, general health, vitality, and role emotional) also showed significantly higher improvements in the DID group than in the standard group.

Diabetes Interactive Diary Study 3

Some questions remained open after the trial, particularly related to the efficacy of the DID versus traditional education on metabolic control when all patients are treated with the same insulin regimen, and its impact on hypoglycemic episodes, glucose variability, and other quality of life measures. Therefore, a new open-label, multicenter, parallel-group, randomized (1:1) clinical trial was developed [14]. The study involved 12 Italian diabetes outpatient clinics. It aimed to compare the effects of DID versus usual care in patients with type 1 diabetes mellitus, all treated with the same insulin regimen (basal:bolus of 1 daily injection of glargine + 3 injections of glulisine).

The primary endpoint was the reduction of HbA_{1c} levels. Secondary endpoints were changes in FBG, glucose variability (expressed as mean amplitude of glucose excursions) [18–20], mean daily doses of basal and prandial insulin, frequency of hypoglycemic episodes, changes in body weight, lipid profile (serum total cholesterol, high-density lipoprotein-cholesterol, low-density lipoprotein-cholesterol, and triglycerides), and blood pressure levels. Quality of life and patient satisfaction were investigated using the DTSQ [16, 17] and the Diabetes Specific Quality of Life Scale (DSQOLS) [21].

Randomization was performed through a telephone call to the coordinating center, and random lists were stratified by the centers. To ensure equal allocation rates within centers, permuted block randomization was used. Data were collected at baseline, and after 3 and 6 months from randomization.

All recruited patients started (if they were not already using) insulin glulisine as a mealtime rapid analogue and insulin glargine as basal insulin. The insulin scheme was the same in both groups: patients had 3 prandial injections per day of insulin glulisine associated with basal insulin glargine. Prandial injections could be performed within 15 min before or up to 20 min after the start of meal, based on doctor judgment and patient needs [22, 23]. Patients were randomized to determine whether the DID system aided carbohydrate counting and the calculation of the most appropriate insulin dose. The experimental group (group A) received the same educational course of the previous study, and the DID was used during the study to estimate the carbohydrate content of the meal and to adjust prandial insulin doses. The control group (group B) received the standard educational approach usually utilized in the center. Insulin doses in group B were adjusted according to the usual practice on the basis of SMBG values reviewed during the doctor office visit.

Overall, 127 individuals were recruited and 15 dropped-out during the study: 7 in the standard group and 8 in the DID group. No drop-out cause was directly related to the DID system or to the insulin treatment. The two groups did not differ in any sociodemographic and clinical characteristic, with the exception of a higher mean age in the DID group (38.4 ± 10.3 years vs. 34.3 ± 10.0; $p = 0.04$). This difference was taken into account in the statistical analysis.

Between- and within-group changes after 6 months showed a reduction in HbA_{1c} levels of 0.5% in both groups. The between-group comparison in the mean changes of HbA_{1c} levels was not statistically significant, but the improvement in metabolic control was statistically significant and clinically relevant within each group. In addition, the use of DID was associated with a 86% lower risk of grade 2 hypoglycemic episodes as compared to the control group.

No additional benefits were found in the other clinical secondary endpoints, such as body weight, FBG, lipid profile, and blood pressure. A nonstatistically significant greater reduction in FBG was detected in the standard group compared to the DID group. Mean daily doses of basal insulin slightly decreased in the DID group (–0.93 ± 0.51 UI) and slightly increased in the control group (0.59 ± 0.50 UI), leading to a statistically significant between-group difference ($p = 0.04$).

The evaluation of mean amplitude of glucose excursions did not show any impact of the DID versus the standard care in reducing glucose variability. However, the compliance with the required frequency of SMBG measurements (7-point glucose profiles) was low, especially for the nocturnal measurement. In fact, only 31 patients correctly performed all the 18 SMBG profiles requested by the protocol.

The use of DID was associated with improvements in several quality of life scales: the 'perceived frequency of hyperglycemic episodes' dimension of the DTSQ and the 'social relations' dimension of the DSQOLS were significantly improved in the DID group compared to the standard group, and the 'fear of hypoglycemia' dimension improved in the DID group but worsened in the standard group, with a borderline statistically significant difference ($p = 0.06$).

In the DID group, 25.0% of the patients required at least one extra visit compared to 31.3% in the control group ($p = 0.43$).

Results obtained with the DID markedly differed among patients: median (minimum; maximum) change was –0.5% (–1.5; +1.3) for HbA_{1c}, 0 kg (–5; +4) for body weight, and +1 (–21; +18) for the DTSQ. The median number of text messages exchanged between patients and healthcare professionals was 20 (0; 135).

The average benefits obtained in the different participating centers also varied substantially: mean HbA_{1c} changes varied from +0.3 ± 0.6 to –1.0 ± 0.4%, mean body weight from +1.7 ± 1.0% to –0.7 ± 1.2 kg, mean text messages exchanged between patient and healthcare professionals ranged between 2 ± 0 and 36 ± 10, and mean DTSQ changes varied from 0.4 ± 4.7 to 9.0 ± 5.2.

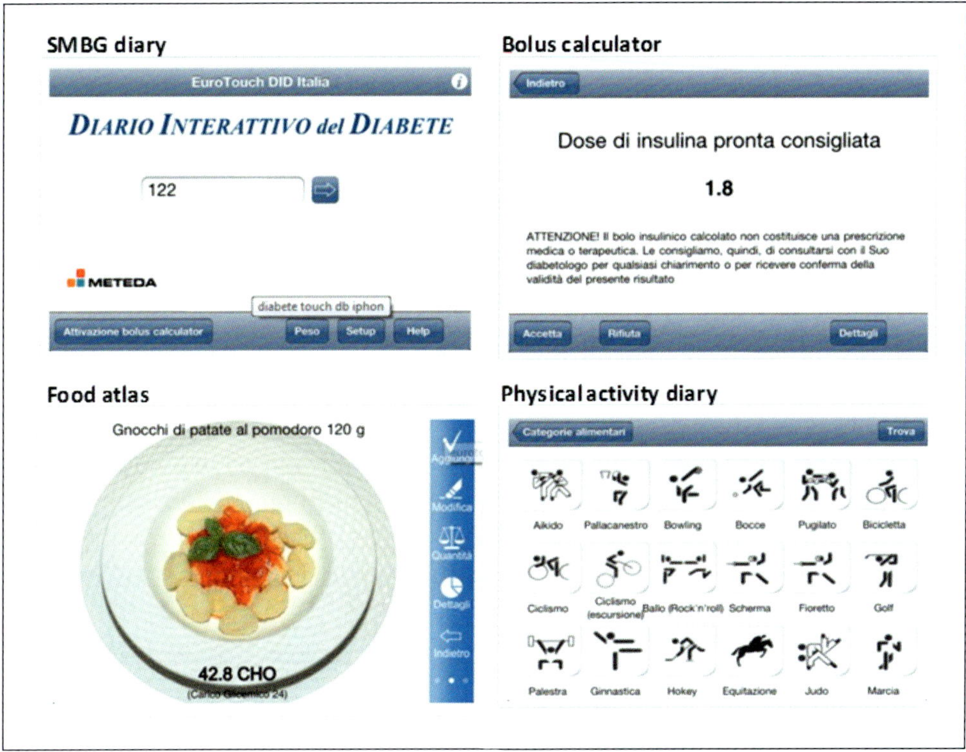

Fig. 2. Updated version of the DID system currently available as an i-Phone free application.

Conclusions

Among telemedicine systems for mobile phones available today, the DID offers the advantage of robust efficacy and safety according to a comprehensive research program including 3 main studies and subanalyses.

Our data show that the DID is a useful device that incorporates several features to help patients promote dietary freedom and flexible insulin bolus. The DID was demonstrated to be as effective as the standard educational approach based on carbohydrate counting in improving metabolic control while ensuring several additional benefits. First, it halved the time dedicated to education and simplified the calculation of carbohydrate content and insulin dose, which could allow more individuals with type 1 diabetes to adopt the flexible regimen. Second, the use of the DID was also associated with an 86% decrease of grade 2 hypoglycemia risk. This result is particularly valuable, considering the heavy impact of hypoglycemia on clinical outcomes, quality of life [24, 25], and costs of diabetes care [26].

Several quality of life scales were significantly improved with the DID, thus suggesting that the use of telemedicine can increase the level of acceptance of insulin treatment and help patients cope with the disease.

Currently, the DID software has been further optimized and is available as a free App for the smart phone (fig. 2).

Benefits on metabolic control and on the other clinical outcomes markedly varied among the different patients and centers. This implies that patient characteristics and healthcare professionals' attitudes and skills can strongly influence the outcomes of care supported by technology. This aspect will need attention in the policies regulating the execution and the reimbursement of technology-based education activities to maximize cost-effectiveness and avoid waste of resources.

In general, carbohydrate counting today represents the most advanced tool for the care of type 1 diabetes; its automation allows a larger utilization in the context of routine clinical practice. It is also important to underline that carbohydrate counting requires cultural and theoretical improvements to increase its efficacy; in fact, it should also take into consideration lipids and proteins intake, the impact of physical activity on blood glucose levels, the parallel titration of basal and prandial insulin, and the calculation of the content of glycemic load and not just of carbohydrates in the meals. A DID app running on a smartphone will help to manage the difficulties related to these potential advancements.

References

1 American Diabetes Association, Bantle JP, Wylie-Rosett J, Albright AL, Apovian CM, Clark NG, Franz MJ, Hoogwerf BJ, Lichtenstein AH, Mayer-Davis E, Mooradian AD, Wheeler ML: Nutrition recommendations and interventions for diabetes: a position statement of the American Diabetes Association. Diabetes Care 2008;31:S61–S78.

2 Franz MJ, Bantle JP, Beebe CA, Brunzell JD, Chiasson JL, Garg A, Holzmeister LA, Hoogwerf B, Mayer-Davis E, Mooradian AD, Purnell JQ, Wheeler M: Evidence-based nutrition principles and recommendations for the treatment and prevention of diabetes and related complications. Diabetes Care 2002;25:148–198.

3 Franz MJ, Monk A, Barry B, McClain K, Weaver T, Cooper N, Upham P, Bergenstal R, Mazze RS: Effectiveness of medical nutrition therapy provided by dietitians in the management of non-insulin-dependent diabetes mellitus: a randomized, controlled clinical trial. J Am Diet Assoc 1995;95:1009–1017.

4 Chiesa G, Piscopo MA, Rigamonti A, Azzinari A, Bettini S, Bonfanti R, Viscardi M, Meschi F, Chiumello G: Insulin therapy and carbohydrate counting. Acta Biomed 2005;76(Suppl 3):44–48.

5 Anderson EJ, Richardson M, Castle G, Cercone S, Delahanty L, Lyon R, Mueller D, Snetselaar L: Nutrition interventions for intensive therapy in the Diabetes Control and Complications Trial. The DCCT Research Group. J Am Diet Assoc 1993;93:768–772.

6 Rabasa-Lhoret R, Garon J, Langelier H, Poisson D, Chiasson JL: Effects of meal carbohydrate content on insulin requirements in type 1 diabetic patients treated intensively with the basal-bolus (ultralente-regular) insulin regimen. Diabetes Care 1999;22:667–673.

7 DAFNE Study Group: Training in flexible, intensive insulin management to enable dietary freedom in people with type 1 diabetes: Dose Adjustment for Normal Eating (DAFNE) randomised controlled trial. BMJ 2002;325:746–757.

8 Hitman GA: Mobile phone intervention for diabetes. Diabet Med 2011;28:381.

9 Liang X, Wang Q, Yang X, Cao J, Chen J, Mo X, Huang J, Wang L, Gu D: Effect of mobile phone intervention for diabetes on glycaemic control: a meta-analysis. Diabet Med 2011;28:455–463.

10 Farmer A, Gibson OJ, Tarassenko L, Neil A: A systematic review of telemedicine interventions to support blood glucose self-monitoring in diabetes. Diabet Med 2005;22:1372–1378.

11 Mair F, Whitten P: Systematic review of studies of patient satisfaction with telemedicine. BMJ 2000;320:1517–1520.

12 Rossi MC, Nicolucci A, Pellegrini F, Bruttomesso D, Bartolo PD, Marelli G, Dal Pos M, Galetta M, Horwitz D, Vespasiani G: Interactive Diary for Diabetes: a useful and easy-to-use new telemedicine system to support the decision-making process in type 1 diabetes. Diabetes Technol Ther 2009;11:19–24.

13 Rossi MC, Nicolucci A, Di Bartolo P, Bruttomesso D, Girelli A, Ampudia FJ, Kerr D, Ceriello A, De La Questa Mayor C, Pellegrini F, Horwitz D, Vespasiani G: Diabetes Interactive Diary: a new telemedicine system enabling flexible diet and insulin therapy while improving quality of life: an open-label, international, multicenter, randomized study. Diabetes Care 2010;33:109–115.
14 Rossi MC, Nicolucci A, Lucisano G, Pellegrini F, Di Bartolo P, Miselli V, Anichini R, Vespasiani G; DID Study Group: Impact of the 'Diabetes Interactive Diary' telemedicine system on metabolic control, risk of hypoglycemia, and quality of life: a randomized clinical trial in type 1 diabetes. Diabetes Technol Ther 2013;15:670–679.
15 Apolone G, Mosconi P: The Italian SF-36 Health Survey: translation, validation and norming. J Clin Epidemiol 1998;51:1025–1036.
16 Nicolucci A, Giorgino R, Cucinotta D, Zoppini G, Muggeo M, Squatrito S, Nicolucci A, Giorgino R, Cucinotta D, Zoppini G, Muggeo M, Squatrito S, Corsi A, Lostia S, Pappalardo L, Benaduce E, Girelli A, Galeone F, Maldonato A, Perriello G, Pata P, Marra G, Coronel GA: Validation of the Italian version of the WHO-Well-Being Questionnaire (WHO-WBQ) and the WHO-Diabetes Treatment Satisfaction Questionnaire (WHO-DTSQ). Diabetes Nutr Metab 2004;17:235–243.
17 Bradley C: Diabetes Treatment Satisfaction Questionnaire (DTSQ); in Bradley C (ed): Handbook of Psychology and Diabetes. Chur, Harwood, 1994, pp 111–132.
18 Service FJ, Molnar GD, Rosevear JW, Ackerman E, Gatewood LC, Taylor WF: Mean amplitude of glycaemic excursions, a measure of diabetic instability. Diabetes 1970;19:644–655.
19 Monnier L, Mas E, Ginet C, Michel F, Villon L, Cristol JP, Colette C: Activation of oxidative stress by acute glucose fluctuations compared with sustained chronic hyperglycemia in patients with type 2 diabetes. JAMA 2006;295:1681–1687.
20 Oyibo SO, Prasad YD, Jackson NJ, Jude EB, Boulton AJ: The relationship between blood glucose excursions and painful diabetic peripheral neuropathy: a pilot study. Diabet Med 2002;19:870–873.
21 Bott U, Muhlhauser I, Overmann H, Berger M: Validation of a diabetes-specific quality-of-life scale for patients with type 1 diabetes. Diabetes Care 1998;21: 757–769.
22 Rave K, Klein O, Frick AD, Becker RHA: Advantage of premeal-injected insulin glulisine compared with regular human insulin in subjects with type 1 diabetes. Diabetes Care 2006;29:1812–1817.
23 Overmann H, Heinemann L: Injection-meal interval: recommendations of diabetologists and how patients handle it. Diabetes Res Clin Pract 1999;43: 137–142.
24 Barnett AH, Cradock S, Fisher M, Hall G, Hughes E, Middleton A: Key considerations around the risks and consequences of hypoglycaemia in people with type 2 diabetes. Int J Clin Pract 2010;64:1121–1129.
25 Holt P: Taking hypoglycaemia seriously: diabetes, dementia and heart disease. Br J Community Nurs 2011;16:246–249.
26 Leese GP, Wang J, Broomhall J, Kelly P, Marsden A, Morrison W, Frier BM, Morris AD; DARTS/MEMO Collaboration: Frequency of severe hypoglycemia requiring emergency treatment in type 1 and type 2 diabetes. Diabetes Care 2003;26:1176–1180.

Dr. Giacomo Vespasiani
Diabetes Unit, Madonna del Soccorso Hospital
Via Silvio Pellico 68
IT–63039 San Benedetto del Tronto (Italy)
E-Mail giacvesp@tiscali.it

Bruttomesso D, Grassi G (eds): Technological Advances in the Treatment of Type 1 Diabetes.
Front Diabetes. Basel, Karger, 2015, vol 24, pp 236–249 (DOI: 10.1159/000363520)

Standardized Information Exchange in Diabetes: Integrated Registries for Governance, Research, and Clinical Practice

F. Carinci[a] · C.T. Di Iorio[a] · M. Massi Benedetti[b]

[a]Serectrix snc, Pescara, [b]Hub for International Health Research, Perugia, Italy

Abstract

To fight diabetes effectively, both local action and global engagement are needed. All of the potential stakeholders are necessary for collating complete data and using the information to improve policy and practice on a daily basis. A substantial contribution is required by those who deliver care regularly to people with diabetes, monitoring the status and progression of the disease with better knowledge of the problem and at a lower cost per contact. As an integral part of a long-term strategy, diabetes registers use information recorded at the point of care to improve quality of care through continuous monitoring of outcomes and prompt identification of subjects at increased risk of developing complications. Modern electronic diabetes registers substantially differ from simple electronic databases, as their role is at the core of a sophisticated network, where anything related to the condition of the individual can be measured with information on all the other levels of the healthcare system. In this chapter, we provide an overview of recent experiences in this field as well as challenges in the implementation of integrated registers, outlining roles and responsibilities of principal stakeholders and providing a snapshot of the best structure required to implement an integrated diabetes register. The chapter closes with a brief presentation of the relevant European legislation and the possible use of the recent achievements delivered by the European Union-funded public health projects BIRO and EUBIROD. The conclusions underpin the importance to follow up all recent experiences concluded positively, with consistent initiatives aimed at engaging governments, health professionals, and the whole community in the safe exchange of diabetes information, which is in everyone's interest.

A modern diabetes register represents the fundamental pillar of regional/national strategies against diabetes. Through the standardized use of electronic medical records and the adoption of evidence-based definitions, registries can feed a continuous quality improvement cycle for the conduction of first class research, efficient healthcare management, and quality-controlled routine care for people with diabetes.

However, developing modern electronic diabetes registers requires substantial organizational efforts and poses significant challenges, as they go well beyond the establishment of computerized databases in medical practice [1]. Their role is central to the automation of a sophisticated network, where all aspects relevant to improving the condition of the individual (structures, processes, and outcomes) are constantly monitored through the adoption of common standards and clear targets for the specific population (epidemiological denominator). Such an integrated framework requires linking information from different sources using clearly defined sets of criteria (metadata), e.g. clinical definitions that can quality-assure the content of databases to be exchanged. For instance, the year of diagnosis and type of diabetes can be set as mandatory for each subject included in a diabetes register.

Electronic registers can be used to rapidly obtain epidemiological measures that only a few years ago required complex and expensive studies. They can produce independent estimates of standardized rates for a range of indicators and may be used to explore the relationship between potential risk factors and different outcomes of interest, taking properly into account the particular clinical and socioeconomic characteristics of the population (case mix).

Over the last 10 years, diabetes registers have been increasingly used to provide robust and timely information on the epidemiology of diabetes and its complications; to monitor the disease across time, interventions, and changes of the environment; to evaluate the quality of care delivered to people with diabetes; to estimate the cost of the disease and the cost-effectiveness of the interventions; to provide a solid platform for diabetes shared care, and offer an essential tool for diabetes research. Typically, a broad range of users may benefit from the existence of integrated information frameworks in diabetes: national decision makers, healthcare policy makers, administrators, and deliverers; diabetes research institutions; people affected by diabetes, and the public. A well-designed register directly involves all members of the patient's health team, including physicians, nurses, other healthcare professionals, and office managers, and can be used in the process of care, as well as to assess quality of care and health services performance. The availability of timely information on high-risk subpopulations may allow the healthcare team to better target their care and evaluate adherence to treatment guidelines in relation to the actual trends observed in their routine activity.

Registers have been key components in numerous diabetes quality initiatives addressing data collection at the point of care and systematic information exchange across a network, most often organized at the regional level. In this chapter, we will examine the main features of recent success stories, highlighting challenges and presenting future perspectives towards the identification of international standards.

An Overview of Best Practices in Diabetes Registers

Diabetes information systems are typically built using a structure similar to that of a cohort study: at a certain date an event, e.g. a visit, examination or even onset, type 1 diabetes triggers the registration of a valid diagnosis. The subject's information is entered into a database in which all personal characteristics (e.g. age, sex), clinical measurements (e.g. blood pressure), processes (e.g. visits, prescriptions, etc.), and intermediate [e.g. glycated hemoglobin (HbA_{1c})] and terminal outcomes (e.g. renal failure, amputations, death) are regularly updated. The extent of coverage of the above registrations from the initial recording to exit from the database (for migration or death) determines the completeness of the diabetes information available for routine care or research, as well as the capacity of the system to produce unbiased indicators for public health monitoring.

Population-based diabetes registers take carefully into account the relationship between individual data and the total cohort registered in the database, estimating results that can be evaluated on a personal basis, rather than a service-oriented approach, for a specified catchment area.

As systems have evolved, it has become increasingly possible to integrate information from different sources through unique IDs shared across a network of centers, including hospitals, outpatient/specialist clinics, primary care, and the government. This way, the performance of healthcare for people with diabetes in a region/country can be measured more comprehensively, reporting results that avoid double counts and minimize selection bias in a systematic way. The advantage is evident if we also consider multimorbidity and the possibility of linking registers from different noncommunicable diseases.

The availability of powerful technology has made it increasingly possible to build population-based registers on top of service-oriented systems through further integration of electronic health records. Perhaps the greatest example of this kind is the SUPREME-DM project [2]. The study included a US network of 11 large health maintenance organizations gathering over 15 million members from their health plans between 2005 and 2009, of whom over 1 million (6.9%) met the criteria for diabetes set through a sophisticated algorithm including diagnoses, tests, and prescriptions. However, as recognized by the same authors, this approach is prone to severe limitations: (1) results may not generalize to patients managed in less integrated settings, in other geographic areas, or to uninsured populations; (2) cases identified could not be validated directly; (3) the type of diabetes could not be precisely identified, and (4) the date of diagnosis was missing in 60% of the diabetes cases.

Population-based diabetes registers aiming to overcome such limitations have been variously realized in the last years through the institutional and regulatory support of local governments.

The simplest (and faster) solution to integrate different information sources is through the linkage of secondary data. Such an approach offers significant cost advantages and can rely on already existing standardized definitions.

In Denmark, a national register covering the entire population of 5.4 million people between 1995 and 2006 was built through linkage of different national registers (Civil Registration System, National Patient Register, and the National Health Service Register) [3]. The register, relying on a reliable personal ID used across the country, allowed the computation of estimates of age- and sex-specific prevalence, incidence rates, mortality rates, and standardized mortality ratios relative to the nondiabetic part of the population. Results showed an increase in prevalence by 6% per year, stable incidence, and a decrease of mortality by 4% per year among subjects with diabetes compared to 2% per year of the residual portion of the population. The mortality rate decreased 40% during the first 3 years after diabetes diagnosis. However, this platform does not integrate clinical data, and indeed is not capable of discriminating between different types of diabetes.

Efforts to integrate clinical and administrative information on a routine basis exist and are more likely to be realized in systems providing universal coverage with a systematic involvement of different levels of healthcare. However, the degree of integration required among service providers and the government is high, and the approach is more feasible in smaller geographical areas or very organized regions.

In New Zealand, the Otago Diabetes Register was established in 1998, as part of the Otago Diabetes Project, to monitor and evaluate diabetes care in the Otago region [4]. Demographic and clinical data, including vital status, type of diabetes and year of diagnosis, diabetes complications, diabetes medication, clinical examination, and biochemistry test results were collected annually from general practice medical records. The register allowed the timely report of the evolution of the disease in the area, and showed how diabetes information was lacking in the official death statistics. Moreover, an evaluation run over 6 years of the program showed a dramatic improvement of processes, and these results are significantly different from those obtained for subjects not enrolled in a centralized register [4].

Perhaps the most genuine experience of a complete population-based register was developed in 1996 in Tayside, Scotland [5], and has been continuously operational since its startup. This initiative, deeply integrated with the local government, supports the provision of clinical practice, research, and governance through performance reporting. The register started as a research project, the Diabetes Audit and Research in Tayside Study (DARTS) [6]. The project progressively grew from the original local catchment area involving the Tayside Regional Diabetes Network (TRDN) to the Scottish Care Information Diabetes Collaboration (SCI-DC), which constitutes the infrastructure of what is today the Scottish Diabetes Register. In the register, information is split between the research reports (analysis) and the clinical services (enhanced information systems).

The register showed similar results to those obtained in Denmark (prevalence in 1996: 1.94% compared with 1.89% in Denmark) with a similar increase (6.7% per year compared with 6.3% per year for men and 6.6% per year for women in Denmark) and decrease in mortality rates [7].

The Tayside register, which is connected to the MEMO database and controls for age, sex, duration of diabetes, blood pressure, cholesterol, HbA_{1c}, smoking, previous hospital admission, and treatment with cardiovascular medication, also investigated the efficacy of pharmaceutical treatment and found that those treated with sulfonylureas only, or combinations of sulfonylureas and metformin, were at higher risk of adverse cardiovascular outcomes than those treated with metformin alone (RR = 1.43; 1.15–1.77 and RR = 1.70; 1.18–2.45, respectively), and at increased risks of cardiovascular hospital admission, mortality, and cardiovascular mortality [8].

The register also explored many other fundamental target endpoints in diabetes, such as hypoglycemia, chronic diabetes complications, and pharmaceutical costs. It allowed the construction of the first validated, population-derived model for prediction of absolute risk of coronary heart disease in people with type 2 diabetes [9]. These algorithms provide decision support tools for clinicians involved in diabetes treatment and indicate appropriate early action to decrease the risk of adverse outcomes.

Data quality of official statistics may also be increased from integrated information, as the Tayside register found similar results to those obtained in Otago [10]: in the Tayside region, diabetes was mentioned on the death certificates of 42.8% and was the underlying cause of death for 6.4%. Male gender was associated with less frequent mention of diabetes, with more frequent mention associated with increasing duration of diabetes, increasing age, and underlying cardiovascular cause of death.

The experience of Tayside shows that information exchanged over a region will never be 100% accurate, but systems may be improved significantly through their routine use and analysis. The Scottish register was born from the bottom up, through the direct participation of clinicians and people with diabetes. The national database is currently updated overnight through a network of operating regional servers, allowing clinicians to benchmark their quality of care on a daily basis and almost in real time.

In a system like the one constructed in Tayside, it is possible for a clinician to instantly access measurements for a person with diabetes across different providers and compare the same parameter across the average scored for the reference population. These results can be returned to the individual, closing the loop of quality of care improvement and person empowerment.

Over the years, strategies encouraging 'clean' clinical recording entry minimized 'dirty' data contamination in the Tayside register. In this case, the evolving nature of the process has been intrinsic to the collaborative integration of different sources, for which 'the job of creating adequate databases will never be finished, but striving to create adequate clinical datasets will always be worth doing' [11].

Complete population-based registers are difficult to implement, but structured information exchange and mandatory reporting may prompt targeted policies of strategic importance. In the USA, the New York Department of Health and Mental Hygiene established in 2006 the first population-based HbA_{1c} registry, the New York City A_{1c} Registry (NYCAR) through a new law that mandated all clinical laboratories in New York City report HbA_{1c} results to the government [12].

Attempts to build national registers may fail to cover the entire population but still be valid to provide estimates of adherence to clinical guidelines and quality of care in real-life conditions.

In Sweden, the Swedish National Diabetes Register was initiated in 1996 by the Swedish Society for Diabetology in response to the demands of the St. Vincent Declaration for Quality Assurance in Diabetes Care. Data represent people with diabetes from 75% of 80 hospital outpatient clinics and 15% of nearly 900 primary healthcare centers collected from all parts of Sweden. The register demonstrated decreasing mean HbA_{1c} and blood pressure levels and the wider use of lipid-lowering drugs in the latter half of the 1990s. Another report showed that the national goals for HbA_{1c} and blood pressure for more than 75,000 people with diabetes were reached with increasing percentages during the period 1996–2003, being achieved by 33 and 71%, respectively, in medical departments, and by 61 and 48% in primary healthcare in 2003. More recently, the register produced risk equations for cardiovascular disease [13], and a stream of reports investigating the level of association between target risk factors and key endpoints in diabetes.

In many cases, diabetes registers are created periodically to deliver public health and systems performance reports. These approaches are mainly based on well structured, standardized administrative data linked to a reliable, validated personal ID that can be repeatedly used over multiple databases.

The province of Alberta, Canada, runs the Alberta Diabetes Surveillance System, which produces an annual report of facts and figures using a system that is similar to the Danish register in terms of demographic capabilities. From 1995 to 2009, the system found an increase in the age-adjusted prevalence rate of 67% among men and 53% in women [14]. All patterns of utilization and health outcomes for people with diabetes are duly reported using structured sources. The same approach is also applied in Manitoba (Canada), where the University of Manitoba is in charge of population-based information systems using very large linked administrative databases. In this case, an important element of health systems analysis is based on data linkage and the application of optimized algorithms that can capture people with diabetes with an adequate balance between sensitivity and specificity [15].

Diabetes registers naturally emerge as the backbone of disease management programs where clinical professionals share an interface either as part of a health plan contract or on a voluntary basis. These types of registers, typical of insurance-based competitive healthcare systems, are only partially population-based, as the denominators are biased by the composition of the served cohort.

The SUPREME-DM project previously described builds upon the experience of Kaiser Permanente (a fully integrated, nonprofit, group practice, prepaid health plan that provides comprehensive medical services to at least 3 million members). Its diabetes register was established in 1993 in California to monitor quality of care and health outcomes for plan members with diabetes [16]. Approximately 30% of the population in the catchment area are Kaiser members. The register has grown from approximately 65,000 to over 200,000 active health plan members with diabetes in 2006. New cases of diabetes are identified annually using a passive surveillance of pharmacy (prescriptions for diabetes medications), laboratory (HbA_{1c} >7.0%), outpatient, emergency room, and hospitalization records listing a diagnosis of diabetes. The register has been validated to be 99% sensitive for detecting members with diabetes. It is purely used for research purposes, and there is no physician accessibility to it for purposes of impacting care.

Various approaches have been attempted to establish links across clinical centers and administrative data, where a structural program for information exchange has not been institutionally supported by governmental programs.

In Umbria, Italy, a regional diabetes register has been based on a 'progressive' approach [17], with diabetes indicators produced in a comprehensive evaluation of regional health services [18].

In many other situations, diabetes registries are developed on top of healthcare databases located in specific settings, e.g. outpatient clinics, specialist services, or primary care centers. In all such instances, databases are built on top of records collected during patient visits. The results that can be obtained without centralized control and structured information exchange (particularly outcomes) may be biased by denominators that are not representatives of the overall population of subjects with diabetes. For example, it would be difficult to estimate indicators, for example the proportion of patients with at least an annual check, given that a significant portion of subjects with diabetes would not be included in the medical database for the reference year.

Challenges of Information Exchange in Diabetes

Cultural and technological barriers pose significant challenges for the realization of structured information exchange in healthcare systems. The scale of the diabetes epidemic, with its burden for the population and implications on the organization of different health services, represent one of the most problematic areas where comprehensive solutions could be organized.

Today, a primary element that cannot be overlooked in the construction of diabetes information platforms is that of individual privacy and data protection. The increasing complexity of the legislation in this field has in fact generated a heterogeneous implementation of fundamental principles, producing in practical situations an imbalance between the right to privacy/data protection and the right to health [19]. A revision of procedures in place in diabetes registers from 18 practices carried out by the EUBIROD project found high heterogeneity in the application of criteria related to anonymization, consent, accuracy, and access to computerized information. Such lack of uniform approaches may generate concern for appropriate safeguard of information in healthcare, which in turn can translate into potential new impediments to information exchange from the revision of relevant legislation.

While it is fundamental that information systems conform to current privacy legislation to ensure their integrity and safe continuation, it is also important that their value for public health and routine care is increasingly recognized, to avoid excessive restrictions being imposed on information exchange and make sure that consent does not become a problematic issue, influenced by mounting concern about threats to personal privacy.

From a scientific perspective, using a computerized integrated register offers new opportunities for research studies based on gold-standard methodology. Sampling plans may be facilitated by the availability of a large or even complete pool of subjects, from which groups of individuals may be enrolled in cohort/observational studies, case-control, or randomized controlled trials.

On the other hand, an evidence-based comparison of the effectiveness of diabetes information systems is hampered by the specificity of their implementation, as it would be difficult to isolate the local conditions from a systematic effect of a particular solution. In fact, it would be impossible to 'randomize' aspects related to the structural organization of health systems, each with a unique culture and specific policies that are associated with the average outcomes. Nonetheless, it would still be possible, although uncommon, to compare different alternatives within similar settings, e.g. routine care against audit and feedback, computerized reminders, mobile healthcare, aid tools for self-care, etc.

Practical challenges emerge from the analysis of specific operational contexts. The task of building a structured platform for information exchange represents a naturally evolving process, which must be tailored to the environment where the system is activated.

Population-based registers, albeit methodologically attractive, may not represent the easiest solution to be implemented at the outset. Computerized data linkage of administrative databases using a unique subject identifier, as well as targeted programs of diabetes monitoring across multiple service units, or a mix of these approaches, may represent convenient alternatives under most practical conditions. By all means, well-planned information infrastructure should be based on the adoption of standardized definitions and is key to avoid catastrophic investments on inadequate frameworks. In this context, the increasing restraints on data protection shall be adequately taken into account.

The brief review of international experiences clearly shows that the creation of national infrastructure for diabetes information is by far the most ambitious endeavor. Even the most advanced health systems struggle to implement large-scale data warehouses, and not only for technological reasons. A more successful strategy would recommend building upon sophisticated systems implemented in regional areas and to extend the approach of direct interaction between all relevant stakeholders (policy makers, health professionals, researchers, and citizens) in a federated fashion. General recommendations should be taken into account in all the above situations.

A diabetes register must be flexible enough to accommodate the evolution of needs, knowledge, and technologies according to the available resources (economical, cultural, and structural). A modern design implies the adoption of a dynamic structure that can embed different sources of information in harmony with the cultural evolution of its own users. Contributors and stakeholders gradually improve their ability to pose sophisticated questions to a system where the overall level of participation is of crucial importance.

An analysis of user perspectives should represent a fundamental element in planning any kind of diabetes register, as in any part of the world the design and evolution of these instruments is heavily influenced by different dimensions of the local culture. At the level of the health system, it is paramount to verify how diabetes care is delivered, and the impact of using modern technology in everyday practice.

Factors outside the healthcare system may considerably interfere with the actual implementation and regular automation of a registry. Interoperability of systems, common semantics, communication technology and software engineering, database implementation (with particular attention to the standardization of classification systems), and, most importantly, the local attitudes towards privacy and security legislation constitute essential elements that must be cautiously evaluated at the outset.

Architecture of an Integrated Diabetes Register

Building an integrated register involves different roles and responsibilities, and multiple actors that would be called to interact continuously with a common system to accomplish different tasks.

An analysis of specific requirements ensuring that short-, medium-, and long-term goals are realized must be performed a priori, taking well into account the vision, mission, and goals of the register. Such requirements are fundamental to define an implementation plan in which all stakeholders participate with a double role of contributor/user, making the information infrastructure sustainable and open to quality improvement.

A taxonomy of roles, responsibilities, and requirements in the use of diabetes information is presented in table 1. All stakeholders involved in a diabetes register are duly represented: citizens, health professionals, healthcare organizations, policy makers, a national/regional ministry of health, academics/scientists, a coordinating center (internal or external to the ministry), and international partners. The architecture of the register derives directly from the efficient organization of all procedures involved in implementing such requirements.

Figure 1 shows a possible structure of an integrated diabetes registry, reflecting the roles and responsibilities of all the above categories of users. A system for structured information exchange should consider data provision from primary care centers, specialist services/outpatient clinics, and acute inpatient care. To be complete, the system should link records contributed by those sources on a daily basis to other archives managed by public entities, whose content is highly sensitive for personal privacy, including

Table 1. Roles, responsibilities, and requirements in diabetes information

Role	General responsibility	Requirements in diabetes information
Citizen	to safeguard personal health and act in ways that protect and promote public health	to contribute to the continuous improvement of diabetes information through the direct provision of accurate clinical information in electronic format; to receive regular reports on quality of care and outcomes in diabetes through an approach that facilitates participation, monitoring of diabetes at the individual and population level, and prevention of diabetes complications
Health professional	to provide the best achievable quality of care to individual citizens	to carefully record and regularly transmit medical records related to people with diabetes to the ministry of health; to access all information related to single individuals affected by diabetes for the optimal provision of health services; to receive regular monthly feedback from the ministry of health in terms of individual reports and group averages
Healthcare organization	to provide the best achievable quality of care to the reference population	to receive feedback from the ministry of health through performance reports and various tools made available for benchmarking, allowing the comparison of quality of care and outcomes delivered by healthcare organizations across the country
Policy maker	to make the best decisions using evidence-based results to continuously improve population health	to receive periodic performance reports on diabetes care and prevention, including evidence-based recommendations and high priority action points to optimize quality of care and outcomes in diabetes, taking into account monitoring of the costs of interventions
Ministry of health	to ensure proper governance to the health system, to coordinate all roles and to optimize access and use of the register	to receive stable political/financial support of the government for the establishment, management, and development of a national information infrastructure for diabetes; to receive expert advice and constant support from the all relevant innovation partners to establish and progressively develop the electronic diabetes register; to establish, maintain, and develop the central register through the activity of a dedicated data linkage unit; to build and maintain an information framework ensuring the highest levels of security and privacy protection; to run complex statistical analyses of diabetes information to provide data to a range of trusted parties, and the regular publication of results; to link all relevant electronic data sources in the country using automated means for the establishment and sustainable maintenance of the central register; to exploit all international collaborations aimed at enhancing the capacity of the register
Academic scientist	to produce new ideas and test new hypotheses, using data to produce new evidence and foster knowledge in diabetes	to access diabetes information that provides substantial input to targeted research studies and investigations in the field of public health
Coordinating center	to act as the leader of research and innovation in diabetes, and as a major hub of scientific development at the international level	to act as the official coordinating center of the register through the formal recognition of the government; to act as the main technological partner in the provision of technology and training in the field of diabetes information; to access an anonymous subset of the diabetes register on a regular basis to run complex customized analysis; to establish and maintain a diabetes research register as an integral part of the diabetes register; to run a wide range of queries and statistical analyses on the register in semiautomated ways that would not require individual consent and/or written approval from the ministry of health; to exchange aggregated information on diabetes with accredited international partners
International partner	to involve the coordinating center in major research initiatives and international public health projects in the field of diabetes	to access and exchange aggregated data for international cooperation and scientific research

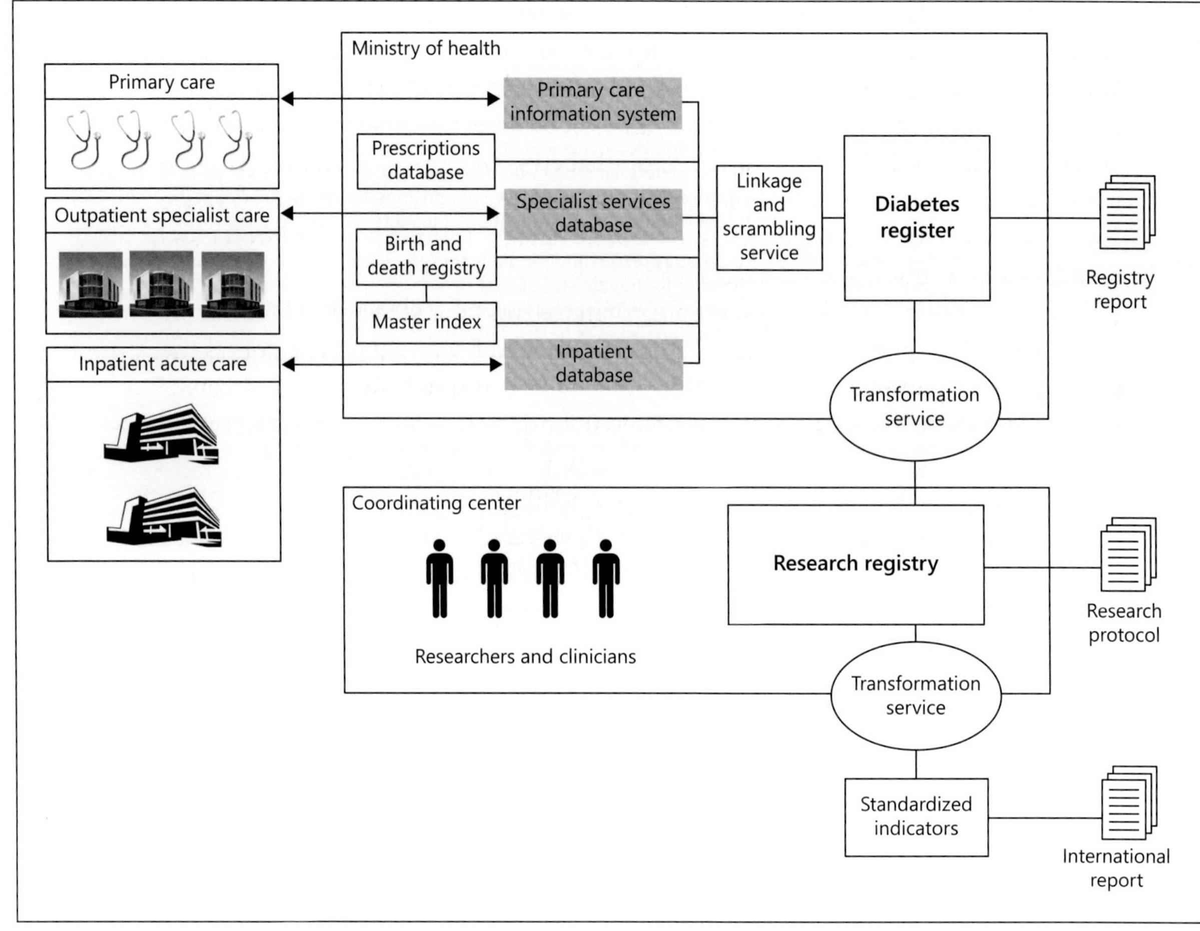

Fig. 1. Structure of an integrated diabetes register.

information on a broad range of personal aspects (residency, socioeconomic status, etc.). A coordinating center may be useful to support the transformation of individual records into a structured dataset that can be used for research and performance reporting. The dataset can be properly anonymized and made available to trusted parties as a research registry, open to collaboration in relevant international activities such as a global diabetes monitoring network. Linkage and transformation services may be established to respect principles of personal privacy and data protection.

International Developments and Future Perspectives

Over the last years, international legislation has become increasingly sensitive to the right of people with diabetes to obtain reliable information on the quality of care they receive against the best available practices, particularly in Europe.

Following the United Nations (UN) Resolution on Diabetes 61/225, the European Union (EU) passed its own Resolution on Diabetes (March 14, 2012), specifying the key action points immediately required to revert the spread of the epidemic. In particular, the Resolution 'calls on the Commission to draw up common, standardised criteria and methods for data collection on diabetes, and, in collaboration with the Member States, to coordinate, collect, register, monitor and manage comprehensive epidemiological data on diabetes, and economic data on the direct and indirect costs of diabetes prevention and management.'

The need consistently follows a number of initiatives funded by the EU during the last 15 years. Two projects, EUDIP and EUCID, defined EU diabetes indicators in the early 2000s. A subsequent project, Best Information through Regional Outcomes (BIRO), 2005–2009, worked out a solution to publish international reports automatically and on a regular basis [20].

The basic principle of the BIRO system is that diabetes information already existing in a fairly standardized form could be rapidly integrated using open standards and privacy-enhanced exchange of aggregate data. In 2009, the project delivered a prototype that allowed collecting 79 indicators from a network of diabetes registers and publishing an international diabetes report in almost real time.

The sequel project, European Best Information through Regional Outcomes in Diabetes (EUBIROD), aimed 'at establishing a European Diabetes Register through the extension of the BIRO network and the use of related technology' [21]. Completed in March 2012, the system delivered fully versatile BIRO software that has been used to successfully collect data and deliver an international diabetes report from 19 countries. The advantages of this approach under different conditions, such as linking data from developed and developing countries, are entirely evident. On the other hand, open source software can be available at no cost, but requires proper training. For this reason, dissemination activities, for example the BIRO Academy, are needed to support a cohesive program.

Other innovative features of EUBIROD also deserve to be highlighted for their general value. A diabetes information system needs to be fully independent, as it must ensure proper use of public funding and publication of health information beyond any conflict of interests and any possible doubt on the credibility of information. Furthermore, information must be rock solid from the point of view of respect for privacy. EUBIROD implemented the fundamental principle of 'privacy by design', an essential element in the secondary use of health data, as highlighted by the recent activities of the EC, and more recently, the OECD [22].

For large-scale data collection, a distributed database is much more efficient than centralized storage of individual data, as it avoids storing/processing huge amounts of data in one place, and by doing so preserves the original data ownership, which in turn guarantees data quality. In EUBIROD, the same clinician involved in the data collection can directly control and correct the data elements at the basis of diabetes indicators. Sound statistical procedures including risk-adjustment methods shall always be applied to help tackle selection bias and deliver standardized comparisons. A common report template should take into account multiple dimensions, including structures, processes, and outcomes. The future legislative trends in the area of integrated diabetes registries make implementations, e.g. EUBIROD, even more urgent.

The EU Directive on the application of patients' rights in cross-border healthcare [23] promotes collaboration between Member States and exchange of information to enable continuity of care and patient safety across borders. According to the Directive, by 2014 a person with diabetes should be able to: (1) access information on the average quality of care provided by accredited centers in Europe, (2) bring personal data to a provider located in a different country and be able to add own data to the local register, and (3) extract personal data from the local registry and be able to transfer its content back to the country of origin. On the other hand, care providers should also be able to reciprocally exchange personal data according to the needs of the patient. These goals can only be achieved by standardization of methods and tools used in different countries. The availability of common guidelines, methodology, and standards to harmonize national registries is the main theme of the EU-funded joint action Cross-Border Patient Registries Initiative (PARENT) started in 2012, of which EUBIROD is an associated project.

Conclusions

Making best use of diabetes information requires concerted efforts at all levels. Approaches proposed by recent initiatives define new avenues to converge towards common definitions and interoperable platforms. However, there is still significant work required to transform the proposed prototypes into stable solutions that can be used on a routine basis.

By all means, structured information exchange can be very useful to improve outcomes, but alone has a limited impact: concrete interventions must be implemented to improve care. For this reason, national diabetes plans have been launched: they can be used as a springboard for further uptake of new information technologies in diabetes.

References

1 Carinci F, Orsini Federici M, Massi Benedetti M: Diabetes registers and prevention strategies: towards an active use of health information. Diab Res Clin Pract 2006;74:S215–S219.

2 Nichols GA, Desai J, Elston Lafata J, Lawrence JM, O'Connor PJ, Pathak RD, Raebel MA, Reid RJ, Selby JV, Silverman BG, Steiner JF, Stewart WF, Vupputuri S, Waitzfelder B; SUPREME-DM Study Group: Construction of a multisite DataLink using electronic health records for the identification, surveillance, prevention, and management of diabetes mellitus: the SUPREME-DM project. Prev Chronic Dis 2012; 9:E110.

3 Carstensen B, Kristensen JK, Marcussen MM, Borch-Johnsen K: The National Diabetes Register. Scand J Public Health 2011;39(Suppl 7):58–61.

4 Coppell KJ, Anderson K, Williams SM, Lamb C, Farmer VL, Mann JI: The quality of diabetes care: a comparison between patients enrolled and not enrolled on a regional diabetes register. Prim Care Diabetes 2011;5:131–137.

5 Morris AD, Boyle DI, MacAlpine R, Emslie-Smith A, Jung RT, Newton RW, MacDonald TM: The Diabetes Audit and Research in Tayside Scotland (DARTS) study: electronic record linkage to create a diabetes register. BMJ 1997;315:524–528.

6 Boyle D, Cunningham S, Sullivan F, Morris A; Tayside Regional Diabetes Network: Technology integration for the provision of population-based equitable patient care: the Tayside Regional Diabetes Network – a brief description. Diabetes Nutr Metab 2001;14:100–103.

7 Evans JM, Barnett KN, Ogston SA, Morris AD: Increasing prevalence of type 2 diabetes in a Scottish population: effect of increasing incidence or decreasing mortality? Diabetologia 2007;50:729–732.

8 Evans JM, Ogston SA, Emslie-Smith A, Morris AD: Risk of mortality and adverse cardiovascular outcomes in type 2 diabetes: a comparison of patients treated with sulfonylureas and metformin. Diabetologia 2006;49:930–936.

9 Donnan PT, Donnelly L, New JP, Morris AD: Derivation and validation of a prediction score for major coronary heart disease events in a UK type 2 diabetic population. Diabetes Care 2006;29:1231–1236.

10 Evans JM, Barnett KN, McMurdo ME, Morris AD: Reporting of diabetes on death certificates of 1872 people with type 2 diabetes in Tayside, Scotland. Eur J Public Health 2008;18:201–203.

11 McAlpine R: Communication to the 1st EUBIROD annual meeting. Kuwait City, May 3, 2009. http://www.eubirod.eu/academy/first_course/lectures/Tayside_mcalpine.html (accessed May 24, 2013).

12 Chamany S, Silver LD, Bassett MT, Driver CR, Berger DK, Neuhaus CE, Kumar N, Frieden TR: Tracking diabetes: New York City's A_{1C} Registry. Milbank Q 2009;87:547–570.

13 Zethelius B, Eliasson B, Eeg-Olofsson K, Svensson AM, Gudbjörnsdottir S, Cederholm J; NDR: A new model for 5-year risk of cardiovascular disease in type 2 diabetes: a report from the Swedish National Diabetes Register (NDR). Diabetes Res Clin Pract 2011;93:276–284.

14 Canada Institute of Health Economics, Alberta. Alberta Diabetes Atlas. 2007. http://www.albertadiabetes.ca/AlbertaDiabetesAtlas2011.php (accessed May 24, 2013).

15 Lix L, Yogendran M, Burchill C, Metge C, McKeen N, Moore D, Bond R: Defining and Validating Chronic Diseases: An Administrative Data Approach. Winnipeg, Manitoba Centre for Health Policy, 2006. http://mchp-appserv.cpe.umanitoba.ca/reference/chronic.disease.pdf (accessed May 24, 2013).

16 Selby JV, Karter AJ, Ackerson LM, Ferrara A, Liu J: Developing a prediction rule from automated clinical databases to identify high-risk patients in a large population with diabetes. Diabetes Care 2001;24:1547–1555.

17 Massi Benedetti M, Carinci F, Orsini Federici M: The Umbria Diabetes Register. Diab Res Clin Pract 2006;74:S200–S204.

18 Documento di Valutazione del Sistema Sanitario regionale (DVSS). http://www.sanita.regione.umbria.it/resources/Risorse/Volume_D_Book.pdf (accessed May 24, 2013).

19 Di Iorio CT, Carinci F: Data protection and health care information systems: where is the balance?; in Carlisle G, Whitehouse D, Penny D (eds): eHealth: Legal, Ethical and Governance Challenges. Berlin, Springer, 2012.

20 Di Iorio CT, Carinci F, Azzopardi J, Baglioni V, Beck P, Cunningham S, Evripidou A, Leese G, Loevaas KF, Olympios G, Orsini Federici M, Pruna S, Palladino P, Skeie S, Taverner P, Traynor V, Massi Benedetti M: Privacy impact assessment in the design of transnational public health information systems: the BIRO project. J Med Ethics 2009;35:753–761.

21 Di Iorio CT, Carinci F, Brillante M, Azzopardi J, Beck P, Bratina N, Cunningham SG, De Beaufort C, Debacker N, Jarosz-Chobot P, Jecht M, Lindblad U, Moulton T, Metelko Ž, Nagy A, Olympios G, Pruna S, Røder M, Skeie S, Storms F, Massi Benedetti M: Cross-border flow of health information: is 'privacy by design' enough? Privacy performance assessment in EUBIROD. Eur J Public Health 2013;23:247–253.

22 Strengthening Health Information Infrastructure for Health Care Quality Governance: Good Practices, New Opportunities and Data Privacy Protection Challenges. Paris, OECD, 2013. http://www.oecd.org/els/health-systems/strengtheninghealthinformationinfrastructure.htm (accessed May 24, 2013).

23 Directive 2011/24/EU of the European Parliament and of the Council of 9 March 2011 on the application of patients' rights in cross-border healthcare. http://eur-lex.europa.eu/LexUriServ/LexUriServ.do?uri=OJ:L:2011:088:0045:0065:EN:PDF (accessed May 24, 2013).

Dr. Fabrizio Carinci, Senior Biostatistician
Serectrix snc
Via Gran Sasso 79
IT–65121 Pescara (Italy)
E-Mail f.carinci@serectrix.eu

Bruttomesso D, Grassi G (eds): Technological Advances in the Treatment of Type 1 Diabetes.
Front Diabetes. Basel, Karger, 2015, vol 24, pp 250–258 (DOI: 10.1159/000363521)

Type 1 Diabetes Care: It's Not All Technology

Gérard Reach

Department of Endocrinology, Diabetes and Metabolic Diseases, Avicenne Hospital APHP, and EA 3412, CRNH-IdF, University of Paris 13, Bobigny, France

Abstract

Type 1 diabetes has always been the realm of tools aimed to replace the missing function: glucose-induced insulin release. During the past decades these tools have been made smaller, more efficient, and more user-friendly, and we are close to the full achievement of a real closed-loop insulin delivery system (artificial pancreas). The aim of this chapter, however, is to suggest that diabetes care should not be reduced to only technology since biopsychosocial factors are also important for diabetes care.

'Please sit down. How are you?'
'On average, as a mean, I can tell you, Doc, that I'm fine.'
' "As a mean", what do you mean?'
'My glycated is 6.2% [laugh].'
A visit of a patient of mine

The Early Years of Diabetes Care

Type 1 diabetes therapy started in the early 1920s, when Banting and Best discovered insulin [1]. Since then, progress has been made to make insulin administration more comfortable: glass syringes were replaced by plastic disposable syringes [2], insulin pens were invented in the mid-1980s [3], and intravenous insulin delivery [4] paved

This text was presented as the keynote lecture opening the 6th International Conference on Advanced Technologies and Treatments in Diabetes (ATTD), held in Paris, February 27, 2013.

the way for subcutaneous continuous insulin infusion (CSII) [5]. In the 1970s, insulins were purified better [6], while at the beginning of the 1980s human insulins became available [7, 8], followed by the development of ultrarapid [9–11] and slow insulin analogues [12, 13].

These advances were accompanied by two developments, conceptual and technological. First, two major publications, by Pirart [14] and Tchobroutsky [15], pointed out the role of chronic hyperglycemia in the development of long-term diabetes complications. Second, daily self-monitoring of blood glucose (SMBG) was made possible by the invention of fingerprick systems [16] and the relationship between 3-month glycemic control and the percentage of glycated hemoglobin (HbA_{1c}) was discovered [17]. These conceptual and technological advances led to 2 major randomized controlled trials in diabetes care: DCCT for type 1 [18], and UKPDS [19] for type 2 diabetes.

Technological Recent Achievements towards a Closed-Loop Insulin Delivery System

Nowadays, a significant percentage of patients, varying from country to country, are treated with CSII [20], and a recent meta-analysis demonstrated the superiority of CSII versus multiple injections to achieve better glycated hemoglobin (HbA_{1c}) control with a reduction in the rate of severe hypoglycemia [21]. Continuous research efforts from the invention by Clark of the oxygen electrode [22] to the development of glucose sensors [23] have led to the development of several systems able to monitor continuously glucose concentration in subcutaneous tissue, with 3 systems commercially available [24–26]. First used as Holter systems [27], they are now able to measure glucose levels in real time, and a number of studies have shown that appropriate use of continuous glucose monitoring (CGM) is associated with an improvement in HbA_{1c} [28–30]. These systems can be coupled to a pump, and the advantage of sensor-augmented pump therapy on HbA_{1c} control has also been demonstrated [31, 32]. Noninvasive measurement of glucose, which for a long time led to nothing but wrong announcements [33], is currently the object of serious investigations [34]. However, the most exciting news concern the development of a real closed-loop insulin delivery system (artificial endocrine pancreas), which is no longer a utopian dream [35].

The aim of this chapter, while recognizing that technology has been of paramount importance to improve the efficacy of diabetes care and the quality of life of patients, is to show that it is necessary to adopt a broader view in the framework of a biopsychosocial model of diseases advocated 30 years ago by George Engel [36]. For this purpose I will critically analyze whether technology indeed improved different diabetes burdens, such as treatment discomfort, diabetes complications, rate of severe hypoglycemia, fear of hypoglycemia, and quality of life.

Technology and Diabetes Discomfort

Technology has provided real benefits to patients, such as the advancements made in needle and fingerprick technology and as a result of modern glucometers becoming smaller, faster, and needing less blood (0.3 µl!). Concerning this last point, this is not a trivial issue: a study showed an inverse relationship between a 'measure of invasiveness' as a reason for skipping SMBG (MISS score) and adherence to SMBG recommendations ($r = -0.47$; $p < 0.01$). The MISS questionnaire used questions such as 'How often do you skip checking your blood sugar level because of frustration with not getting enough blood on the strip, having to "milk" the fingertip for blood, having to prick several times to get enough blood?', and so forth [37]. On the other hand, technology success may be limited by discomfort: among the reasons cited by patients for stopping CGM are tape/adhesive issues, the sensor being too bulky, and alarms that are too loud or are triggered too often [38].

Technology and Advancements in the Prevention of Complications

Clearly, complications may severely hinder patient quality of life, but luckily there has been a major decrease in the incidence rate of complications in type 1 diabetes over the last decades [39]. However, this may not be due to technological progresses, but rather to a better definition of the strategy which was established in the late 1970s [14, 15]. This decrease in the rate of complications may also be the consequence of patient education starting in the same period [40, 41]: patient education is a powerful tool to improve HbA_{1c} and to decrease the rate of hospitalization and severe hypoglycemia in patients with type 1 diabetes [42].

Technology and the Prevention of Severe Hypoglycemia

Severe hypoglycemia is the most feared complication of insulin therapy [43], and indeed, fear of hypoglycemia can prevent patients from intensifying insulin therapy [44] and increasing insulin doses when needed [45]. The DCCT trial showed that attempts at improving HbA_{1c} control may be linked to an increase in the rate of severe hypoglycemia [18], and it is a major aim of patient education to succeed in improving HbA_{1c} and in *reducing* the rate of hypoglycemia. Certainly, the use of technology in the form of continuous insulin infusion and of patient education may help to reach this goal [21].

The effect of using CGM on the risk of severe hypoglycemia is more controversial. There is no doubt that CGM use is associated with a decrease in the time spent in hypoglycemia, for instance below 65 mg/dl [46]. However, there is no evidence that it has an impact on the rate of severe hypoglycemia: there was no effect specifically in the JDFI trial [28] or in a recent meta-analysis [47]. However, one may argue that patients with a history of severe hypoglycemia are often excluded from these studies, thus making the number of events smaller and giving the studies low power to show such an effect. In one study, however, severe hypoglycemic events occurred even more frequently in the pump arm than in the control group (11 vs. 3 episodes, $p = 0.04$) [48]. This shows that patient selection and education is important before introducing CGM in the treatment of a diabetic patient.

The fear of hypoglycemia is an important issue. Indeed, in a recent study in 4- to 9-year-old children, CGM use was not associated with an improvement in HbA_{1c} [49]. The authors attributed this result in part to the fact that parental fear of hypoglycemia was not reduced. Concerning the impact of CGM use on the fear of hypoglycemia, one study showed that it is associated with a decrease in the fear of hypoglycemia and in the fear of needing help to treat severe hypoglycemia [38]; however, a more recent study using a specific questionnaire indicated that there was no reduction in the fear of hypoglycemia [50]. These conflicting data suggest that there is a need for prospective studies to address this important issue because the reduction in the fear of hypoglycemia is perceived by patients as a main advantage of CGM.

Technology and Quality of Life

Continuous Subcutaneous Insulin Infusion

In the 5-Nations crossover trial, there were fewer episodes of severe hypoglycemia under SCII, and the overall daily quality of life score was significantly higher for CSII at the end of treatment compared with multiple daily insulin injections (75 vs. 71, $p < 0.001$) [51]. However, a critical review of the literature pointed out the fact that most of the studies are often flawed, making judgment difficult and stressing the need for large-scale multicenter patient preference controlled trials focusing specifically on quality of life issues surrounding insulin pump therapy. It also appeared necessary to clarify what quality of life really means: increased independence, greater freedom, greater flexibility, easier management of diabetes, better control, etc. [52].

Continuous Glucose Monitoring and Quality of Life

Data here are also conflicting. In a retrospective study of 43 patients (children and young adults), improvement in quality of life (78%) was among the most common reported benefits (answers to a questionnaire), and after 4 weeks of use, only 4 patients (12%) decided *against* long-term use, even if covered by their insurer [53]. However, in a retrospective study comparing 162 patients using RT-CGM/CSII and 149 patients using SMBG + CSII, neither improvement nor deterioration in quality of life was observed [54].

As for any new technology, introduction of CGM use may induce stress [38]. Indeed, any technology such as RT-CGM has benefits (e.g. getting continuous data, trend info, warnings of hypo- and hyperglycemia, etc.) as well as hassles (e.g. size of the device, pain at sensor insertion, too many alerts, skin irritation, etc.) [55]. Interestingly, a study showed the relationship between the perception of hassles and benefits and the real use of the system: persons who use the device infrequently focus more on the hassles than the benefits [56].

The Issue of Adherence to Technology

This observation is of paramount importance since there is a large body of evidence that the frequency of CGM use has an impact on its ability to improve HbA_{1c} [28]. In his meta-analysis, Pickup et al. [47] showed that every 1-day increase of sensor usage per week increased the effect of CGM compared with SMBG by 0.150% HbA_{1c} (–0.194 to –0.106%).

Interestingly, sensor usage was *unrelated* to the effect of CGM on the time spent in hypoglycemia. Pickup et al. [47] hypothesized that CGM may result in a decrease in hypoglycemia, not (as expected) by patients' adjusting their insulin dosage or taking extra carbohydrates based on CGM data, but instead through an indirect effect, such as general behavioral changes like an increase in the general confidence to manage diabetes. According to these authors, 'continuous glucose monitoring is a highly complex therapy that involves interacting behaviours, learning and decisions. Effective sensor use is likely to be a combination of frequency of sensor use, amount and quality of education and training, and ability of patients to use the data' [47].

Conclusion: It's Not All Technology

> If somebody says that a task is mechanical, it does not mean that people are incapable of doing the task; it implies, though, that only a machine could do it over and over, without ever complaining, or feeling bored.
> *Douglas R. Hofstadter*; in *Gödel, Escher, Bach: An Eternal Golden Braid*

Thanks to technology, considerable progress has been made in the treatment of diabetes, both in terms of efficacy of care and of comfort. However, the aim of this chapter was to suggest that a purely biomedical approach would miss the psychosocial component of diabetes as a chronic disease. Technology can only be a part of the solution for several reasons. First, one must consider the patients who will not have access to technology due to economic reasons or issues such as poor health literacy or numeracy [57]. Second, other factors may be involved in the improvement of HbA_{1c} and the prevention of hypoglycemia, i.e. human factors, such as patient education, motivation, and adherence. In addition, blood glucose does not depend entirely on the patient's behavior [58], as countless other factors – some known, some unknown, and some unknowable – have a role to play.

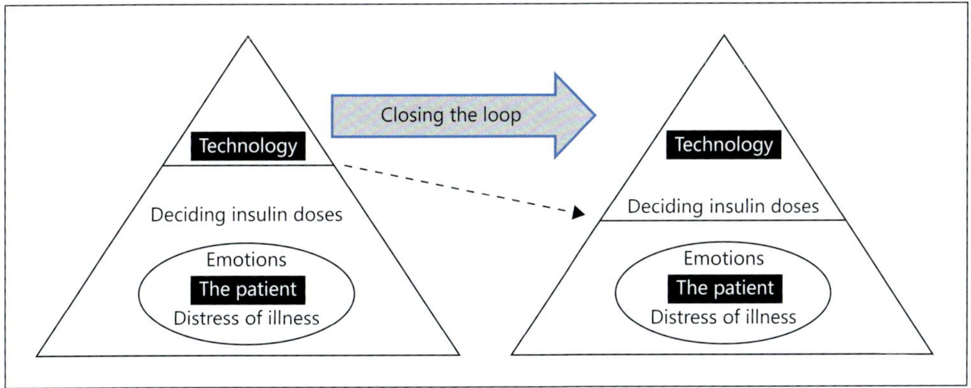

Fig. 1. How closing the loop (deciding insulin doses, one of the diabetes burdens, becomes a part of the technology) may represent a breakthrough. Emotions and the distress of illness, however, will remain.

However, the considerations presented herein may help in understanding why closed-loop systems are so appealing. Their appeal is they may convey the perception that decisions no longer must be taken by the patient and that the hurdle of deciding the dosing of insulin can be transferred to a machine for good (fig. 1).

Finally, we should always remember that technology is a biomedical, not biopsychosocial, solution to diabetes burdens. The distress linked to the life event represented by a chronic disease will remain: according to philosopher-physician Georges Canguilhem, 'no cure is a return to biological innocence' [59].

Disclosure Statement

Participation to symposia organized by Novo-Nordisk, Lilly, Novartis, Sanofi-Aventis, Merck-Serono, GSK, Ipsen, Abbott-Pharma, BMS, Pfizer, Roche-Pharma, Roche-Diagnostics, Abbott-Diagnostics, Lifescan, Bayer-Diagnostics, Dexcom. Advisory boards for Lifescan, Bayer Diagnostics, Lilly, Sanofi-Aventis, Novo-Nordisk Grant from Lifescan for the evaluation of a tool used in functional insulin therapy.

References

1 Bliss M: The Discovery of Insulin. Chicago, University of Chicago Press, 1982.
2 Haler D: Disposable syringes. Lancet 1973;1:1130.
3 Jefferson IG, Marteau TM, Smith MA, Baum JD: A multiple injection regimen using an insulin injection pen and pre-filled cartridged soluble human insulin in adolescents with diabetes. Diabet Med 1985;2:493–495.
4 Slama G, Hautecouverture M, Assan R, Tchobroutsky G: One to five days of continuous intravenous insulin infusion on seven diabetic patients. Diabetes 1974;23:732–738.
5 Pickup JC, Keen H, Parsons JA, Alberti KG: Continuous subcutaneous insulin infusion: an approach to achieving normoglycaemia. Br Med J 1978;1:204–207.

6 Heller S, Kozlovski P, Kurtzhals P: Insulin's 85th anniversary – an enduring medical miracle. Diabetes Res Clin Pract 2007;78:149–158.

7 Keen H, Glynne A, Pickup JC, Viberti GC, Bilous RW, Jarrett RJ, Marsden R: Human insulin produced by recombinant DNA technology: safety and hypoglycaemic potency in healthy men. Lancet 1980;2: 398–401.

8 Morihara K, Oka T, Tsuzuki H: Semi-synthesis of human insulin by trypsin-catalysed replacement of Ala-B30 by Thr in porcine insulin. Nature 1979;280: 412–413.

9 Howey DC, Bowsher RR, Brunelle RL, Woodworth JR: [Lys(B28), Pro(B29)]-human insulin. A rapidly absorbed analogue of human insulin. Diabetes 1994; 43:396–402.

10 Mudaliar SR, Lindberg FA, Joyce M, Beerdsen P, Strange P, Lin A, Henry RR: Insulin aspart (B28 asp-insulin): a fast-acting analog of human insulin: absorption kinetics and action profile compared with regular human insulin in healthy nondiabetic subjects. Diabetes Care 1999;22:1501–1506.

11 Dailey G, Rosenstock J, Moses RG, Ways K: Insulin glulisine provides improved glycemic control in patients with type 2 diabetes. Diabetes Care 2004;27: 2363–2368.

12 Bolli GB, Di Marchi RD, Park GD, Pramming S, Koivisto VA: Insulin analogues and their potential in the management of diabetes mellitus. Diabetologia 1999;42:1151–1167.

13 Heinemann L, Sinha K, Weyer C, Loftager M, Hirschberger S, Heise T: Time-action profile of the soluble, fatty acid acylated, long-acting insulin analogue NN304. Diabet Med 1999;16:332–338.

14 Pirart J: Le diabète sucré et ses complications. Une étude prospective de 4400 patients suivis entre 1947 et 1973. Diabete Metab 1977;3:97–107, 173–182, 245–256.

15 Tchobroutsky G: Relation of diabetic control to development of microvascular complications. Diabetologia 1978;15:143–152.

16 Sönksen PH, Judd SL, Lowy C: Home monitoring of blood glucose. Method for improving diabetic control. Lancet 1978;8067:729–732.

17 Koenig RJ, Peterson CM, Jones RL, Saudek C, Lehrman M, Cerami A: Correlation of glucose regulation and hemoglobin A_{1c} in diabetes mellitus. N Engl J Med 1976;295:417–420.

18 The Diabetes Control and Complications Trial Research Group: The effect of intensive treatment of diabetes on the development and progression of long-term complications in insulin-dependent diabetes mellitus. N Engl J Med 1993;329:977–986.

19 UK Prospective Diabetes Study (UKPDS) Group: Intensive blood-glucose control with sulphonylureas or insulin compared with conventional treatment and risk of complications in patients with type 2 diabetes (UKPDS 33). Lancet 1998;352:837–853.

20 Pickup J: Insulin pumps. Int J Clin Pract Suppl 2011; 170:16–19.

21 Pickup JC, Sutton AJ: Severe hypoglycaemia and glycaemic control in type 1 diabetes: meta-analysis of multiple daily insulin injections compared with continuous subcutaneous insulin infusion. Diabet Med 2008;25:765–774.

22 Reach G, Wilson GS: Can continuous glucose monitoring be used for the treatment of diabetes? Anal Chem 1992;64:381A–386A.

23 Reach G, Choleau C: Continuous glucose monitoring: physiological and technological challenges. Curr Diabetes Rev 2008;4:175–180.

24 Bode BW, Gross TM, Thornton KR, Mastrototaro JJ: Continuous glucose monitoring used to adjust diabetes therapy improves glycosylated hemoglobin: a pilot study. Diabetes Res Clin Pract 1999;46:183–190.

25 Garg SK, Schwartz S, Edelman SV: Improved glucose excursions using an implantable real-time continuous glucose sensor in adults with type 1 diabetes. Diabetes Care 2004;27:734–738.

26 Csöregi E, Schmidtke DW, Heller A: Design and optimization of a selective subcutaneously implantable glucose electrode based on 'wired' glucose oxidase. Anal Chem 1995;67:1240–1244.

27 Reach G: Continuous glucose monitoring, a critical appraisal. Diabetes Technol Ther 2008;10:69–80.

28 Juvenile Diabetes Research Foundation Continuous Glucose Monitoring Study Group: Continuous glucose monitoring and intensive treatment of type 1 diabetes. N Engl J Med 2008;359:1464–1476.

29 Riveline JP, Schaepelynck P, Chaillous L, Renard E, Sola-Gazagnes A, Penfornis A, Tubiana-Rufi N, Sulmont V, Catargi B, Lukas C, Radermecker RP, Thivolet C, Moreau F, Benhamou PY, Guerci B, Leguerrier AM, Millot L, Sachon C, Charpentier G, Hanaire H; EVADIAC Sensor Study Group: Assessment of patient-led or physician-driven continuous glucose monitoring in patients with poorly controlled type 1 diabetes using basal-bolus insulin regimen. Diabetes Care 2012;35:965–971.

30 Battelino T, Conget I, Olsen B, Schütz-Fuhrmann I, Hommel E, Hoogma R, Schierloh U, Sulli N, Bolinder J; SWITCH Study Group: The use and efficacy of continuous glucose monitoring in type 1 diabetes treated with insulin pump therapy: a randomized controlled trial. Diabetologia 2012;55: 3155–3162.

31 Bergenstal RM, Tamborlane WV, Ahmann A, Buse JB, Dailey G, Davis SN, Joyce C, Peoples T, Perkins BA, Welsh JB, Willi SM, Wood MA; STAR 3 Study Group: Effectiveness of sensor-augmented insulin-pump therapy in type 1 diabetes. N Engl J Med 2010; 363:311–320.
32 Hermanides J, Nørgaard K, Bruttomesso D, Mathieu C, Frid A, Dayan CM, Diem P, Fermon C, Wentholt IM, Hoekstra JB, DeVries JH: Sensor-augmented pump therapy lowers HbA_{1c} in suboptimally controlled type 1 diabetes. A randomized controlled trial. Diabet Med 2011;28:1158–1167.
33 Wentholt IM, Hoekstra JB, Zwart A, DeVries JH: Pendra goes Dutch: lessons for the CE mark in Europe. Diabetologia 2005;48:1055–1058.
34 Vashist SK: Non-invasive glucose monitoring technology in diabetes management: a review. Anal Chim Acta 2012;750:16–27.
35 Cobelli C, Renard E, Kovatchev B: Artificial pancreas, past, present, future. Diabetes 2011;60:2672–2682.
36 Engel GL: The need for a new biomedical model: a challenge for biomedicine. Science 1977;196:129–135.
37 Wagner J, Malchoff C, Abbott G: Invasiveness as a barrier to self-monitoring of blood glucose in diabetes. Diabetes Technol Ther 2005;7:612–619.
38 Halford J: Determining clinical and psychological benefits and barriers with continuous glucose monitoring therapy. Diabetes Technol Ther 2010;12:201–205.
39 Bojestig M, Arnqvist HJ, Hermansson G, Karlberg BE, Ludvigsson J: Declining incidence of nephropathy in insulin-dependent diabetes mellitus. N Engl J Med 1994;330:15–18.
40 Miller LV, Goldstein J: More efficient care of diabetic patients in a county-hospital setting. N Engl J Med 1972;286:1388–1391.
41 Lacroix A, Assal JP: L'Education thérapeutique des patients: nouvelles approches de la maladie chronique. Paris, Editions Vigot, 1998.
42 Sämann A, Mühlhauser I, Bender R, Hunger-Dathe W, Kloos C, Müller UA: Flexible intensive insulin therapy in adults with type 1 diabetes and high risk for severe hypoglycemia and diabetic ketoacidosis. Diabetes Care 2006;29:2196–2199.
43 McCrimmon RJ, Frier BM: Hypoglycaemia, the most feared complication of insulin therapy. Diabetes Metab 1994;20:503–512.
44 Thompson CJ, Cummings JF, Chalmers J, Gould C, Newton RW: How have patients reacted to the implications of the DCCT? Diabetes Care 1996;19:876–879.
45 Reach G: A psychophysical account of patient non-adherence to medical prescriptions. The case of insulin dose adjustment. Diabetes Metab 2013;39:50–55.
46 Battelino T, Phillip M, Bratina N, Nimri R, Oskarsson P, Bolinder J: Effect of continuous glucose monitoring on hypoglycaemia in type 1 diabetes. Diabetes Care 2011;34:795–800.
47 Pickup JC, Freeman SC, Sutton AJ: Glycaemic control in type 1 diabetes during real time continuous glucose monitoring compared with self monitoring of blood glucose: meta-analysis of randomised controlled trials using individual patient data. BMJ 2011; 343:d3805.
48 Hirsch IB, Abelseth J, Bode BW, Fischer JS, Kaufman FR, Mastrototaro J, Parkin CG, Wolpert HA, Buckingham BA: Sensor-augmented insulin pump therapy: results of the first randomized treat-to-target study. Diabetes Technol Ther 2008;10:377–383.
49 Mauras N, Beck R, Xing D, Ruedy K, Buckingham B, Tansey M, White NH, Weinzimer SA, Tamborlane W, Kollman C; Diabetes Research in Children Network (DirecNet) Study Group: A randomized clinical trial to assess the efficacy and safety of real-time continuous glucose monitoring in the management of type 1 diabetes in young children aged 4 to <10 years. Diabetes Care 2012;35:204–210.
50 Davey RJ, Stevens K, Jones TW, Fournier PA: The effect of short-term use of the Guardian RT continuous glucose monitoring system on fear of hypoglycaemia in patients with type 1 diabetes mellitus. Prim Care Diabetes 2012;6:35–39.
51 Hoogma RP, Hammond PJ, Gomis R, Kerr D, Bruttomesso D, Bouter KP, Wiefels KJ, de la Calle H, Schweitzer DH, Pfohl M, Torlone E, Krinelke LG, Bolli GB; 5-Nations Study Group: Comparison of the effects of continuous subcutaneous insulin infusion (CSII) and NPH-based multiple daily insulin injections (MDI) on glycaemic control and quality of life: results of the 5-Nations trial. Diabet Med 2005;23: 141–147.
52 Barnard KD, Lloyd CE, Skinner TC: Systematic literature review: quality of life associated with insulin pump use in type 1 diabetes. Diabet Med 2007;24: 607–617.
53 Cemeroglu AP, Stone R, Kleis L, Racine MS, Postellon DC, Wood MA: Use of a real-time continuous glucose monitoring system in children and young adults on insulin pump therapy: patients' and caregivers' perception of benefit. Pediatr Diabetes 2010; 11:182–187.
54 Rubin RR, Peyrot M: Treatment satisfaction and quality of life for an integrated continuous glucose monitoring/insulin pump system compared to self-monitoring plus an insulin pump. J Diabetes Sci Technol 2009;3:1402–1410.
55 Ramchandani N, Arya S, Ten S, Bhandari S: Real-life utilization of real-time continuous glucose monitoring: the complete picture. J Diabetes Sci Technol 2011;5:860–870.

56 Tansey M, Laffel L, Cheng J, Beck R, Coffey J, Huang E, Kollman C, Lawrence J, Lee J, Ruedy K, Tamborlane W, Wysocki T, Xing D; Juvenile Diabetes Research Foundation Continuous Glucose Monitoring Study Group: Satisfaction with continuous glucose monitoring in adults and youths with type 1 diabetes. Diabet Med 2011;28:1118–1122.

57 White RO, Wolff K, Cavanaugh KL, Rothman R: Addressing health literacy and numeracy to improve diabetes education and care. Diabetes Spectr 2010; 23:238–243.

58 Wolpert HA, Anderson BJ: Metabolic control matters: why is the message lost in the translation? The need for realistic goal-setting in diabetes care. Diabetes Care 2004;24:1301–1303.

59 Canguilhem G: The Normal and the Pathological. New York, Zone Books, 1989, p 228.

Prof. Gérard Reach
Service d'Endocrinologie, Diabétologie, Maladies Métaboliques
Hôpital Avicenne APHP, 125 route de Stalingrad
FR–93000 Bobigny (France)
E-Mail gerard.reach@avc.aphp.fr

Author Index

Subject Index